Manual of
SALIVARY GLAND DISEASES

Manual of
SALIVARY GLAND DISEASES

Editor

B Sivapathasundharam MDS
Principal and Head
Department of Oral and Maxillofacial Pathology
Meenakshi Ammal Dental College and Hospital
(A Constituent College of Meenakshi Academy of
Higher Education and Research)
Chennai, Tamil Nadu, India

Foreword

K Ranganathan

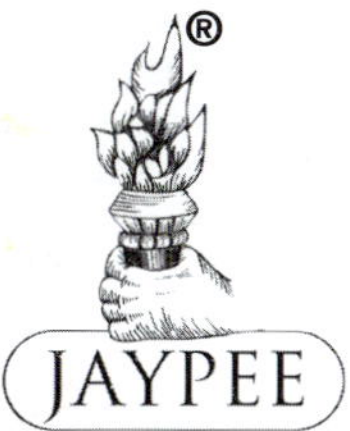

JAYPEE BROTHERS MEDICAL PUBLISHERS (P) LTD

New Delhi • London • Philadelphia • Panama

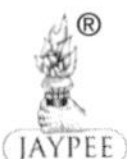 **Jaypee Brothers Medical Publishers (P) Ltd.**

Headquarters

Jaypee Brothers Medical Publishers (P) Ltd.
4838/24, Ansari Road, Daryaganj
New Delhi 110 002, India
Phone: +91-11-43574357
Fax: +91-11-43574314
Email: jaypee@jaypeebrothers.com

Overseas Offices

J.P. Medical Ltd.
83, Victoria Street, London
SW1H 0HW (UK)
Phone: +44-2031708910
Fax: +02-03-0086180
Email: info@jpmedpub.com

Jaypee Medical Inc.
The Bourse
111, South Independence Mall East
Suite 835, Philadelphia, PA 19106, USA
Phone: +267-519-9789
Email: joe.rusko@jaypeebrothers.com

Jaypee Brothers Medical Publishers (P) Ltd.
Shorakhute, Kathmandu
Nepal
Phone: +00977-9841528578
Email: jaypee.nepal@gmail.com

Jaypee-Highlights Medical Publishers Inc.
City of Knowledge, Bld. 237, Clayton
Panama City, Panama
Phone: +507-301-0496
Fax: +507-301-0499
Email: cservice@jphmedical.com

Jaypee Brothers Medical Publishers (P) Ltd.
17/1-B, Babar Road, Block-B, Shaymali
Mohammadpur, Dhaka-1207
Bangladesh
Mobile: +08801912003485
Email: jaypeedhaka@gmail.com

Website: www.jaypeebrothers.com
Website: www.jaypeedigital.com

Manual of Salivary Gland Diseases

First Edition: **2014**

ISBN: 978-93-5090-695-8

Printed at Sanat Printers, Kundli

Dedicated to

My wife—Dr S Rohini

Contributors

AR Raghu MDS PhD
Professor and Head
Department of Oral Pathology
Manipal College of Dental Sciences
Manipal, Karnataka, India

B Sivapathasundharam MDS
Principal and Head
Department of Oral and Maxillofacial Pathology
Meenakshi Ammal Dental College and Hospital
(A Constituent College of Meenakshi Academy of
Higher Education and Research)
Chennai, Tamil Nadu, India

Einstein T Bertin A MDS
Professor and Head
Badu Banarasi Das College of Dental Sciences
Lucknow, Uttar Pradesh, India

G Sriram MDS
Research Scholar
Faculty of Dentistry
National University of Singapore
Singapore

Geetha Prakash MD
Professor and Head
Department of Pathology
Meenakshi Medical College and
Research Institute
Kanchipuram, Tamil Nadu, India

Harsha Vardhan BG MDS
Professor
Department of Oral Medicine and Radiology
Meenakshi Ammal Dental College and Hospital
Chennai, Tamil Nadu, India

Kanthimathi Sekhar MD
Professor
Department of Pathology
Meenakshi Medical College and
Research Institute
Kanchipuram, Tamil Nadu, India

R Rajendran MDS PhD
Professor
Division of Oral Pathology
College of Dentistry
King Saud University, Riyadh, Saudi Arabia

Vinod Narayanan MDS FDSRCS
Professor and Head
Department of Oral and Maxillofacial Surgery
Saveetha Dental College
Chennai, Tamil Nadu, India

Foreword

There have been tremendous advantages in our understanding of the pathogenesis of diseases of the oral and maxillofacial region in the recent years. One of the prime reasons for this, is the introduction and widespread use of molecular techniques, such as immunohistochemistry, *in situ* hybridization and polymerase chain reaction, as diagnostic tools. Despite these great strides, identification and classification of salivary gland lesions are still a challenge. This is because of the wide spectrum of pathological changes, similarities in the pathological features among different groups of lesions and the absence of specific immunohistochemical markers in many of the salivary gland neoplasms.

The book is timely, concise and lucid. It elegantly explains our current understanding and concepts in diagnosis and management with relevant topical examples. It is noteworthy that the contributors have taken troubles to incorporate cases from developing countries, thus making the text relevant to the dental students across the country.

The structured text is to be used as an easy-to-read reference for graduate students of all three specialties: oral and maxillofacial pathology, oral medicine and oral and maxillofacial surgery. It comprehensively discusses the basics of salivary gland development, anatomy functions and investigative techniques in disease and their management.

The contributors are to be commended to have collectively brought out this well-written text on salivary gland pathology in a format that is an easy-to-read, grasp and translate into practice. This text should prove to be a valuable addition to the growing times in the field of oral and maxillofacial pathology.

K Ranganathan MDS MS (USA) PhD
Professor and Head
Department of Oral and Maxillofacial Pathology
Ragas Dental College and Hospital
Chennai, Tamil Nadu, India

Preface

Incidences of salivary gland diseases are relatively higher than we expect in practice. Understanding of salivary gland pathology is still not concluded, since the newer diagnostic techniques are evolving continuously, which dictate the modified approach to their management. *Manual of Salivary Gland Diseases* is confluence of the anatomy, physiology, pathology of salivary glands and their diagnosis and management.

There are few books available in the market on salivary gland tumors, but there is not a single book dealing with the entire salivary gland diseases and their management available at present. The book will be the first of this kind, to serve the postgraduates and teaching faculties in the field of oral pathology, oral medicine and oral surgery, and the practitioners and general surgeons.

Contributors for the book are stalwarts in their respective field with more than two decades of professional experience and made an attempt to the readers to understand the pathology and diagnosis through the basic sciences. A balance is maintained between the basics and the advanced concepts.

Clinical, histopathological photographs and an easy-to-understand line diagrams are added, wherever necessary.

B Sivapathasundharam

Acknowledgments

I wish to acknowledge with gratitude, the continuous help and support by the way of providing photographs, proof corrections and typing by the following friends and colleagues: Divya, Girija Sanjay, Karthiga Kannan, Manjunath, I Ponniah, Preethi, D Spencer Lilly and Sunitha.

In addition, I would like to thank my wife, Dr S Rohini, for her never-ending support and encouragement.

Finally, I would like to express my gratitude to Shri Jitendar P Vij (Group Chairman), Mr Ankit Vij (Managing Director), Mr Tarun Duneja (Director-Publishing), Mr KK Raman (Production Manager) and other staff of M/s Jaypee Brothers Medical Publishers (P) Ltd, New Delhi, India, for their guidance in making the book.

Contents

6. Histogenesis and Molecular Pathogenesis of Salivary Gland Tumors   67
G Sriram, Geetha Prakash

7. Benign Tumors of Salivary Glands   84
Einstein T Bertin A, B Sivapathasundharam

8. Malignant Tumors of the Salivary Glands   115
Kanthimathi Sekhar, B Sivapathasundharam

1

Introduction

B Sivapathasundharam

Salivary glands are important exocrine glands and their prime function being secretion of saliva. Saliva has many protective functions. The health and function of the oral cavity depends on the secretion, composition, and flow of the saliva which inturn may be affected in various salivary gland diseases.

Saliva protects the mouth in many ways. Due to its fluid nature it flushes away the non-adherent bacteria and other debris. Apart from its role in maintaining the integrity of the tooth, it also helps in digestion, taste perception and tissue repair. By its buffering action it protects the tooth from dental caries.

Failure of salivary secretion results in dry mouth, known as xerostomia, which is distressing and leads to the imbalance of the oral ecological system. A decrease in salivary volume and altered composition leads to the development of dental caries and makes the oral soft tissues more susceptible for infections. Movements of the oral soft tissues and swallowing become difficult and painful if the mouth is dry.

Salivary glands may be affected by a number of diseases, both local and systemic.

For the sake of discussion diseases of the salivary glands are usually categorized into neoplastic and non-neoplastic.

Diagnosis of salivary gland diseases is difficult in many times. Clinicians' diagnostic skills are often challenged in case of non-neoplastic lesions, since reactive, metabolic, autoimmune, infectious, and iatrogenic factors may produce almost similar clinical signs and symptoms. In contrast, neoplastic lesions of the salivary glands though have a similar clinical presentation, as either an asymptomatic mass or ulcer, may have varied and confusing histological patterns and their histomorphology being complex and diverse. Neoplasms of major and minor glands do differ in the frequency, rate of malignancy, and management.

Though most of the salivary gland neoplasms are arising from the epithelial parenchyma, a significant minority of them are from the non-parenchymal tissues. Even a thorough history and clinical examination may not suffice to derive a correct diagnosis. Laboratory tests, special diagnostic aids, or an incisional biopsy, coupled with the knowledge of pathology may be required for clenching the correct diagnosis.

Non-neoplastic salivary gland diseases occur throughout the world. However, certain types of diseases like sialadenitis, cysts of the parotid glands, and sialosis of metabolic etiology are seen more frequently in tropical regions when compared to rest of the world. It is not clear whether to ascribe this to a geographical or etiological predisposition.

Perception of salivary gland pathology passed through a substantial modification of terminology, histogenesis, pathogenesis, investigative procedures, and treatment modalities over a time. Till today our understanding of salivary gland pathology has not concluded, since this area is ever-changing and evolving. Here an attempt is made to present the current understanding of the diseases of the salivary glands, to be readily usable as a reference by the pathologists, physicians and surgeons.

2

Anatomy of Human Salivary Gland

B Sivapathasundharam, AR Raghu

INTRODUCTION

Glands are organized a rrangements of secretory cells. They are broadly classified as exocrine and endocrine glands. Those glands that pour their secretions directly on to the epithelial surface or through ducts are called *exocrine glands*. The glands which do not have ducts but elaborate their secretion directly into the blood stream are called the *endocrine glands.* Exocrine glands may be *unicellular,* as in goblet cells which are interspersed among other non-secretory cells or *multicellular* which have two major epithelial components, the *secretory units and ducts.* The secretory units produce glandular secretion, and the ducts convey the secretions to the surface.

Exocrine gland may be *simple gland* if it has a single unbranched duct (e.g. sweat gland) or *compound* gland if it has branched duct system emerging from a number of secretory units, (e.g. liver and pancreas).

On the basis of structural modification of secretory units, glands may be classified as *tubular, alveolar (acinar),* or *tubuloalveolar* (having both the tubular and alveolar secretory units) (Figs 2.1A to C). Based on the nature of secretion, glands may be *mucous, serous* or *mixed.* Mucous glands produce viscous glycoprotein secretion while the serous glands secrete a watery, proteinaceous secretion. Mixed glands produce both mucous and serous secretions.

Exocrine glands can also be classified based on the manner in which their secretions *are expelled out of the cells. In a merocrine* gland, the secretion

is released by exocytosis, where the membranous walls of secretory vesicles fuse with the cell membrane, keeping the cell intact. Most exocrine glands are *merocrine.* In *apocrine* glands, the apical portion of the cell is lost during the release of their secretion (e.g. mammary glands). In *holocrine* gland the entire cell is lost while producing its secretion (e.g. sebaceous glands).

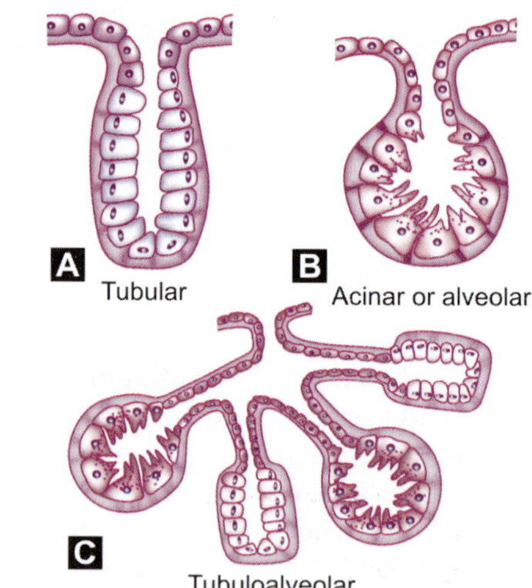

Figures 2.1A to C: Diagrammatic representation of three different arrangements found in exocrine glands. Simple gland has a duct that does not branch (A and B). Compound glands have a branching duct system (C). The glands may have tubular (A) or acinar or alveolar (B) secretory units. Compound glands possess both types of secretory units tubuloalveolar (C)

SALIVARY GLANDS

Salivary glands are compound tubuloalveolar glands whose secretions enter into the oral cavity through ducts. They secrete a complex fluid called saliva which has digestive, lubricating and immunologic functions among many others. In humans and most other mammalian species, there are three paired glands (*major*) namely the parotid, submandibular and sublingual located extra-orally and about 600 to 1000 small glands (*minor*) distributed in the mucosa and submucosa of the oral cavity and oropharynx. Figures 2.2A and B shows the histological section of developing salivary glands.

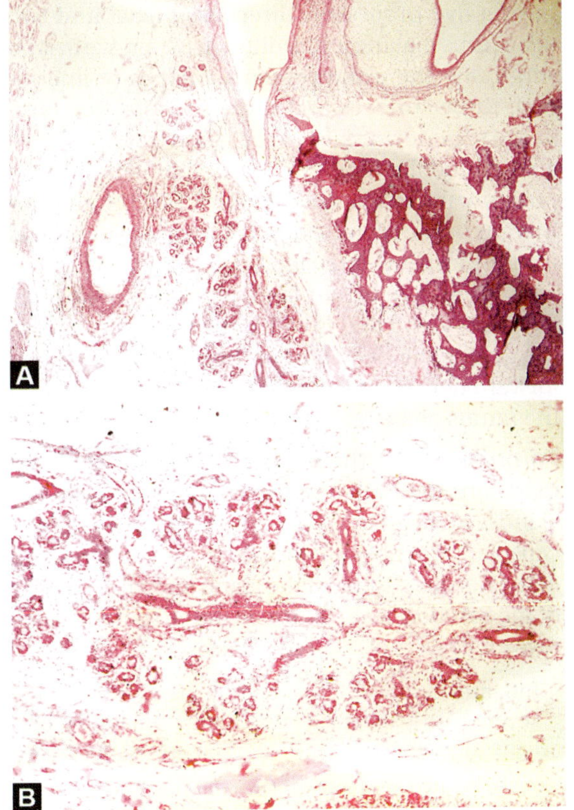

Figures 2.2A and B: Histological section of developing salivary glands. (A) Developing salivary acini and ductal system of minor salivary glands in the buccal vestibule (4 X), (B) Shows the same in higher magnification (10 X)

Embryology

The major salivary glands develop from the 6th-8th week of intrauterine like as outpouchings of oral ectoderm into the surrounding mesenchyme. They arise bilaterally as a result of epithelial-mesenchymal interaction between the oral ectoderm and underlying neural crest induced mesenchyme (ectomesenchyme).

All salivary glands develop similarly as initial discrete thickenings of the epithelium of the oral ectoderm that is adjacent to the condensed mesenchyme. This thickening undergoes proliferation and invades the underlying mesenchyme in the form of a cord of cells similar to dental lamina. This cord of cells is called *primary cord*. At the distal end of this primary cord is a *terminal bulb*. The distal terminal bulb undergoes branching and each branch leads to *secondary epithelial cords* that terminate in one or two solid end bulbs. The epithelial cords undergo canalization to form the ducts. Canalization occurs either by differential growth of peripheral and central cells or through apoptosis of the central cells. Similarly the terminal end bulbs also undergo luminalization which transforms the end bulbs into *terminal tubules*. The distal most part of the terminal tubules do not canalize and are called *terminal saccules*.

The inner cells of the terminal saccules differentiate into mucous and serous cells while the outer cells differentiate into myoepithelial cells. The inner/central cells of the tubules differentiate into specialized cells that characterize the excretory, striated, and intercalated ducts.

With the epithelial ingrowth, the ectomesenchyme differentiates to form the connective tissue component that supports the parenchyma of the gland. This component consists of a fibrous capsule and a septa that divide the gland into lobes and lobules. During the development of the gland, the autonomic nervous system involvement is crucial; sympathetic nerve stimulation leads to acinar differentiation while parasympathetic stimulation is needed for overall glandular growth. The minor salivary glands develop after the development of major glands and arise from the oral ectoderm and nasopharyngeal endoderm.

The *parotid gland* anlage in the human embryo may be observed in the 8 mm embryo stage as a furrow of tissue that projects dorsally between the maxillary and mandibular processes of the developing mandibular arch. The groove, which is later converted into a tube, loses its connection with the epithelium of the mouth except at its ventral end and grows dorsally into the substance of the cheek. The tube persists as parotid duct and its blind end proliferates into the mesenchyme to form the gland. Eventually, the fully developed parotid gland surrounds the facial nerve and become encapsulated after the lymphatics develop, resulting in its unique anatomy with entrapment of lymph nodes in the parenchyma of the gland. The parotid ducts are canalized at 10 weeks post conception, the terminal buds are canalized at 16 weeks, and secretions commence at 18 weeks.

> The salivary epithelial cells included within these lymph nodes, are thought to play a role in the development of Warthin's tumor and lymphoepithelial cyst within the parotid gland.

The *submandibular gland* primordium may be observed in the 13 mm embryo stage as an epithelial outgrowth into the mesenchyme from the floor of the linguogingival groove. It increases in size rapidly and gives off numerous branching processes which later acquire lumina and maintain its connection with the oral cavity lateral to the tongue. Later the duct is shifted forwards till it is below the tip of the tongue, close to the median plane.

> The differentiation of serous acini starts at 12 weeks; serous secretory activity starts at 16 weeks, increases until the 28th week, and then diminishes. The serous secretions during the 16th to 28th week contribute to the amniotic fluid and contain amylase and possibly nerve and epidermal growth factors.

The *sublingual gland* arises in the 20 mm stage of the embryo as small epithelial thickenings in the linguogingival groove and adjacent to the area where the submandibular gland develops. Each thickening canalizes separately and several sublingual ducts open separately on the summit of the sublingual fold while others join the submandibular duct.

MAJOR SALIVARY GLANDS

Parotid Gland

The parotid gland represents the largest salivary gland and it is situated below the external auditory meatus and lies in a deep hollow behind the ramus of the mandible and infront of the sternocleidomastoid muscle (Fig. 2.3). The gland measures about 5.8 cm in the craniocaudal dimension, and 3.4 cm in the ventrodorsal dimension. The average weight of the parotid gland is about 14.28 g. It has an irregular, inverted pyramidal form, with its base above and apex below behind the angle of mandible.

The facial nerve and its branches pass forward within the parotid gland and divide it into superficial and deep part. The parotid has been described as having five processes (three superficial and two deep) thus making it very difficult to remove *in-toto* surgically. The gland presents an apex or inferior end, three surfaces and three borders. The base or the superior surface of the gland extends above and behind the temporomandibular joint into the posterior part of the mandibular fossa. The anterior margin of the gland extends forwards superficial to the masseter muscle and a small part of the anterior margin of the gland may be separate from the main gland and is called the accessory part of the gland. The deep part of the gland may extend forward between the medial pterygoid muscle and the ramus of the mandible.

Parotid capsule: The parotid gland is a lobulated mass surrounded by a connective tissue capsule. The gland is invested by an inner true and an outer false capsule. True capsule is formed by the condensation of the fibrous stroma of the gland and false capsule or the parotid sheath is formed by the splitting of the investing layers of deep cervical fascia.

> Inflammation within the parotid gland can cause severe pain just infront of the temporomandibular joint due to stretching of the capsule and stimulation of the greater auricular nerve.

Structures within the parotid gland: The structures within the parotid gland from lateral to medial are the facial nerve, retromandibular vein, and external carotid artery. A part of the auriculo-

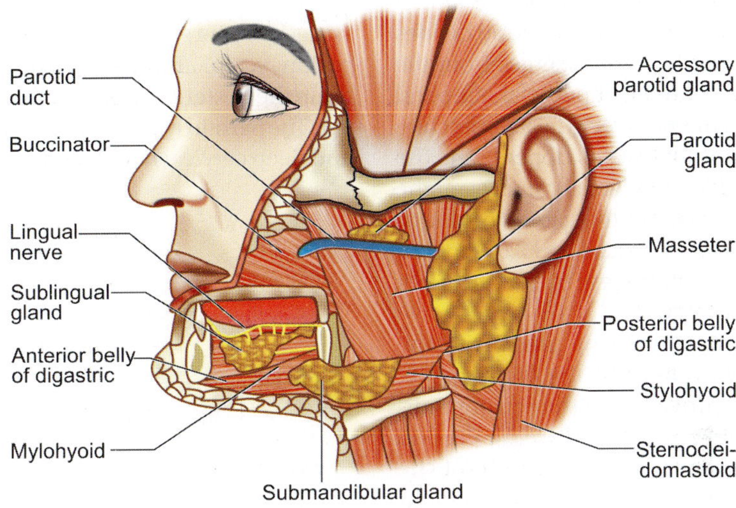

Figure 2.3: Diagram illustrating the relations of major salivary glands

temporal nerve winds round behind and lateral to the neck of the mandible and traverses the deep part of the base of the gland.

The most superficial portion of the parotid gland makes up the neural compartment, containing facial nerve, the auriculotemporal nerve, and the greater auricular nerve. Facial nerve is intimately associated with the parotid gland, dividing it into two surgical zones (the superficial and deep lobe). It emerges from the base of the skull via the stylomastoid foramen (styloid process-medially, mastoid process-laterally). Facial nerve turns laterally to enter the parotid gland at its posteromedial surface. Within the gland, the nerve courses forwards for about 1 cm superficial to the retromandibular vein and the external carotid artery and then divides into *temporofacial* and *cervicofacial trunks*. The temporofacial trunk turns abruptly upwards and subdivides into *temporal and zygomatic* branches. The cervicofacial trunk passes downwards and forwards and then subdivides into *buccal, marginal mandibular and cervical branches*. The five terminal branches radiate like the goose's foot through the anterior border of the gland and

supplies the facial muscles. Hence, this branching pattern is known as the *pes anserinus* (goose's foot).

Of note, branches of the facial nerve are more superficial at the anterior border of the parotid gland, and are therefore more prone to injury.

The auriculotemporal nerve, a branch of trigeminal nerve, runs anterior to the external acoustic meatus, paralleling the superficial temporal artery and the vein. This nerve carries parasympathetic postganglionic fibers from the otic ganglion to the parotid gland. In addition, the auriculotemporal nerve provides sensory innervation to the parotid capsule, skin of the auricle and the temporal region. As a result, referred pain from parotitis can involve the auricle, external auditory meatus, temporomandibular joint and the temple.

When the parasympathetic postganglionic fibers from the otic ganglion are injured intraoperatively, aberrant parasympathetic innervation to the skin results in Frey's syndrome (i.e. gustatory sweating). This nerve may be resected intentionally to prevent Frey's syndrome.

The arterial compartment sits in the deep portion of the gland containing the external carotid artery, which enters the posteromedial surface and divides into the maxillary artery, which emerges from the anteromedial surface and the superficial temporal artery which gives off its transverse facial branch in the gland and ascends to leave its upper limit. The posterior auricular artery may also branch from the external carotid artery within the gland, leaving at its posteromedial surface (Figs 2.4 and 2.5). Arterial supply is provided by the transverse facial artery from the superficial temporal artery.

The venous compartment is present in the middle of the parotid, deep to the facial nerve. Venous drainage is provided by the retromandibular vein. This vein runs lateral to the carotid artery, and emerges at the inferior pole of the parotid gland (Figs 2.4 to 2.6). The retromandibular vein joins the posterior auricular vein to form the external jugular vein and the anterior facial vein to form the common facial vein, which empties into the internal jugular vein.

Lymphatic drainage of the parotid gland is by paraparotid and intraparotid nodes. The paraparotid nodes are more numerous and drain the temporal region, scalp, and auricle. The intraparotid nodes drain the posterior nasopharynx, soft palate, and the ear. The parotid lymphatics drain into the superficial and deep cervical lymph nodes.

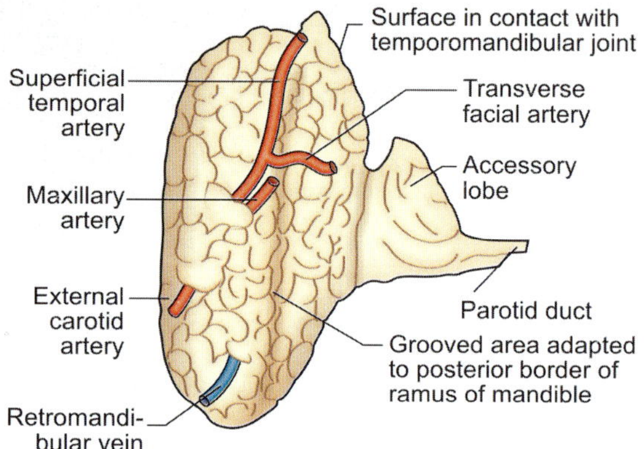

Figure 2.4: Anteromedial aspect of left parotid less gland

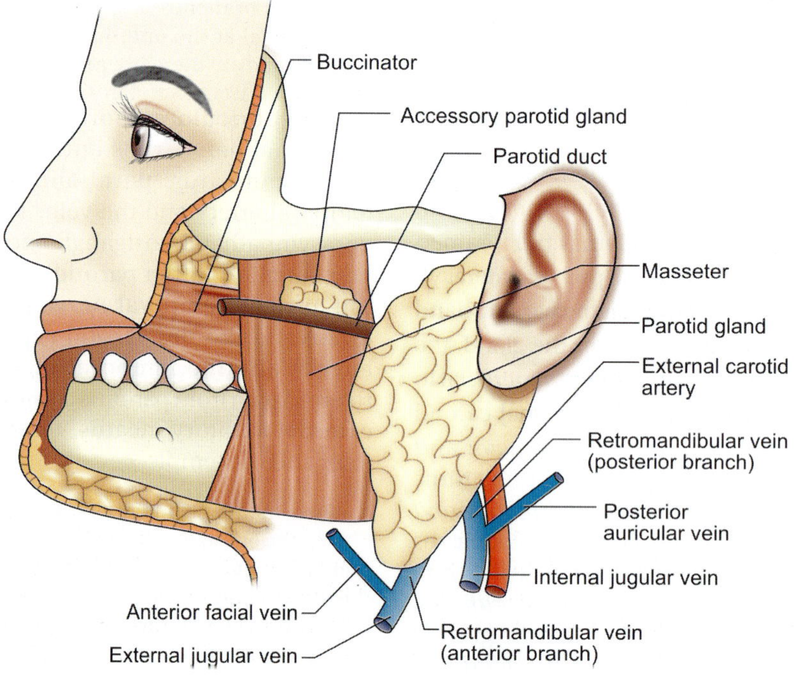

Figure 2.5: Diagram illustrating the structures related to parotid gland

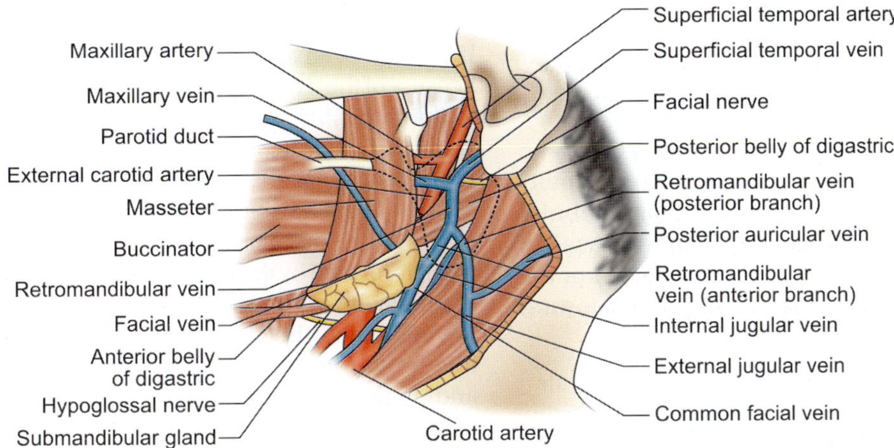

Figure 2.6: Immediate deep relations of parotid gland.
The outline of parotid gland is indicated by the interrupted black line

Relations of the parotid gland: The structures that are intimately related to the deep surface of the gland are sometimes called the parotid bed.

The relationship of the gland to the *apex or the lower end* overlaps the posterior belly of digastric and appears in the carotid triangle. Prominent structures passing through the apex of the gland are the cervical branches of the facial nerve and anterior division of the retromandibular vein along with the formation of the external jugular vein (Figs 2.5 and 2.6).

The *base of the gland* is related to the external acoustic meatus and posterior part of TMJ. Structures passing through the base of the gland include temporal branch of the facial nerve, superficial temporal vessels and the auriculo-temporal nerve.

The *superficial surface* or the lateral aspect of the gland is related to the superficial lamella of the parotid sheath, posterior fibers of platysma, superficial fascia and the skin. The *anteromedial surface* relations are the posterior border of the ramus of the mandible, the capsule of temporomandibular joint, the posteroinferior part of masseter and the medial pterygoid muscle, near its insertion. The posteromedial surface comes in contact with the

mastoid process, sternocleidomastoid muscle and the posterior belly of digastric, the styloid process and its attachment, carotid sheath with the internal carotid artery, the internal jugular vein, and the vagus, glossopharyngeal, accessory, hypoglossal and facial nerves. The *anterior border* is related to the rest of the masseter and the structures radiating deeper to this border are the zygomatic branch of the facial nerve, transverse facial vessels, upper buccal branch of the facial nerve, accessory parotid gland and its duct, parotid duct, lower buccal branch of the facial nerve; marginal mandibular branch of facial nerve from above downwards. The *posterior border* rests on sternomastoid, posterior auricular branch of facial nerve and posterior auricular vessels that pass upward and backward beneath this border. The *medial border* separates the anteromedial from posteromedial surfaces and at times it comes in contact with the wall of pharynx, and is known as the pharyngeal border.

About 80% of the gland overlies the masseter muscle and the mandible. In addition, the stylomandibular ligament separates the parotid from the submandibular gland. This portion of the gland lies in the prestyloid compartment of the para pharyngeal space.

A tumor of the deep lobe can push the tonsillar fossa and soft palate anteromedially. Parotid tumors that involve the parapharyngeal space are referred to as *dumb-bell tumors.*

The isthmus of the parotid gland runs between the mandibular ramus and the posterior belly of the digastric to connect the retromandibular portion to the remainder of the gland. The tail of the parotid overlies the upper one-fourth of the sternocleidomastoid muscle and extends toward the mastoid process.

Patients with parotitis frequently have pain with mastication because the gland becomes trapped between the mandible and mastoid process upon opening the mouth.

Parotid duct: Also called stensen's duct (parotid duct) arises from the anterior border of the parotid and parallels the zygomatic arch, 1.5 cm (approximately one finger breadth) inferior to the inferior margin of the arch. It is about five centimeters in length and three millimeters in width. The duct emerges through the anterior border of the upper part of the gland and passes horizontally across masseter, then turns medially at its anterior border to pierce the buccal pad of fat and buccinator muscle and opens into the vestibule of the mouth as a small papilla, into the oral cavity at the level of the second maxillary molar. The oblique course of the duct anteriorly between the mucous membrane and the buccinator serves as a valve and prevents inflation of the duct system during forceful blowing. Stensen's duct lies midway between the zygomatic arch and the corner of the mouth along the line between the upper lip philtrum and the tragus. The buccal branch of the facial nerve runs with the parotid duct. An accessory parotid gland along with its duct is noted in 20% of the people. The accessory gland is typically found overlying the masseter, and the accessory duct typically lies cranial to the Stensen's duct.

The parotid is invested in its own fascia (capsule), which is continuous with the superficial layer of deep cervical fascia. Of note, parotid tissue can herniate through the stylomandibular membrane. Thus, deep parotid tumors can present as parapharyngeal masses.

Submandibular Gland

It is often referred to as the submaxillary gland because of the tendency of British anatomists to refer to the mandible as the 'submaxilla'. It is a paired gland, irregular in shape and having the size of a walnut and measures about 10 to 20 g in weight. It is a mixed gland having a predominantly serous type of secretion. This gland lies in the submandibular triangle formed by the anterior and posterior bellies of the digastric muscle and the inferior margin of the mandible. The gland is positioned medial and inferior to the mandibular ramus partly superior and partly inferior to the base of the posterior half of the mandible. The gland forms a 'C' around the anterior margin of the mylohyoid muscle, which divides the submandibular gland into a superficial and deep lobe. Thus each gland consists of a large *superficial part* and a small *deep part*, both of which are continuous with each other.

Superficial Part

The superficial part of the gland is related anteriorly to the anterior belly of digastric and posteriorly to the stylomandibular ligament. Above it extends medial to the body of the mandible and below it usually overlaps the intermediate tendon of digastric and the insertion of stylohyoid. The superficial gland thus presents two ends—the anterior and posterior and three surfaces—inferior, lateral and medial.

Medially the gland is extensive and is divided into three parts—anterior, intermediate and posterior. Anterior part is related to the mylohyoid, from which it is separated by the mylohyoid nerve and vessels and the branches of submental vessels. The intermediate part rests on the hyoglossus muscle and the lingual and hypoglossal nerve while the posterior part is related to styloglossus, and stylopharyngeus muscle, the glosso-pharyngeal and nerve, the posterior belly of digastric and middle constrictor of pharynx.

Laterally, the gland lies in contact with the submandibular fossa on the medial surface of the mandible. Inferolaterally, it is covered by the investing layer of deep cervical fascia, the platysma and skin. The investing layer of deep cervical fascia splits into two layers to cover the inferior and medial surfaces of the gland, and is attached respectively to the lower border of the body of mandible and to the mylohyoid line.

The inferior surface is covered by the skin, superficial fascia, platysma and deep cervical fascia and is crossed by the facial vein and cervical branch of the facial nerve. Near the mandible, submandibular group of lymph nodes may be in contact and some may even be embedded within it.

The posterior end presents a groove for the lodgement of ascending limb of the cervical loop of facial artery.

Deep part: The deep part of the gland extends forward in the interval between the mylohoid and the hyoglossus up to the posterior end of the sublingual salivary gland. The deep lobe comprises the majority of the gland. The deep part of the gland is related anteriorly to the sublingual gland, posteriorly to the stylohyoid, the posterior belly of the digastric and the parotid gland, medially to the hyoglossus and styloglossus and laterally to the mylohyoid muscle and the superficial part of the gland. Superiorly it is related to the lingual nerve and the submandibular ganglion; it is covered by the mucous membrane of the floor of the mouth inferiorly to the hypoglossal nerve (Fig. 2.7). As is the case with the parotid gland, the submandibular gland is invested in its own capsule, which is also continuous with the superficial layer of deep cervical fascia.

Submandibular duct (Wharton's duct): It is about five centimeters long and thinner than the parotid duct. It begins from numerous tributaries in the superficial part of the gland and emerges from the medial surface of this part of the gland behind the posterior border of the mylohoid. It traverses the deep part of the gland, passes at first up and slightly back for about five millimeters and then forwards between mylohyoid and hyoglossus. It passes next between the sublingual gland and genioglossus to open in the floor of the mouth on the summit of the sublingual papilla at the side of the frenulum of tongue. The duct presents an intimate relationship with the lingual nerve. At first the nerve lies above the lingual nerve and then crosses its lateral side and finally ascends medially winding round the lower border of the duct (Fig. 2.7).

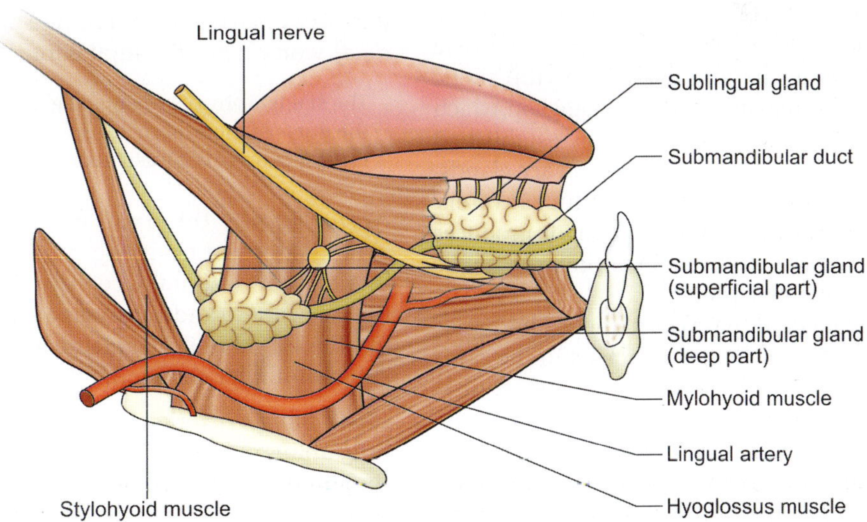

Figure 2.7: Relations of the submandibular and sublingual gland

Blood supply: The submandibular gland is supplied by the branches of facial and lingual arteries. The veins correspond to the arteries and drain into the internal jugular veins. The facial artery forms a groove in the deep part of the gland, and then curves up and around the inferior margin of the mandible to supply the face. The facial artery and vein are the first blood vessels encountered when resecting the submandibular glands as they cross superficially over the inferior border of the mandible. Venous drainage is provided by the anterior facial vein, which lies deep to the marginal mandibular branch of facial nerve.

One method of preserving the marginal mandibular nerve is to identify and ligate the facial vein two to three centimeters inferior to the mandible and elevate the vein and all superior tissue superiorly.

Lymphatic drainage: The lymph vessels drain into the submandibular and deep cervical group of lymph nodes. Perivascular lymph nodes near the facial artery are often involved with malignant tumors originating in the submandibular gland, and these nodes should be removed with submandibular resection.

Nerve supply: Innervation to the submandibular gland is derived from two important sources: Sympathetic innervation from the superior cervical ganglion via the lingual artery, and parasympathetic innervation from the submandibular ganglion, which is fed by the lingual nerve. It is now established that both are secretomotor to the salivary glands. Parasympathetic stimulation produces watery secretion whereas sympathetic stimulation produces a sticky mucus rich fluid. In addition, the sympathetic provides vasomotor supply.

The preganglionic parasympathetic fibers arise from the superior salivatory nucleus in the pons and pass successively through the facial, chorda tympani and lingual nerves and terminate in the submandibular ganglion. Postganglionic fibers from the ganglion directly supply the submandibular gland, and reach the sublingual gland via the lingual nerve.

The sympathetic nerves reach the gland around the facial artery and convey postganglionic fibers from the superior cervical ganglion of the sympathetic trunk.

The submandibular salivary gland is a common site of sialolith formation. Examination of the floor of the mouth will reveal absence of ejection of saliva from the orifice of the duct of the affected gland.

Sublingual Gland

This is the smallest of the major salivary glands. Each gland is narrow, flat, shaped like an almond and weighs about four grams. The gland lies just deep to the floor of mouth mucosa between the mandible and genioglossus muscle. It is bounded inferiorly by the mylohyoid muscle. Wharton's duct and the lingual nerve pass between the sublingual gland and genioglossus muscle (Fig. 2.7). Unlike the parotid and submandibular glands, the sublingual gland has no true fascial capsule.

Sublingual ducts: Unlike the parotid and submandibular glands, the sublingual gland lacks a single dominant duct. Instead, it is drained by approximately ten small ducts (the *Ducts of Rivinus*), which exit the superior aspect of the gland and open along the sublingual fold on the floor of mouth. Occasionally, several of the more anterior ducts may join to form a common duct (*Bartholin's duct*), which typically empties into Wharton's duct.

The sialography of sublingual glands is difficult as the ducts of the sublingual glands are too small for the injection of contrast media.

Nerve supply: Innervation of the sublingual gland is derived from two sources: Sympathetic innervation is from the cervical chain ganglia via the facial artery and parasympathetic innervation, like the submandibular gland, is derived from the submandibular ganglion.

Blood supply: Arterial supply to this gland is from the sublingual branch of the lingual artery, and the submental branch of the facial artery. Accompanying veins from the gland drain into the facial and lingual veins. Lymphatic drainage is into the submandibular nodes and deep cervical lymph nodes.

MINOR SALIVARY GLANDS

Unlike the major salivary glands, the minor salivary glands lack a branching network of draining ducts. Instead, each salivary unit has its own simple duct. The minor salivary glands are concentrated in the buccal, labial, palatal, and lingual regions. In addition, minor salivary glands may be found at the superior pole of the tonsils *(Weber's glands)*, tonsillar pillars, base of the tongue *(von Ebner's glands)*, paranasal sinuses, larynx, trachea, and bronchi.

The labial and buccal glands contain both mucous and serous elements. The palatoglossal glands are mucous glands and are located around the pharyngeal isthmus. The palatal glands are mucous glands and occur in both the soft and hard palate. The anterior and posterior lingual glands are mainly mucous. The anterior glands are embedded within the muscle near the ventral surface of the tongue and open by means of four or five ducts near the lingual frenum and posterior glands are located in the root of the tongue. The deep posterior lingual glands are predominantly serous glands found around the circumvallate papillae.

Most of the minor glands receive parasympathetic innervation from the lingual nerve, except for the minor glands of the palate, which receive parasympathetic fibers from the palatine nerves, through the sphenopalatine ganglion.

Tumors of the minor salivary gland most commonly arise from palate, upper lip and buccal mucosa.

MICROSTRUCTURE OF THE SALIVARY GLANDS

The structural framework of the three major salivary glands are similar. There are only minor differences in details of histology and cytology. Both the major and minor salivary glands are composed of invested parenchymal elements and supported by connective tissue. The blood and lymph vessels and nerves that supply the gland are contained within the connective tissue. The connective tissue forms a capsule around the major glands and extends into it dividing the secretory portion of the gland into lobes and lobules. Each lobule has a single duct, whose branches terminate as dilated secretory "end piece" which are tubular or acinar in shape. The parenchymal compartment of salivary gland consists of the acinus, myoepithelial cells, the intercalated duct, the striated duct, and the excretory duct.

The basic structure of salivary gland is a blind ending acini that forms the secretory component. An acinus (from Latin, grape) is a small ball of secretory epithelial cells containing a tiny central lumen [Acini are sometimes called *alveoli*, from Latin-*small cavity*].

Each individual acinus is an ovoid or tubular structure that consists of a single layer of specialized cells, surrounding the central lumen. The lumen of each acinus is continuous with the ductal system. The cells that make up an acinus or terminal end piece are known as the "acinar secretory cell". They are generally classified as "serous acinar cells" and "mucous acinar cells". Acini, that are responsible for producing the primary secretion, are divided into three types: Serous (protein-secreting); Mucous (mucin-secreting); and Mixed or predominantly mucous acinar cells capped by a few serous acinar cells (serous demilunes) (Figs 2.8 to 2.11).

The serous acini, which contain only serous cells are generally spherical; Mucous acini, which contain only mucous cells are usually more tubular. Mixed acini contain both serous and mucous cells.

Serous Cells

Secretory end pieces that are composed of serous cells are typically spherical and consist of 8 to 12 cells surrounding a central lumen. A typical serous cell is pyramidal in shape with a basally located ovoid nucleus. It has a broad base resting on basal lamina and narrow apex bordering the lumen. These are the cells specialized for the synthesis, storage and secretion of proteins. The so called serous cells in humans also secrete demonstrable amounts of polysaccharide and they have been more appropriately termed as *sero-mucous cells*. The adjacent secretory cells are joined together by junctional complexes consisting of *zonula occludens* (tight junctions); *zonula adherens* (adhering junctions), desmosomes and gap junctions.

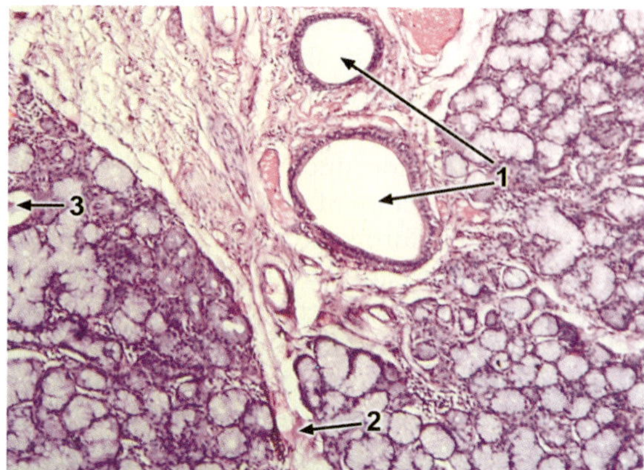

Figure 2.8: Photomicrograph showing the lobes and lobules of mixed salivary gland and interlobular septa (2) with interlobular ducts (1). (H and E, 10x)

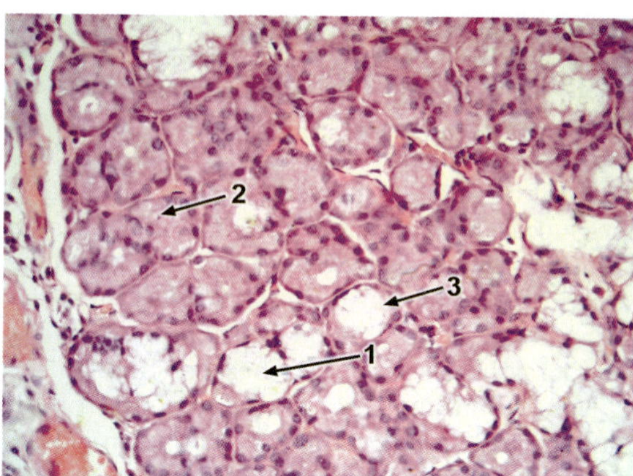

Figure 2.10: Photomicrograph of a mixed salivary gland showing mucous acini (1), serous acini (2) and serous demilunes (3). (H and E, 20x)

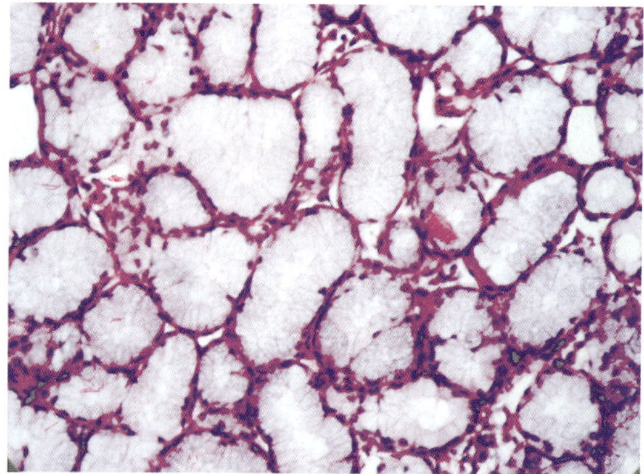

Figure 2.9: Photomicrograph of a mucous salivary gland showing mucous acini with basally placed, flattened nucleus and basophilic cytoplasm. (H and E, 40x)

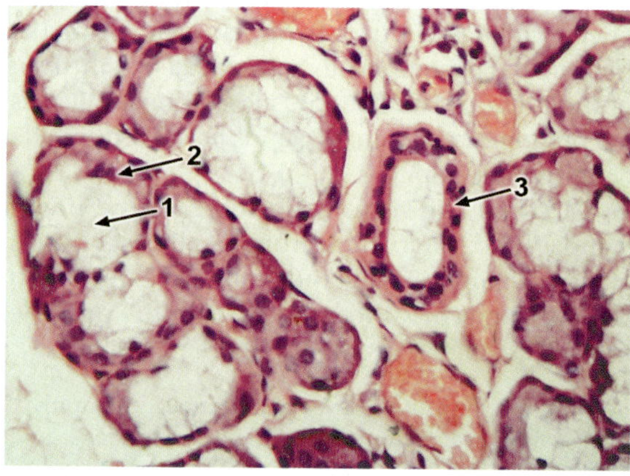

Figure 2.11: Photomicrograph showing mucous acini (1), with serous demilunes (2). Also seen is a striated duct (3). (H and E, 40x)

H and E stained paraffin sections of serous cell in light microscopy, has an extremely basophilic basal cytoplasm and fairly granular acidophilic apical cytoplasm. Three subclasses of serous cells have been described:

1. *The serous cell:* Secretes a watery proteinaceous material.
2. *The sero-mucous cell:* An intermediate cell with characteristics of both the serous cell and mucous cell.

3. *Special serous cell:* It is similar to the serous cell by histochemistry but differ in its ultrastructure.

Ultrastructural Features

The fine structure of serous cell is similar to that of other protein synthesizing cells. It contains abundant basally located rough endoplasmic reticulum (rER) and imparts the infra nuclear basophilia in H and E stained sections, indicating the presence of ribosomal RNA and regular arrangement of flattened cisternae. In the more active cell, the cisternae are frequently dilated and contain an electron dense material. A well developed Golgi complex consisting of multiple stacks of smooth walled membranous saccules is located lateral or apical to the nucleus. Free ribosomes are found throughout the cytoplasm and are associated with the synthesis of non-secretory cellular proteins. Mitochondria is spread throughout the cell. The mitochondria contain the enzymes of citric acid cycle, electron transport, and oxidative phosphorylation. Lysosomes and peroxisomes are generally seen in the apical cytoplasm. Lysosomes contain potent hydrolytic enzymes and function to destroy foreign materials taken up by the cell as well as portions of the cells themselves, such as worn out mitochondria or other membranous organelles. Peroxisomes or microbodies are small organelles containing the enzyme catalase and other oxidative enzymes, and they participate in lipid metabolism. Serous cells also possess well developed cytoskeleton of microtubules and microfilaments. The most prominent feature of serous cell is the presence of secretory granules which occupy the greater portion of apical cytoplasm (Fig. 2.12).

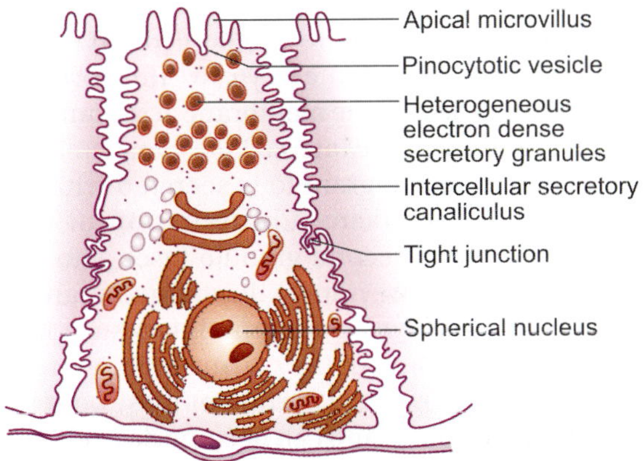

Figure 2.12: Schematic diagram of ultrastructure of a serous cell

Secretory Granules

These are the spherical granules delineated by a single unit membrane. They measure about a micrometer in diameter. The granules may be apposed to one another but in an unstimulated state they do not fuse. They may range from being granular and electron-lucent to being homogenous and electron dense. Granules contain one or more of the following enzymes such as amylase, peroxidase, lactoperoxidase, lysozyme, DNAse, RNAse and lipase in addition to growth factors such as nerve growth factor and epidermal growth factor. The secretory granules are discharged from the apical aspect of the cell by a calcium dependent mechanism called *exocytosis*. The limiting membrane of the granules fuses with the apical plasmalemma of the serous cell. The contents of the secretory granules are ultimately released into the central lumen of the acinus.

In a seromucous end piece, the cells are supported by a basement membrane that separates the parenchyma from the connective tissue. The space between the basement membrane and basal plasma membrane may be increased by the complex folding of basal plasma membrane especially when the cell is not distended with secretory granules. The plasmalemma of a typical serous cell has certain complex specialization necessary for fluid and electrolyte transport. These specializations include basal infoldings, lateral plication, apical microvilli and apical canalicular system. The canalicular system allows the lumen to extend as far as the basal lamina and results in the formation of a stellate shaped lumen. In the submandibular salivary gland the seromucous cells possess a more complicated basal specialization than in parotid gland. The plasma membrane is thrown into a series of tail narrow basal folds extending beyond the lateral border of the cell. This specialization is estimated to increase the basal region of the cell by 60 times. Laterally the adjacent serous cells are attached to each other by apical junctional complexes, which consist of tight junctions, intermediate junctions (*zonula adherens*), and desmosomes (*macula adherens*). The tight junctions help to maintain cell surface domains and regulate the passage of material from the lumen to the intercellular spaces and vice versa. They exhibit selective permeability, allowing the passage of certain ions and water. The adhering junctions and desmosomes found elsewhere along the lateral surfaces serve to hold adjacent cells together. The secretory cells are attached to basal lamina and the underlying connective tissue by hemidesmosomes. Through interactions with cytoplasmic proteins and cytoskeletal elements, these cell to cell and cell to matrix junctions also function in signaling events. Adhering junctions linking the cytoplasm of adjacent cells allow the passage of small molecules between cells, such as ions, metabolites and cyclic adenosine monophosphate (cAMP).

In cells that produce large amounts of protein for secretion, the rER is well developed and arranged in parallel stacks, basally lateral to the nucleus. A closed system of membranous sacs or cisternae, comprised of ribosome studded endoplasmic reticulum fill the basal portion of cytoplasm. The ribosomes then translate the encoded message upon direction from mRNA within the nucleus, and add appropriate amino acids in the protein being synthesized. These initially synthesized secretory proteins known as pre-proteins having an amino terminal extension of about 30 amino acids are called the *signal sequence*. Soon the specific proteins in the rER recognize the signal sequences emerging from the ribosome and bring about the attachment of ribosome on to its membrane. This newly synthesized protein reaching the cisternal space of rER is soon detached of its signal sequence by a proteolytic enzyme called the signal peptidase and the protein assumes its three dimensional structure. The signal sequences also aid in transfer of the growing polypeptide chain across the rER membrane.

The second system of membranous cisternae located apically and lateral to the nucleus are the Golgi apparatus. The Golgi apparatus consists of four to six smooth surface saccules with the concave or trans face towards the secretory surface of the cell. The Golgi apparatus is functionally interconnected with the rER through vesicles budding from the ends of the rER cisternae that approach the *cis* or convex face of the Golgi apparatus. These small vesicles

facilitate the transport of the newly synthesized secretory proteins within the rER to the Golgi apparatus. It is believed that in most instances, the vesicles fuse with *cis* Golgi saccule and the proteins apparently move through the Golgi saccules toward the *trans* face of the Golgi apparatus, where they are packaged into vacuoles of variable size and density. These vacuoles which are the forming secretory granules are called the *immature granules* or *prosecretory granules*. The smaller secretory granules have a light flocculent content and increase in size as their content becomes concentrated.

Generally, most of the proteins undergo modification prior to their secretion and the most common covalent modification of salivary proteins is *glycosylation*, in that there is addition of carbohydrate side chains to the amino acids asparagine, serine and threonine in the proteins. Glycosylation is a multistep process that begins in the rER and is completed in the Golgi apparatus. Other modifications of the secretory proteins may include phosphorylation, sulfation and proteolysis to produce the final secretory product.

The proteins are located in the basally located rER and are subsequently transferred to the apically located Golgi saccules through transitional vesicles. Modification of nascent protein takes place in the Golgi apparatus by glycosylation, involving glycosyl transferase present in the Golgi saccules. Final packaging for export takes place in the Golgi apparatus as well.

The final secretory proteins are stored in the apical cytoplasm and are discharged out of the cell by a process called *exocytosis*. This involves the fusion of the granule membrane at the luminal surface or towards the intercellular canaliculi and in this manner the granule is secreted without any loss of cytoplasm. Continuation of this process, where a second granule fuses with the membrane of a previously discharged granule is termed *compound exocytosis*. This results in a greater enlargement of the plasma membrane at the secretory surface. A portion of these vesicles fuse with lysosomes and can become degraded or they may return to the Golgi apparatus where the membrane may be reutilized for the formation of new secretory granules.

- During exocytosis, secretory granules fuse together to form long chain of secretory granules
- Exocytosis increases the surface area of the acinar lumen
- When discharge is complete, the acinar lumen is gradually decreased in size by membrane uptake process involving pinocytosis.
- In this way specific membrane fragments are recycled.

Mucous Acini

The mucous acini which contain only mucous cells are usually more tubular. Mucous cells are usually cuboidal to columnar in shape; their nuclei are oval and pressed towards the base of the cells. Usually a mucous cell is larger than a serous cell. Unlike the serous acini, mucous acini are characterized by the presence of highly vacuolated, foamy appearing, pale staining apical cytoplasm in H and E stained sections (see Figs 2.8 and 2.9). This appearance and staining is due to the presence of abundant carbohydrate containing moieties in the supranuclear compartment. On the contrary, the cells stain strongly with carbohydrate stains (e.g. mucicarmine stain), which indicates that mucous acini contain carbohydrate content. Functionally, the mucous cells are involved in the complexing of carbohydrate to proteins to form the mucoproteins which are the secretory product of mucous acini. It is imperative that special stains that reveal sugar moieties or acidic groups such as PAS or Alcian blue stains are used to demonstrate the mucous tubules.

Ultrastructural Features

The morphology of mucous cell is variable and depends on the specific stage of the secretory cycle. By transmission electron microscopy, a typical mucous cell is shown to have well developed Golgi complexes, which are located adjacent to or between the nucleus and the secretory droplets (Fig. 2.13). In addition, rER, mitochondria and other cellular organelles are generally confined

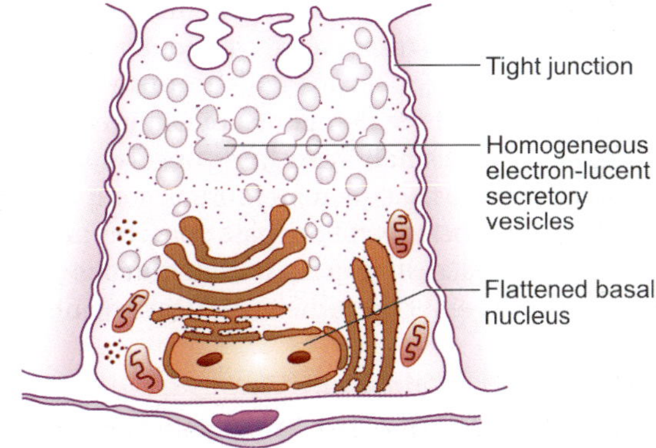

Figure 2.13: Schematic diagram of ultrastructure of mucous cell

to the base and lateral aspects of the cell. The secretory product of the mucous cell differs from the serous cell in three important aspects.
1. They have little or no enzymatic activity
2. Their sole function is that of lubrication
3. The ratio of carbohydrate to protein is greater and larger amounts of sialic acid and occasionally sulphated sugar residues are also present

Secretory product of a mucous cell is stored in the form of mucous droplets unlike the serous acini in which the secretory product is stored in membrane delimited secretory granules. Mucous secretory droplets are larger and more irregularly shaped than serous secretory droplet. Adjacent mucous droplets are separated by thin strands of cytoplasm and these droplets get disrupted during tissue processing. At the ultra- structural level they possess a limiting membrane.

PLASMA MEMBRANE MODIFICATIONS

The interdigitations between the adjacent mucous cells tend to be fewer than serous cell and intercellular canaliculi are found leading to demilunes. Apparently, in the major salivary glands there exists a complex system of basal folds, whereas minor salivary glands exhibit well developed, lateral interdigitations.

In addition to serous and mucous secretory units, the mucous tubules are frequently capped with a collection of serous cells to form serous demilunes, called the demilunes of Gianuzzi (See Fig. 2.11). These small aggregates of serous cells are located in the basement membrane complex of mucous acini. These secretions pass down the lateral intercellular spaces between adjacent mucous cells and eventually enter the lumen of mucous acini.

Mucous Cell at Different Stages of Secretion has Different Appearances

1. The mucous cell at the beginning of secretion may stain well with H and E and closely resemble a seromucous cell
2. With the deposition of mucous droplets in the apical cytoplasm, the cell becomes pale.

Secretion of Mucous Droplets

- The protein synthesis takes place within the rER located in the infranuclear compartment
- The formed proteins are shuttled to various saccules of Golgi apparatus
- Carbohydrate complexing in the Golgi apparatus results in the formation of mucoproteins
- Golgi saccules at the secretory products becomes dilated and give rise to mucous droplets.

Mechanism of Mucous Secretion is not Clearly Known

- Some have advocated an apocrine secretory mechanism involving the luminal release of entire apical cytoplasmic mass
- However, the others believe that mucous cell secretion is similar to serous cell and thus involves a merocrine secretion.

MYOEPITHELIAL CELL

Myoepithelial cells are the contractile cells with numerous processes associated with salivary glands. These are non-secretory cells found in close association with terminal secretory end piece and intercalated ducts. They occupy the space between the basement membrane and the basal plasma membrane of terminal secretory units. Generally, there is usually one myoepithelial cell per secretory end piece. These cells are not evident on the routine H and E preparation however at times only the nucleus is visible. Special histochemical techniques and immunofluorescent techniques will reveal their presence.

The myoepithelial cells have a flattened central body from which five to eight processes radiate to embrace the long axis of the secretory unit (Fig. 2.14). Myoepithelial cells, surrounding serous acini are highly branched cells reminiscent of a basket cradling the secretory unit and are thus called the "basket cells". Those associated with mucous tubules and intercalated ducts are spindle shaped and have far fewer processes and lie parallel to the length of the duct and are not present along the striated duct.

Desmosomal attachments are present between myoepithelial cell and the overlying secretory cell to provide structural stability and prevent the processes from sliding over the acinar or duct cell during contraction (Fig. 2.14). The processes contain many microfilaments or myofilaments that frequently aggregate to form dark bodies along the course of these processes. The normal cytoplasmic organelles found in any cell are mainly located in the perinuclear region of the cell. The structural surface of the cell has many invaginations and contains neural elements that influence the cell's function.

Ultrastructural features of myoepithelial cell are similar to those of a smooth muscle cell. Because of this similarity the function of myoepithelial cell is related to its ability to contract.

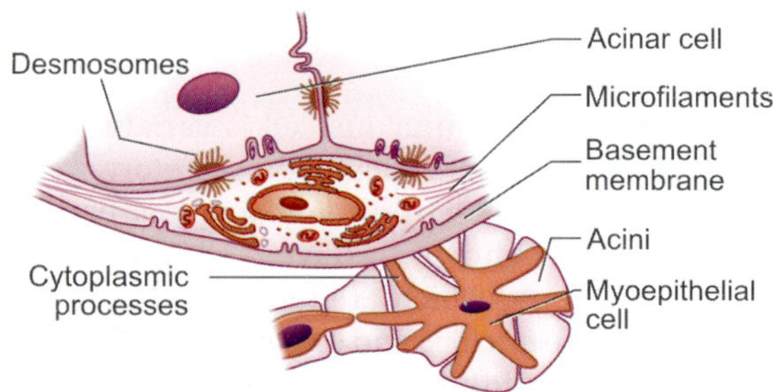

Figure 2.14: Schematic diagram of ultrastructure of myoepithelial cell

Numerous micropinocytic vesicle/caveolae are located on the plasma membrane of myoepithelial cell. The origin of myoepithelial cell has not yet been determined. The cells are generally considered to be of epithelial origin, derived from intercalated duct reserve cell. They are always situated between the parenchymal cell and the basement membrane. Myoepithelial cells demonstrate numerous processes around the proximal ductal system near the intercalated duct.

Myoepithelial cell functions in expelling saliva from the lumen of secretory units and intercalated duct. They support the secretory cells by preventing its over distension as the secretory products accumulate within its cytoplasm. Myoepithelial cells contract and widen the diameter of intercalated duct thus lowering or raising their resistance to overflow. They may also aid in the rupture of acinar cells packed with mucous secretion and lastly may prevent the backward flow of saliva into the gland.

Parotid gland: Purely serous salivary gland. It is unique in that it contains many fat cells; the adipocyte to acinar cell ratio in the parotid is 1:1.

Submandibular gland: It is a mixed salivary gland, but predominantly serous. Ten percent of its acini are mucinous.

Sublingual gland: It is mixed, but predominantly mucous.

DUCT SYSTEM

Among the major salivary glands, the sublingual gland utilizes a simple system of transport, whereas the parotid and submandibular glands involve elaborate networks of ducts. The lumen of the acinus is continuous with the duct system—made up of the intercalated duct, the striated duct, and the excretory duct (from proximal to distal Fig. 2.15).

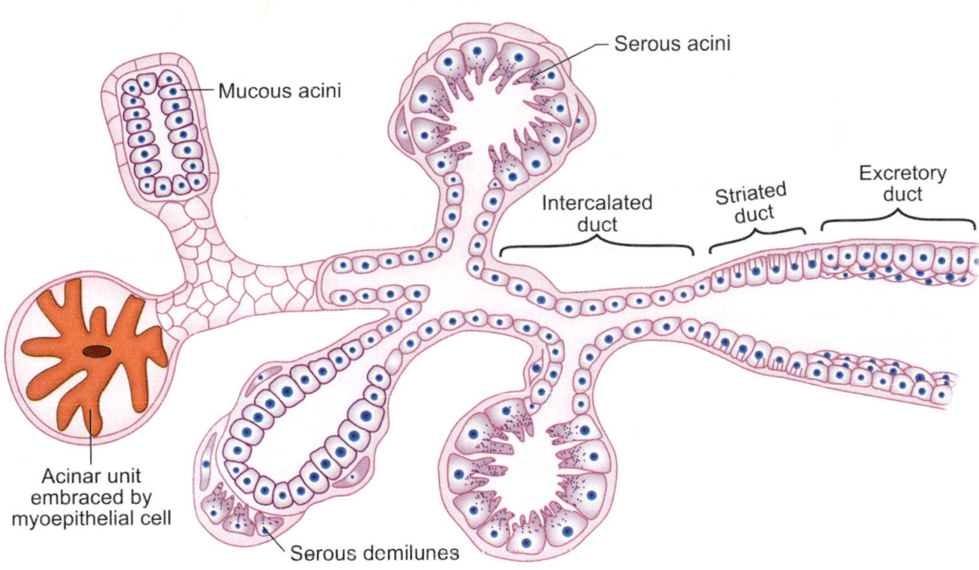

Figure 2.15: Diagrammatic representation of ductal system of the salivary gland

Intercalated Duct

The secretions of the terminal end pieces passes through the intercalated ducts (ICDS). The ducts have smaller diameter and consists of a single row of low columnar cells ranging in shape from low columnar to cuboidal (Fig. 2.16A). It is often difficult to identify them under light microscopy because they are compressed between the secretory units of serous acini. The intercalated duct cells lack the structural specialization suggestive of their passive role in the transport of water and electrolytes or both.

Ultrastructurally, they contain a large centrally located nucleus, few scattered mitochondria, poorly developed rER and a small Golgi complex. These cuboidal cells have a few microvilli projecting into the duct and their lateral border interdigitate with each other by means of junctional complexes situated apically. Some intercalated duct cells contain small secretory granules especially close to the secretory end pieces. Myoepithelial cells are associated with the basal aspect of intercalated duct cells (Fig. 2.16B).

The functional activities of intercalated duct is poorly understood. The intercalated duct is rich in carbonic anhydrase. These cells secrete bicarbonate into the ductal lumen and absorb chloride from the lumen. Intercalated ducts are found in salivary glands having a watery secretion and therefore occur quite frequently in parotid gland. The length of intercalated duct is variable being quite long in parotid; very short in submandibular gland and absent in sublingual salivary gland. From their morphology it is obvious that the cells of intercalated duct do not participate in the activities involving the transport of water and electrolytes. Some investigators have speculated that the cells of intercalated duct represent a population of undifferentiated cells that differentiate into acinar cells, myoepithelial cells, and striated duct cells.

Striated Duct (Intralobular Ducts)

Secretions from the intercalated duct pass directly into the striated duct. The cells of striated duct show abrupt changes in their morphology. They

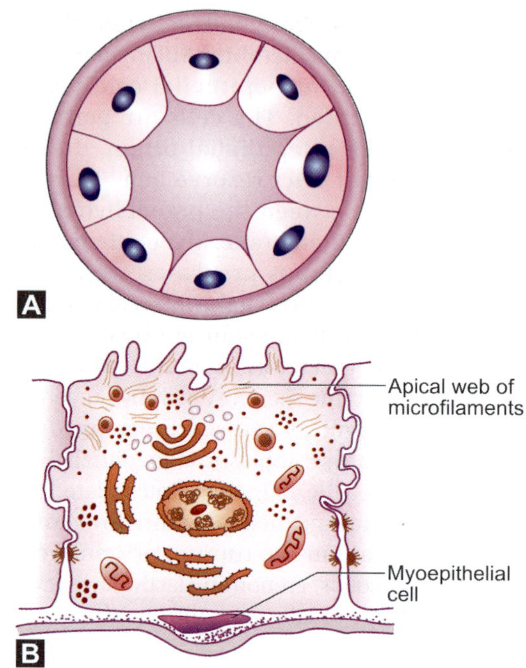

Figures 2.16A and B: (A) Schematic diagram of intercalated duct exhibiting cuboidal cells with centrally placed nucleus. (B) Schematic diagram of the ultrastructure of intercalated duct cell

are essentially made up of tall columnar cells with an eosinophilic cytoplasm having basal striations. In human the striated duct consist primarily of tall columnar epithelial cells, centrally placed ovoid nucleus, scattered rER and Golgi complex (supra nuclear). H and E stained sections of striated duct cell under light microscopy exhibit high degree of eosinophilia, as well as prominent basal striations and thus termed as striated duct (Fig. 2.17A). With transmission electron microscope, striations are seen to consist of basally located elongated mitochondria which alternate with basal infoldings of plasma membrane.

Basal Specializations

The basal indentations extend beyond the lateral boundaries of a single duct cell. As a result, the basal foldings are characterized by a complex series of interlocking basal folds. The net effect of this basal infoldings is an increase in the surface area of basal plasma membrane. In addition, the infoldings in close proximity to the mitochondria facilitate active transport. Micropuncture studies on isolated striated ducts have demonstrated that these structures are responsible for sodium reabsorption from saliva, thus rendering saliva hypotonic with respect to blood plasma.

Such reabsorption is an active process requiring energy in the form of ATP. The ATP is supplied by the numerous mitochondria (Fig. 2.17B) In contrast to these saliva formed in salivary glands that lack striated duct is isotonic to blood plasma. The luminal plasma membrane demonstrates short

stubby microvilli as well as occasional bulbous process known as blebs. The adjacent cells are united by junctional complexes and desmosomes. Striated ducts are always surrounded by a number of longitudinally oriented small blood vessels. Interspersed between the cells of ductal epithelium of both intercalated duct and striated duct are cells described simply as clear cells. They are thought to be of two types, one macro-phage-like and the other lymphocyte-like, and both are involved in immune surveillance. Striated duct demonstrates a few light cells and dark cells containing numerous mitochondria termed oncocytes. The striated duct in parotid gland is described as "pink necklace" permeating the gland. They stain intensely with H and E. *Striated ducts are the sites of reabsorption of Na^+ from the primary secretion and secretion of K^+ and HCO_3^- into the secretion.* The diameter of the striated ducts often exceeds that of the secretory acinus. Striated ducts are located in the parenchyma of the glands (intralobular ducts) but may be surrounded by small amounts of connective tissue in which blood vessels and nerves can be seen running in parallel with the duct.

Terminal Excretory Duct (Interlobular Ducts)

Saliva passes from striated duct into the terminal excretory duct. Salivary fluid is secreted into the oral cavity through the excretory duct. The histology of these ducts varies as they course from striated duct to oral cavity. Near the striated ducts they are lined by pseudostratified epithelium consisting of tall columnar cells admixed with small basal cells and goblet cells. As the excretory duct approaches the oral cavity, the epithelium changes to a true stratified epithelium, merging with that of the oral epithelium. These duct cells lack the basal striations and other specializations seen in the striated duct. However, lateral boundaries show numerous membranous folds or lateral plications. Numerous mitochondria are found scattered through the cytoplasm. The apical cytoplasm contains large electron dense lysosomes as well as small Golgi complex. The confluence of multiple excretory ducts forms the main excretory

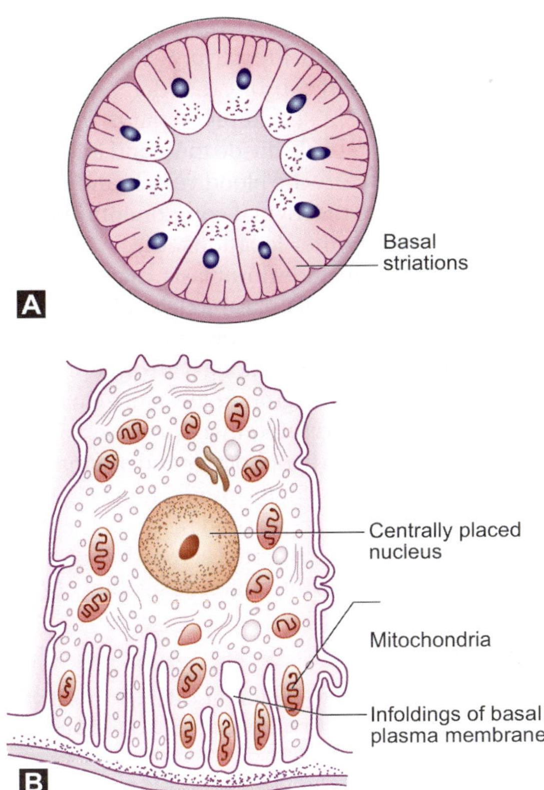

Figures 2.17A and B: (A) Schematic diagram of light microscopic structure of striated duct depicting the columnar cells with basal striations. (B) Schematic diagram of the ultrastructure of a striated duct cell

duct. The main excretory duct modifies the final saliva by altering the electrolyte concentration and also by adding the mucoid component.

> The intercalated duct is short and poorly developed in mucous glands, while the striated duct is nonexistent in mucous glands. However, both of these ducts are well developed in serous glands, where the secretion is heavily modified. Mucous glands, in contrast, do not significantly modify the primary secretion.

FUNCTIONS OF SALIVARY DUCT

The main function of the salivary duct is to convey the primary saliva secreted by the terminal secretory units to the oral cavity. Ducts actively modify primary saliva by secretion and reabsorption of electrolytes and secretion of proteins. In intercalated ducts, the cells contain secretory granules in their apical cytoplasm and two antibacterial enzymes of saliva namely the lysozyme and lactoferrin. The striated duct cells contain kallikrein, an enzyme found in saliva and synthesize secretory glycoproteins which are stored in the apical granules. Studies have shown that both intercalated duct and striated duct cells are capable of absorbing proteins from the lumen by endocytic mechanism. The structure of striated duct cells of basal foldings and mitochondria is typical of cells or tissues involved in water and electrolyte transport such as kidney tubules.

1. *Conveys the primary secretion from the terminal secretory unit* to the oral cavity.
2. *Antibacterial enzymes secreted* by intercalated duct *cell are lactoferrin and lysozyme* and those by the striated duct cells are kallikrein.
3. The structural specialization in the cells of striated duct facilitates *electrolyte transportation* as well as bring about the reabsorption of electrolytes.

The basal cells of the intercalated duct and the excretory duct are capable of giving rise to fully differentiated ductal epithelial cells. This is a significant feature with respect to the bicellular theory of tumorigenesis, which states that all tumors of the salivary glands arise either from the intercalated duct stem cells (Pleomorphic adenoma, Warthin's, oncocytoma, acinic cell carcinoma, adenoid cystic carcinoma, oncocytic carcinoma) or the excretory duct stem cells (Squamous cell carcinoma, mucoepidermoid carcinoma). The bicellular theory, however, has been more or less abandoned in favor of the multicellular theory of tumorigenesis, which states that salivary gland tumors arise from the differentiated cells of the salivary gland unit (i.e., acinar cells, striated duct epithelium, excretory duct epithelium, intercalated duct epithelium, and myoepithelial cells).

CONNECTIVE TISSUE STROMA OF THE SALIVARY GLAND

The connective tissue of the salivary glands includes a variably developed capsule, that demarcates the gland from adjacent structures, septa that extend inward from the capsule divide the gland into lobes and lobules and carry the blood vessels and nerves that supply the parenchymal components and the main duct. As in other locations, the cells of the connective tissue include fibroblasts, macrophages, dendritic cells, mast cells, plasma cells, adipose cells, and occasionally, granulocytes and lymphocytes. Collagen and elastic fibers along with glycoproteins and proteoglycans of the ground substance constitute the extracellular matrix of connective tissue. Salivary gland stroma is rich in lymphocytes and plasma cells, which are responsible for the production of IgA. IgA that fuses with the secretory end piece on the basal membrane, is then transported across the epithelial cell, and released into the lumen as secretory IgA.

BIBLIOGRAPHY

1. Ambudkar IS. Regulation of calcium in salivary gland secretion. Crit Rev Oral Biol Med 2000;11: 4-25.
2. Batsakis JG. Tumors of the head and neck: Clinical and pathological considerations, 2nd edn. Baltimore MD. Williams and Wilkins, 1979.
3. Beahrs OH, Adson MA. The surgical anatomy and technique of parotidectomy. Am J Surg 1958; 95(6):885-96.

4. Crawford EA. Minor salivary glands as a major source of secretory immunoglobulin A in the human oral cavity. Science 1975;190:1206-9.

5. Denny PC, Ball WD, Redman RS. Salivary glands: A paradigm for diversity of gland development. Crit Rev Oral Biol Med 1997;8:51-75.

6. DiGiuseppe JA, Corio RL, Westra WH. Lymphoid infiltrates of the salivary glands: pathology, biology, and clinical significance. Curr Opin Oncol 1996;8:232-7.

7. Dubrull EL. Sicher and DiBrul's oral anatomy. 8th edn. AITBS publishers, New Delhi 1996.

8. Gartner LP, Hiatt JL. Colour textbook of histology. WB Saunders, Pennsylvania 1997.

9. Gray H, Williams LP, Bannister LH. Gray's anatomy: the anatomical basis of medicine and surgery. 38th edn, Elsevier 1995.

10. Klijanienho J, Vielh P. Salivary gland tumours: Monographs in clinical cytology. Karger: Basel 2000;15.

11. Lafrenie RM, Yamada KM. Integrins and matrix molecules in salivary gland cell adhesion, signalling, and gene expression. Ann NY Acad Sci 1998;842:42-8.

12. Nanci A. Ten Cate's oral histology: development, structure, and function, 7th edn, Mosby 2007.

13. Redman RS. Myoepithelium of salivary glands. Microsc Res Tech 1994;27:25-45.

14. Riva A, Tandler B, Testa Riva F. Ultrastructural observations on human sublingual gland. Am J Anat 1988;181:385.

15. Sperber GH. Craniofacial embryology. 4th edn. Wright, Oxford 1993.

16. Stevens A, Lowe J. Human histology. 2nd edn. Mosby, London 1997.

17. Tandler B. Structure of mucous cells in salivary glands. Microsc Res Tech 1993;26:49-56.

18. Tandler B. Structure of serous cells in salivary glands. Microsc Res Tech 1993;26:32-48.

19. Tandler B. Structure of the duct system in mammalian major salivary glands. Microsc Res Tech 1993;26:57-74.

20. Turner RJ. Mechanisms of fluid secretion by salivary glands. Ann NY Acad Sci 1993;694:24-35.

21. Young B, Heath JW. Wheeters' functional histology. 4th edn. Churchill Livingstone, Toronto 2000.

3

Classification of Salivary Gland Diseases

B Sivapathasundharam

Salivary gland diseases vary in their incidence in different parts of the world, and are usually classified into neoplastic and non-neoplastic lesions. A more detailed classification based on their etiology, pathogenesis, histopathology, and management is given below.

CLASSIFICATION OF NON-NEOPLASTIC SALIVARY GLAND DISEASES

Developmental

- Aplasia
- Hypoplasia
- Atresia
- Sialectasia
- Aberrancy (Heterotopia)
- Accessory salivary duct
- Diverticuli
- Polycystic disease of the parotid gland
- Adenomatoid hyperplasia.

Infectious and Inflammatory

- Bacterial
  - Acute sialadenitis
  - Chronic sialadenitis
- Viral
  - Mumps
  - Cytomegalic sialadenitis
  - HIV associated salivary gland disease
  - EBV infection
  - Coxsackie A infection
  - Echo virus infection
  - Parainfluenza type 1, 3 infections.

Obstructive and Traumatic Lesions

- Sialolithiasis
- Extravasation cysts
- Retention cysts
- Fistula
- Other obstructive sialadenopathies (stenosis of ducts, strictures, congenital atresia trauma to parotid papilla due to cheek biting, ill-fitting dentures)
- Necrotizing sialometaplasia
- Radiation induced sialadenitis
- Pneumoparotitis
- Anesthetic mumps.

Functional Disorders

- Xerostomia
- Sialorrhea
- Cystic fibrosis.

Allergic and Immunologic Disorders

- Allergic sialadenitis
- Sjögren's syndrome
- Mikulicz's disease
- Sarcoidosis
- Uveoparotid fever.

Metabolic and Hormonal Disorders

- Sialosis (or sialadenosis)
- Iodide mumps
- Acromegaly.

Ageing

Oncocytosis.

Idiopathic

- Necrotizing sialometaplasia
- Benign cysts of parotid glands
- Angiolymphoid hyperplasia with eosinophilia
- Kimura disease
- Cheilitis glandularis.

CLASSIFICATION OF SALIVARY GLAND NEOPLASMS

Salivary gland neoplasms are remarkable for their histologic diversity. These neoplasms include benign and malignant tumors of epithelial, mesenchymal, and lymphoid origin. Salivary gland tumors pose a great challenge to the histopathologist primarily because of the complexity of the classification and the rarity of several entities, which may exhibit a broad spectrum of morphologic diversity in individual lesions, thus making differentiating benign from malignant tumors difficult.

In the past 50 years, various classifications for salivary gland tumors have been proposed, but none of them appear to be universally accepted. Most of these classification systems follow the general outline proposed by Foote and Frazell (1954) in the first AFIP classification (Table 3.1). In this classification system, the tumors were divided into five specific types of benign tumors and four types of carcinomas, including six subtypes of adenocarcinoma.

The first WHO classification of salivary glands (Thackeray and Sobin) was published in 1972. (Table 3.2) In this classification, there were some major changes, which include:

1. Introduction of the term 'monomorphic adenoma'
2. Change in terminology of papillary cystadenoma lymphomatosum to adeno-lymphoma
3. Change in terminology of acinic cell adenocarcinoma to acinic cell tumor

But within two years, Thackeray and Lucas (1974) modified the WHO classification and was published in the second AFIP atlas of tumor pathology (Table 3.3). In this system, they defined other specific types of monomorphic adenomas, which were not defined in the first WHO classification.

Many of the shortcomings of the above two classification systems were addressed in the second edition of WHO classification (1991) (Table 3.4). The term monomorphic adenoma was a term used to clump all apparently benign lesions that were morphologically homogeneous. In fact it became a diagnostic term for a wide range of lesions that did not meet the criteria for pleomorphic adenoma and included clearly monomorphic entities such as basal cell adenoma but also Warthin's tumor, which is not monomorphic. Additionally, this imprecise term implied that all monomorphic lesions were adenomas which had lead to misclassify monomorphic malignancies such as some adenoid cystic carcinomas, basal cell adenocarcinoma and clear cell carcinoma as monomophic adenomas. Hence, in the second edition, the term 'monomorphic adenoma' was eliminated, as many of the lesions described under monomorphic adenoma category in the first WHO classification, were neither monomorphic nor monocellular. So, the individual tumors were separated and were categorized separately. Also, adenolymphoma was renamed as Warthin's tumor, as the previous terminology had a lymphoma connotation.

In the 1972 WHO classification, two carcinomas were termed tumors, muco-epidermoid tumor and acinic cell tumor. Both were known to have the potential to metastasize, but debate at the time made their true nature uncertain. Hence tumor was used, with the result that clinicians may have regarded these lesions as benign. Recognizing that all of these tumors have the ability to metastasize, in the second edition acinic cell and mucoepidermoid 'tumors', were included in the carcinoma category. Additional new tumors include polymorphous low-grade adenocarcinoma, sebaceous carcinoma, basal cell

Table 3.1: Classification of salivary gland neoplasms by Foote and Frazell (1954)

Benign
- Pleomorphic adenoma (mixed tumor)
- Papillary cystadenoma lymphomatosum
- Oxyphil adenoma
- Sebaceous cell adenoma
- Benign lymphoepithelial lesion
- Unclassified

Malignant
- Malignant mixed tumor
- Mucoepidermoid tumor, low grade and high grade
- Squamous cell carcinoma
- Adenocarcinoma
  - Adenoid cystic (Trabecular or solid)
  - Anaplastic
  - Mucous cell
  - Pseudoadamantine
  - Acinic cell
- Unclassified

Table 3.2: Classification of salivary gland neoplasms by the World Health Organization (Thackeray and Sobin, 1972)

Epithelial tumors
Adenomas
- Pleomorphic adenoma
- Monomorphic adenoma
  - Adenolymphoma
  - Oxyphilic adenoma
  - Other

Mucoepidermoid tumor
Acinic cell tumor
Carcinomas
- Adenoid cystic carcinoma
- Adenocarcinoma
- Epidermoid carcinoma
- Undifferentiated carcinoma
- Carcinoma ex pleomorphic adenoma

Nonepithelial tumors
Unclassified tumors
Allied conditions
- Benign lymphoepithelial lesion
- Sialosis
- Oncocytosis

Table 3.3: Classification of salivary gland neoplasms by Thackeray and Lucas (1974)

Adenomas
Pleomorphic adenoma
Monomorphic adenoma
- Adenolymphoma
- Oxyphilic adenoma
- Tubular adenoma
- Clear cell adenoma
- Basal cell adenoma
- Trabecular adenoma
- Sebaceous adenoma
- Sebaceous lymphadenoma

Mucoepidermoid tumor
Acinic cell tumor
Carcinomas
- Adenoid cystic carcinoma
- Adenocarcinoma
- Epidermoid carcinoma
- Undifferentiated carcinoma
- Carcinoma ex pleomorphic adenoma
- Malignant lymphoepithelial lesion

Connective tissue and other tumors
Benign
- Hemangioma
- Lymphangioma
- Lipoma
- Neurinoma

Malignant
- Sarcoma
- Lymphoma

Metastatic tumors

adenocarcinoma, epithelial-myoepithelial carcinoma (previously termed as clear cell adenoma), salivary duct carcinoma, small cell and undifferentiated carcinomas, oncocytic carcinoma, and malignant myoepithelioma.

All the above classification systems were based on morphology. These systems are simple lists of tumor types divided by their microscopic appearance based on recognizable morphological patterns. These classification systems were challenged, particularly by surgeons, who felt that a list based on pattern matching has little to commend itself in modern onco-surgical practice. With few exceptions, the terminologies used in the

Table 3.4: Revised classification of salivary gland neoplasms by the World Health Organization (Seifert and Sobin, 1991)

Adenomas
- Pleomorphic adenoma
- Myoepithelioma (myoepithelial adenoma)
- Basal cell adenoma
- Warthin's tumor (adenolymphoma)
- Oncocytoma (oncocytic adenoma)
- Canalicular adenoma
- Sebaceous adenoma
- Ductal papilloma
  - Inverted ductal papilloma
  - Intraductal papilloma
    Sialadenoma papilliferum
- Cystadenoma
  - Papillary cystadenoma
  - Mucinous cystadenoma

Carcinomas
- Acinic cell carcinoma
- Mucoepidermoid carcinoma
- Adenoid cystic carcinoma
- Polymorphous low-grade adenocarcinoma (terminal duct adenocarcinoma)
- Epithelial-myoepithelial carcinoma
- Basal cell adenocarcinoma
- Sebaceous carcinoma
- Papillary cystadenocarcinoma
- Mucinous adenocarcinoma
- Oncocytic carcinoma
- Salivary duct carcinoma
- Adenocarcinoma
- Malignant myoepithelioma (myoepithelial carcinoma)
- Carcinoma in pleomorphic adenoma (malignant mixed tumor)
- Squamous cell carcinoma
- Small cell carcinoma
- Undifferentiated carcinoma
- Other carcinomas

Nonepithelial tumors
Malignant lymphomas
Secondary tumors
Unclassified tumors
Tumor-like lesions
- Sialadenosis

Contd...

Contd...

- Oncocytosis
- Necrotizing sialometaplasia (salivary gland infarction)
- Benign lymphoepithelial lesion
- Salivary gland cysts
- Chronic sclerosing sialadenitis of submandibular gland (Kuttner tumor)
- Cystic lymphoid hyperplasia in acquired immunodeficiency syndrome

classifications do not give an indication of tumor grade or behavior.

Considering the clinical usefulness of the classification systems, in 1990 Ellis and Auclair devised a new classification scheme which divided all malignant tumours into low, medium and high grade (AFIP, 1990) (Table 3.5). Clinicians, in particular, found this useful, but the main disadvantage is that some tumors (for example, mucoepidermoid carcinoma, adenoid cystic carcinoma) were categorised in more than one category. Pathologists found it difficult to place an individual tumor into a specific grouping. Pathologists also found that the tumor behavior may be unpredictable and giving a lesion a label of low grade might result in inappropriately conservative management of a malignancy that still retains the potential to metastasize.

In 1996, the most recent AFIP atlas of salivary gland tumor pathology, written by Ellis and Auclair, was published. Their classification system was almost identical to the 1991 WHO system, with only a few differences (Table 3.6). They clarified the group of tumors classified under the term carcinoma in pleomorphic adenoma by subdividing the malignant mixed tumor group into three entities: the more common carcinoma ex pleomorphic adenoma and the much rarer carcinosarcoma and metastasizing mixed tumor. In addition, they included a separate category of clear cell carcinoma that was distinct and different from epithclial-myoepithelial carcinoma and they placed the sebaceous lymphadenoma group of neoplasms

Table 3.5: Classification of salivary gland neoplasms by Ellis and Auclair (1990)

Primary Epithelial Neoplasms

Benign
- Mixed tumor (pleomorphic adenoma)
- Papillary cystadenoma lymphomatosum (Warthin's tumor)
- Oncocytoma
- Cystadenoma
- Basal cell adenoma
- Canalicular adenoma
- Ductal papillomas
    - Sialadenoma papilliferum
    - Inverted ductal papilloma
    - Intraductal papilloma
- Myoepithelioma
- Sebaceous adenomas
    - Sebaceous adenoma
    - Sebaceous lymphadenoma
- Adenoma, not otherwise specified

Malignant

Low-grade
- Mucoepidermoid carcinoma, low-grade
- Acinic cell adenocarcinoma
- Polymorphous low-grade adenocarcinoma (terminal duct carcinoma)
- Basal cell adenocarcinoma
- Adenocarcinoma, not otherwise specified, low-grade
- Metastasizing mixed tumor

Intermediate-grade
- Mucoepidermoid carcinoma, intermediate-grade
- Adenoid cystic carcinoma, cribriform-tubular
- Epithelial-myoepithelial carcinoma
- Adenocarcinoma, not otherwise specified, intermediate-grade
- Clear cell carcinoma
- Cystadenocarcinoma
    - Papillary
    - Nonpapillary
- Sebaceous carcinomas
    - Sebaceous carcinoma
    - Sebaceous lymphadenocarcinoma
- Mucinous adenocarcinoma

Contd...

Contd...

High-grade
- Mucoepidermoid carcinoma, high-grade
- Adenoid cystic carcinoma, solid
- Malignant mixed tumor
    - Carcinoma ex-mixed tumor
    - Carcinosarcoma
- Adenocarcinoma, not otherwise specified, high-grade
- Squamous cell carcinoma
- Undifferentiated carcinoma
    - Small cell carcinoma
    - Lymphoepithelial carcinoma (malignant lymphoepithelial lesion)
    - Others
- Oncocytic carcinoma
- Adenosquamous carcinoma
- Salivary duct carcinoma
- Myoepithelial carcinoma

Nonepithelial Neoplasms of the Major Salivary Glands
- **Benign mesenchymal**
    - Hemangioma
    - Schwannoma
    - Neurofibroma
    - Lipoma
    - Others

Sarcomas
- Hemangiopericytoma
- Malignant schwannoma
- Fibrosarcoma
- Malignant fibrous histiocytoma
- Rhabdomyosarcoma
- Others

Lymphomas
- Non-Hodgkin's lymphoma
- Hodgkin's disease

Metastatic Neoplasms
- Malignant melanoma
- Squamous cell carcinoma
- Renal cell carcinoma
- Thyroid carcinoma
- Others

Table 3.6: Classification of salivary gland neoplasms by Ellis and Auclair (1996)

Benign epithelial neoplasms
- Mixed tumor (pleomorphic adenoma) Myoepithelioma
- Warthin's tumor
- Basal cell adenoma
- Canalicular adenoma
- Oncocytoma
- Cystadenoma
- Ductal papillomas
  - Sialadenoma papilliferum
  - Inverted ductal papilloma
  - Intraductal papilloma
- Lymphadenomas and sebaceous adenomas
- Sialoblastoma

Malignant epithelial neoplasms
- Mucoepidermoid carcinma
- Adenocarcinoma
- Acinic cell adenocarcinoma
- Adenoid cystic carcinoma
- Polymorphous low-grade adenocarcinoma
- Malignant mixed tumors
  - Carcinoma ex mixed tumor
  - Carcinosarcoma
  - Metastasizing mixed tumor
- Squamous cell carcinoma
- Basal cell adenocarcinoma
- Epithelial-myoepithelial carcinoma
- Clear cell adenocarcinoma
- Cystadenocarcinoma
- Undifferentiated carcinomas
  - Small cell undifferentiated carcinoma
  - Large cell undifferentiated carcinoma
  - Lymphoepithelial carcinoma
- Oncocytic carcinoma
- Salivary duct carcinoma
- Sebaceous adenocarcinoma and lymphadenocarcinoma
- Myoepithelilal carcinoma
- Adenosquamous carcinoma
- Mucinous adenocarcinoma

Mesenchymal neoplasms
- Benign
- Sarcomas

Malignant lymphomas
Metastatic tumors
Non-neoplatic tumor-like conditions

Table 3.7: Revised classification of salivary gland neoplasms by the World Health Organization (2005)

Malignant epithelial tumors
- Acinic cell carcinoma
- Mucoepidermoid carcinoma
- Adenoid cystic carcinoma
- Polymorphous low-grade adenocarcinoma
- Epithelial-myoepithelial carcinoma
- Clear cell carcinoma, not otherwise specified
- Basal cell adenocarcinoma
- Sebaceous carcinoma
- Sebaceous lymphadenocarcinoma
- Cystadenocarcinoma
- Low-grade cribriform cystadenocarcinoma
- Mucinous adenocarcinoma
- Oncocytic carcinoma
- Salivary duct carcinoma
- Adenocarcinoma, not otherwise specified
- Myoepithelial carcinoma
- Carcinoma ex pleomorphic adenoma
- Carcinosarcoma
- Metastasizing pleomorphic adenoma
- Squamous cell carcinoma
- Small cell carcinoma
- Large cell carcinoma
- Lymphoepithelial carcinoma
- Sialoblastoma

Benign epithelial tumors
- Pleomorphic adenoma
- Myoepithelioma
- Basal cell adenoma
- Warthin tumor
- Oncocytoma
- Canalicular adenoma
- Sebaceous adenoma
- Lymphadenoma
  - Sebaceous
  - Non-sebaceous
- Ductal papillomas
  - Inverted ductal papilloma
  - Intraductal papilloma
  - Sialadenoma papilliferum
- Cystadenoma

Soft tissue tumors
- Hemangioma

Hematolymphoid tumors
- Hodgkin's lymphoma
- Diffuse large B-cell lymphoma
- Extranodal marginal zone B-cell lymphoma

Secondary tumors

into the category of 'lymphadenomas', which encompassed tumors with and without sebaceous differentiation.

In 2005, the third revision of WHO classification of salivary gland neoplasms was published (Table 3.7). This classification system is a listing of all the tumors and adds no information to the clinician regarding clinical behavior. Pathologists suggest that, classification systems should not dictate the treatment protocol, especially for the malignant neoplasms. Instead, the TNM/ TNMp staging should be used by the clinicians to plan the treatment.

BIBLIOGRAPHY

1. Barnes L, Eveson JW, Reichart P, Sidransky D. World Health Organization Classification of Tumours. Pathology and Genetics of Head and Neck Tumours. Salivary glands. Lyon, IARC Press, 2005;5.
2. Batsakis JG, Luna MA, el-Naggar AK. Basaloid monomorphic adenomas. Ann Otol Rhinol Laryngol 1991;100:687-90.
3. Batsakis JG. Tumors of the head and neck: Clinical and pathological considerations, 2nd edn. Baltimore, MD: Williams and Wilkins, 1979.
4. Cawson RA, Odell EW. Neoplastic and non-neoplastic diseases of salivary glands. In: Cawson's essentials of oral pathology and oral medicine, 7th edn. Churchill Livingstone 2002;18:255-74.
5. Di Palma S, Simpson RHW, Skalova A, Leivo I. Major and minor salivary glands. In: Cardesa A, Slootweg PJ (Eds). Pathology of the head and neck. Springer Verlag, 2006;5:132-7.
6. Ellis GL, Auclair PL. Classification of salivary gland neoplasms. In: Ellis GL, Auclair PL, Gnepp DR (Eds). Surgical Pathology of the Salivary Glands. Philadelphia, Saunders 1991.pp.35-64.
7. Ellis GL, Auclair Pl. Major Salivary Glands. In: Silverberg SG, DeLellis RA, Frable WJ (Eds). Principles and Practice of Surgical Pathology and Cytopathology, 3/e (Vol 2), Churchill Livingstone, 1997.
8. Ellis GL, Auclair PL. Tumours of the salivary glands. 3rd edn. Armed Forces Institute of Pathology: Washington, 1996.
9. Foote FW Jr, Frazell EL. Atlas of Tumor Pathology. Tumors of the Major Salivary Glands. 1st Series, Fascicle II, Washington, DC: Armed Forces Institute of Pathology, 1954.
10. Harris MD, McKeever P, Robertson JM. Congenitals of the salivary gland: A case report and review. Histopathology 1990;17(2):155-7.
11. Lundeberg D. Non-neoplastic disorders of the parotid gland. West J Med 1983;138:589-95.
12. Mandel L, Surattanont F. Bilateral parotid swelling: A review. Oral Surg Oral Med Oral Pathol Oral Radiol Endod 2002;93:221-37.
13. McQuone SJ. Acute viral and bacterial infections of the salivary glands. Otolaryngol Clin North Am 1999;32:793-811.
14. Rice DH. Noninflammatory, non-neoplastic disorders of the salivary gland. Otolaryngology Clinics of North America 1999;32(5):835-42.
15. Rice DH. Salivary gland disorders: Neoplastic and Non-neoplastic. Medical Clinics of North America 1999;83(1):197-218.
16. Seifert G, Brocheriou C, Cardesa A, Eveson JW. WHO International Histological classification of tumors. Tentative histological classification of salivary gland tumors. Pathol Res Pract 1990;186; 555-81.
17. Seifert G, Miehlke A, Haubrich J, Chillar R. Disease of the salivary glands. Stuttgart: George Thieme, 1986.
18. Seifert G, Sobin LH. Histological typing of salivary gland tumors. World Health Organization international histological classification of tumors. 2nd edn. New York: Springer-Verlag 1991.
19. Seifert G, Sobin LH. The World Health Organization's Histological classification of salivary gland tumors. A commentary on the 2nd edn. Cancer 1992;70:379-85.
20. Seifert G. Tumor-like lesions of salivary glands. The new WHO classification. Pathol Res Pract 1992;188:836-46.
21. Sobin LH, Wittekind C. TNM. Classification of Malignant Tumours. 6th edn. John Wiley & Sons: New York, 2002.
22. Thackray AC, Lucas RB. Tumors of the Major Salivary Glands. Fascicle 10, 2nd Series, Atlas of Tumor Pathology, Washington DC, Armed Forces Institute of Pathology, 1974.
23. Thackray AC, Sobin LH. Histological Typing of Salivary Gland Tumours. Geneva, World Health Organization, 1972.

4

Non-neoplastic Diseases of Salivary Glands

B Sivapathasundharam

DEVELOPMENTAL DISORDERS

Aplasia

Salivary gland aplasia refers to the failure of development of the salivary glands. Congenital absence of the major salivary glands is very rare. Any one of the glands or group of glands may be missing, unilaterally or bilaterally. Parotid gland agenesis has been reported in conjunction with several congenital conditions, including hemifacial microsomia, mandibulofacial dysostosis, cleft palate, lacrimoauriculodentodigital syndrome, Treacher Collins syndrome, and anophthalmia. Enamel hypoplasia, and anodontia are other oral manifestations related to salivary agenesis.

Hypoplasia

It refers to under development of any of the major gland and can be a feature of Melkersson-Rosenthal syndrome or ectodermal dysplasia.

Atresia

Absence or marked narrowing of the excretory duct of the salivary gland is known as atresia. Atresia may lead to mucous retention or xerostomia. It is thought to be due to a congenital malformation of the first branchial arch.

Aberrant Salivary Gland

Salivary gland tissue located in sites other than normal anatomic distribution of the major salivary glands, oral mucosa, and pharynx is referred to as *heterotopic salivary gland, ectopic salivary gland,* or *salivary gland choristoma.*

Etiology

The embryogenesis of heterotopic salivary gland tissue is unclear and is more related to the anatomic site of occurrence. *Willis* has proposed three explanations for heterotopia:
1. Abnormal persistence and development of vestigeal structures,
2. Dislocation of a portion of a definite organ rudiment during mass movement of development, and
3. Heteroplasia or abnormal differentiation of the local tissues.

Clinical Features

Most of the heterotopic salivary glands are seen to occur in the head and neck region, but few cases have been reported in the remote areas of the body. The most common locations include paraparotid lymph nodes, the middle ear, and the lower neck. Less frequent sites include upper neck, mandible, external auditory canal, mediastinum, cerebellopontine angle, pituitary gland, prostate gland, vulva, rectum, thyroglossal duct, thyroid gland, and parathyroid capsules.

Salivary gland tissue is occasionally found associated with mandible either in an intraosseous location or in crypt-like invaginations of the lingual surface. Basically, they do not represent heterotopic tissue, because they are most often extensions of indigenous salivary gland tissue of submandibular salivary gland. The most common location for this type of involvement is the posterior mandible and is referred to as the *Stafne's bone cavity or cyst.* It is usually located between the angle of the mandible and the first molar below the level of the inferior alveolar nerve. The gland is usually asymptomatic and appears on radiographs as a round unilocular well-circumscribed radiolucency.

Intraorally many cases of salivary gland choristomas have been reported in the gingiva. Clinically, they are seen as yellow swellings at the mucogingival junction and are composed of seromucous or pure mucous glands. They possibly arise from pluripotent gingival epithelium or results from a mechanical disturbance during development.

Lobules of parotid salivary tissues that are separated from the main gland is known as *accessory parotid gland*. They drain into the stensen's duct, by one or more accessory ducts. Masseter muscle (bound to the fascia of the masseter) is the common site for the occurrence of accessory parotid tissue. Clinically they present themselves as masses in the cheek, anterior to the tragus of the ear. They are usually asymptomatic except for the cosmetic problem.

Accessory or ectopic glandular tissues are susceptible to the same diseases that may affect the main gland. Failure to recognize the accessory gland during clinical evaluation could result in inadequate treatment and may be the reason for recurrence in some instances.

Polycystic Disease of the Parotid Gland

Polycystic disease of parotid gland is considered to be a development malformation of the ductal system. It shows a prominent female predilection and is most often bilateral. It is characterized by recurrent, painless swelling of the parotid glands, but salivation is usually not affected. It manifests in childhood or manifestation may be delayed until adulthood. Involvement is most often bilateral.

Histologically, this lesion is characterized by honeycombed or lattice-like pattern, produced by many epithelium lined cysts, and these cysts replace the lobules and cause their distension. Lumen of the cyst may contain eosinophillic material and few macrophages. Concentric eosinophilic bodies resembling spherolith is seen in many cystic lumen. Occasional ducts open into

the cysts and some acinar units communicate with these cysts suggesting their origin from the intercalated ducts. Residual acinar cells may be seen as islands between the cysts. There is lack of inflammatory reaction in the involved gland.

Care should be taken to differentiate polycystic disease from, salivary gland tumors, having multicystic pattern, such as mucoepidermoid carcinoma, acinic cell adenocarcinoma, and adenoid cystic carcinoma.

ADENOMATOID HYPERPLASIA

Giansanti et al in 1971 first described this uncommon entity. It represents a hamartomatous proliferation or reactive hyperplasia, of the mucous glands of the palate.

Clinically, it mimics benign salivary gland neoplasm and appears as firm, sessile, painless mass having normal or bluish color. Though hard palate is the most common site of involvement, followed by soft palate, and junction of hard and soft palate, cases have been reported in retromolar area, buccal mucosa, labial mucosa, and ventral tongue.

Microscopically, the glandular lobules are enlarged with presence of normal appearing mucous acini and ducts. The amount of acinar cells is more than normal and appears crowded to justify acinar hyperplasia. The overlying epithelium may show pseudoepitheliomatous hyperplasia. Inflammation is usually absent.

Since it cannot be clinically differentiated from the salivary gland neoplasms, it is imperative that the lesion be excised for histologic examination.

Accessory Salivary Ducts

Accessory ducts are common and do not require treatment. The most frequent location being superior and anterior to the normal location of Stensen's duct.

Diverticuli

A diverticulum is a pouch or sac protruding from the wall of a duct. Diverticuli in the ducts of the major salivary glands lead to pooling of saliva and recurrent sialadenitis. Diagnosis is made by sialography.

INFECTIONS AND INFLAMMATORY DISORDERS (SIALADENITIS)

Inflammation of the salivary gland is known as sialadenitis and that of the duct is sialodochitis. These may be caused by microorganisms including bacteria, mycobacteria, viruses, fungi, parasites, and protozoa, trauma, irradiation, and allergic conditions.

Bacterial Sialadenitis

Acute Bacterial Sialadenitis

Etiology: Acute bacterial sialadenitis also called as *acute suppurative sialadenitis* is usually caused by ascending infection from the oral cavity, especially in patients with reduced salivary gland function. The reduction of salivary flow results in diminished mechanical flushing, which allows bacteria to colonize the oral cavity and then to invade the salivary duct and cause acute bacterial infection.

This condition was previously referred to as 'surgical parotitis' because postsurgically patients often experienced gland enlargement from ascending bacterial infections. This was thought to be related to the markedly decreased salivary flow during anesthesia (as a result of administered anticholinergic drugs and relative dehydration due to restricted fluids). With the administration of prophylactic antibiotics and routine perioperative hydration, this condition now occurs much less frequently.

The parotid gland is the most frequently involved. This may be the consequence of long and narrow anatomy of Stensen's duct compared to short and wide submandibular and sublingual duct. It is also theorized that the submandibular glands may be protected by the high level of mucin in the saliva, which has potent antimicrobial activity. Additionally, the orifice of Stensen's duct is located adjacent to the molars, where heavy bacterial colonization occurs.

The various predisposing factors include congenital malformation of ducts, a decreased rate of secretion, stasis, alteration in composition of the saliva and development of antibiotic-resistant bacteria. Coagulase-positive *Staphylococcus aureus* and *Streptococcus viridans* are the most common causative bacteria, and less commonly *Escherichia coli*, *Streptococcus pneumoniae* and *Haemophilus influenzae.*

Clinical features: Acute suppurative sialadenitis is usually unilateral. The affected gland is swollen and tender, and systemic symptoms, such as fever, malaise, regional lympadenopathy and leukocytosis, are common. The excretory duct is indurated, and pus can usually be expressed from its orifice. In case of parotitis, it manifests as a sudden onset of pain at the angle of the mandible, which worsens when the jaws are opened for eating or speaking. Examination reveals a tender, enlarged gland, with the overlying skin characteristically warm and red.

Histopathology: Histopathology reveals edema, hyperemia, and acute inflammatory infiltrate. A periductal and intraductal polymorphonuclear leukocytic infiltrate is associated with destruction of the ductal epithelium. Acini are lost and parenchymal microabscesses form as the inflammatory process progresses. Bacterial colonies may be seen in the ducts.

Chronic Bacterial Sialadenitis

Etiology: The various etiological factors include mechanical, physical, microbial, and immunologic factors. Mechanical obstruction of the duct (sialolith, strictures, stenosis, extrinsic duct compression), decreased salivary flow, increased salivary viscosity, and ascending infection all play a potential role in chronic sialadenitis. Ascending infection is a potential complication of ductal obstruction. Long-standing obstruction leads to chronic sialadenitis with acinar atrophy and fibrosis. The fibrotic change in the end-stage is referred to as *chronic sclerosing sialadenitis* or *Kuttner tumor.* The affected glands are stony hard and clinically simulate tumors.

Chronic (juvenile) recurrent parotitis is a disorder primarily affecting children and has exhibited autosomal dominant inheritance in some cases. Patients with cystic fibrosis are predisposed to developing chronic sialadenitis, particularly of the sublingual and minor (mucus-rich) salivary glands. Other causes include radiotherapy and granulomatous inflammation. Radiotherapy commonly leads to sialadenitis especially of the parotid glands.

Granulomatous sialadenitis is a form of chronic sialadenitis with many potential causes. It is most commonly caused by obstructive disease, with extravasation of duct contents and a subsequent foreign body reaction. An infectious etiology is much less common. The various infectious agents responsible for granulomatous inflammation include mycobacteria, fungi, and the agent of cat-scratch disease. Up to 6% of patients with sarcoidosis have parotid involvement.

Clinical features: Chronic recurrent sialadenitis is characterized by recurrent painful swelling of salivary glands, usually the parotid. It may or may not be bilateral. Pus can be expressed from the excretory duct, and the organisms most frequently cultured are *staphylococci* and *streptococci.* Fever and leucocytosis are absent or mild. Symptom-free periods last from weeks to months. After several recurrences, the glandular parenchyma may undergo fibrosis and result in decreased salivary flow.

Chronic (juvenile) recurrent parotitis is a long-standing disorder characterized by bilateral fluctuating parotid enlargement, as frequent as every 3 to 4 months. *Streptococcus pneumoniae* and *Haemophilus influenzae* are frequently recovered in these cases. Boys are affected more commonly than girls, and the disease commonly becomes asymptomatic at puberty.

Histopathology: Chronic sialadenitis is characterized by fibrosis, with acinar atrophy and chronic inflammation. Inflammation tends to aggregate periductally. Lymphoid aggregates with germinal center formation are common. Acinar atrophy may be marked so that acini are completely lacking. The ductal epithelium is prone to metaplastic changes, including squamous cell, mucous cell, and ciliary cell metaplasia. Oncocytic change is common in inflamed minor salivary glands.

A granulomatous inflammatory response may be seen, with extravasation of saliva secondary to duct rupture. The Kuttner tumor is characterized by periductal lymphoplasmacytic inflammation with incorporation of the interlobular and intralobular ducts in thick fibrous trabeculae. Chronic (juvenile) recurrent parotitis shows dilatation of interlobular ducts with marked periductal lymphocytic infiltration. Exocytosis of lymphocytes into the hyperplastic ductal epithelium is typical.

Viral Sialadenitis

Several viruses have been causally associated with viral sialadenitis, including paramyxovirus (mumps), coxsackievirus, lymphocytic-chorio-meningitis virus, herpes virus, cytomegalovirus, influenza A, parainfluenza and adenovirus. Of these, the paramyxovirus due to its common association is also called as the sialoadenotropic virus.

Mumps (Epidemic Parotitis)

Clinical Features

Mumps is an acute, contagious, self-limiting viral infection that predominantly affects children. It is caused by droplet infection of the upper respiratory tract. Viremia develops during an incubation period usually lasting 16 to 18 days, following which pain and rapid swelling in one or both of the parotid glands becomes evident. The salivary gland continues to enlarge for 2 to 3 days, and returns to normal size in 7 to 10 days. The rubbery or elastic swelling is located below the ear, and displaces the ear lobe upward and outward. It is accompanied by fever, malaise, and anorexia. Citrus fruits that stimulate salivation intensify the pain. Diagnosis is usually made on clinical grounds and is supported by the serologic findings.

Saliva expressed from the Stensen's duct appears normal (in contrast to bacterial sialadenitis).

Pathogenesis

Droplet infection with the virus is followed by replication of the virus in the respiratory epithelial cells. It spreads from the respiratory tract to regional lymph nodes and subsequently leads to viremia. The affected area shows perivascular and interstitial mononuclear cell infiltrates with edema. Necrosis of acinar and epithelial duct cells are seen in salivary glands and in the germinal epithelium of seminiferous tubules.

Complications

The viremia that develops during the course of the disease can infect other organs, and may cause orchitis, meningoencephalitis, pancreatitis, and arthritis. It may lead to sterility in males (sequela to orchitis) and deafness (sequela to encephalitis).

Cytomegalic Inclusion Disease (Salivary Gland Inclusion Disease)

Cytomegalic inclusion disease is an infection with Cytomegalovirus (CMV) which could occur in one of the four forms: congenital infection, perinatal infection, CMV mononucleosis in immunocompetent and immunocompromised individuals.

Clinical Features

Cytomegalovirus (CMV) infection occurs in a newborn trans-placentally and manifests as an acute illness. It is associated with petechiae, thrombocytopenia, hepatosplenomegaly, chorioretinitis, and microcephaly. The virus can be isolated from various body fluid or cells, including saliva, urine, semen, feces, breast milk and cervical secretions.

Detection of CMV infections in pregnant women is extremely important as transplacental transmission of CMV can result in prematurity, low-birth weight, and various congenital malformations. Infected newborns and young children suffer from hepatitis, myocarditis, hematologic abnormalities, pneumonitis, and nervous system damage. The infection is often fatal; those children who do survive frequently experience permanent nerve damage resulting in mental retardation and seizure disorders.

In AIDS, CMV is the most common cause of life-threatening opportunistic infection. CMV infection can result in gastrointestinal distress (gastritis, colitis); visual loss (retinitis); non-productive cough (pneumonitis); and abnormal liver, kidney and adrenal function tests.

Pathologic Features

The CMV-infected cells are large (almost twice that of normal cell), with characteristic amphophilic large nuclear and smaller cytoplasmic inclusions and eccentrically placed nuclei, resulting in an 'owl-eye' appearance.

HIV Associated Salivary Gland Disease (HIV-SGD)

HIV infected individuals may manifest enlargement of the salivary glands due to AIDS-related tumors, Kaposi's sarcoma, and lymphoma. In addition, a Sjögren's like syndrome of unknown etiology causes xerostomia and salivary gland enlargement in AIDS patients.

Clinical Features

The HIV-SGD is associated with a cluster designation-8 (CD8) cell lymphocytosis of the salivary glands and with diffuse infiltrative lymphocytosis syndrome (DILS). In this condition, lymphocytic infiltration is found in the salivary glands, lungs, gastrointestinal tract and liver. The parotid gland is involved in 98% of cases, and is bilateral in 60% of cases. The main clinical sign noted in children and in earlier stage of disease is parotid enlargement, which is bilateral and concomitant with cervical lymphadenopathy. As HIV progress, as a result of altered immunomodulation, the salivary glands are infiltrated with CD8 lymphocytes leading to diffuse infiltrative lymphocytosis syndrome, which leads to enlargement of the salivary gland. This group of patients are at risk of B cell lymphoma.

The xerostomia could be due to drugs (anti-retrovirals, antifungals, chemotherapeutics, antihistaminics, mood altering drugs, multi-vitamins), oral diseases (candidiasis) or as a part of the progression of the HIV disease.

Pathological Features

Biopsy of labial minor salivary glands shows lymphocytic infiltration similar to Sjögren's syndrome, but with a predominance of T8 lymphocytes (in Sjögren's syndrome T4 lymphocytes predominate). Biopsy of the involved salivary gland show that the enlargement is due to a combination of hyperplastic lymph nodes, lymphocytic infiltrates, and cystic cavities.

OBSTRUCTIVE AND TRAUMATIC DISORDERS

Obstructive disorders are some of the most common disorders of the major and minor salivary glands. They can occur as a result of traumatic severance of salivary gland ducts, stasis of salivary secretions in ducts, and partial or complete blockage of the excretory ducts. Many conditions may cause enlargement of salivary glands or cessation of salivary flow and, thus, mimic or promote the development of an obstructive disorder. The primary means by which these disorders cause a reduction or cessation of salivary flow are tabulated in Flow chart 4.1. The effects of these disorders are often interrelated (Flow chart 4.2).

Sialolithiasis

Sialoliths are calcified and organic matter that forms within the secretory system of the major salivary glands.

Etiology

The various factors that contribute to stone formation include inflammation, irregularities in the duct system, local irritants, and anticholinergic medications. These factors may cause pooling of saliva within the duct, which is thought to promote stone formation.

The most accepted theory is that stone formation is the result of deposition of salts around a nidus of debris accumulated within the lumen of the duct. The debris may include bacteria, exfoliated ductal epithelial cells, mucous plugs, foreign bodies, dried secretions or other cellular debris.

Variations in serum calcium and phosphorus levels do not have any relationship to the formation of sialolith.

Flow chart 4.1: Various disorders that cause a reduction or cessation of salivary flow

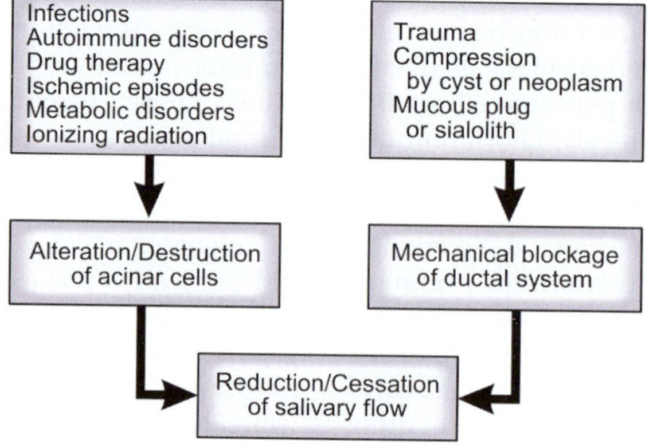

Flow chart 4.2: Inter-relationship of various factors that cause stasis of salivary secretion

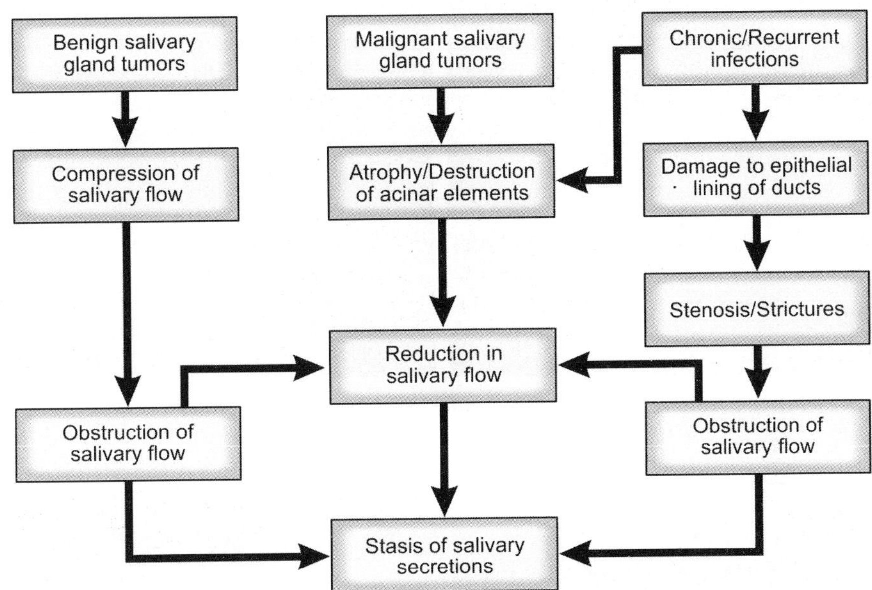

Composition

Sialoliths are crystalline and are primarily composed of hydroxyapatite. The chemical composition is calcium phosphate and carbon, with trace amounts of magnesium, potassium chloride and ammonium.

> Eighty percent of parotid gland sialoliths and 20% of submandibular gland sialoliths are poorly calcified. This is clinically significant because such sialoliths are not radiographically detectable.

Location

Eighty to ninety percent of sialoliths occur in the submandibular gland (Figs 4.1 to 4.3). Less than 20% occur in the parotid gland. The sublingual gland accounts for approximately 1%, and the minor salivary glands for even fewer. When salivary calculi do involve minor salivary glands, they usually occur in the glands of the upper lip and buccal mucosa. The higher rate of sialolith formation in the submandibular gland is attributed to the tortuous course of Wharton's duct; higher pH, mucin content, calcium and phosphate levels of submandibular saliva; and the dependent position of the submandibular glands, which leave them prone to stasis.

Calculi may be present both within the ducts and within the parenchyma of the gland. Intraparenchymal stones are uncommon and usually asymptomatic.

Clinical Features

Sialolithiasis occurs most often in middle age and is slightly more common in men. Occurrence in children is quite rare. Patients with sialoliths most commonly present with a history of acute, intermittent swelling and postprandial pain of the affected major salivary gland. The degree of symptoms depends on the extent of ductal obstruction and the presence of secondary infection. Complete or partial blockage of salivary flow causes salivary pooling within the ducts and gland. Since, the glands are encapsulated and there is little space for expansion, the enlargement causes pain. In case of partial blockage of the duct, the swelling subsides as salivary stimulation is removed and output decreases, and saliva seeps past the partial obstruction.

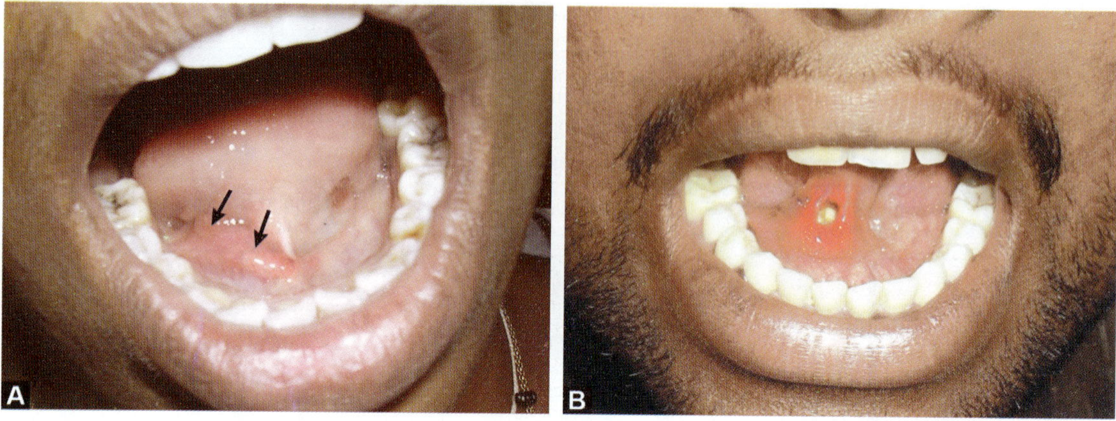

Figures 4.1A and B: Sialolith of submandibular duct

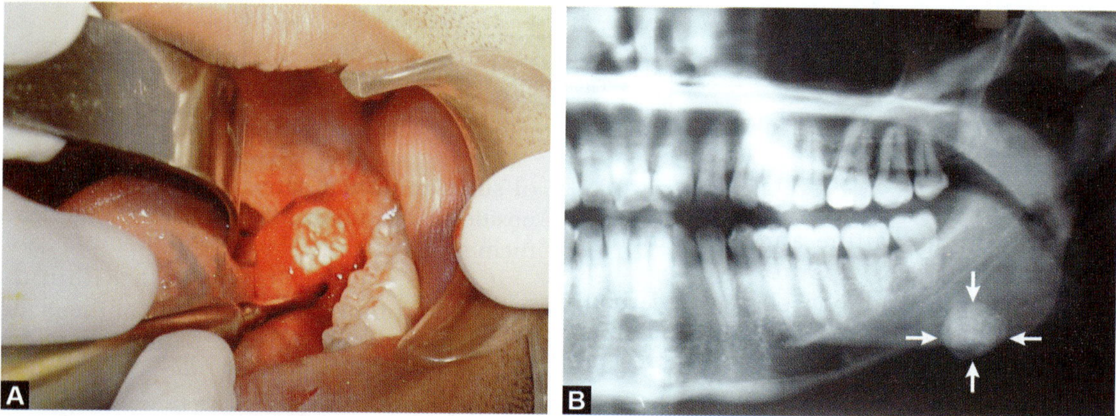

Figures 4.2A and B: Sialolith of posterior part of left submandibular duct. The yellowish mass with irregular surface is seen on exposure of the duct (A). The radiograph of the same case showing a circular radiopaque mass superimposed on the angle of the mandible (B)

Bacterial infections may or may not be superimposed and are more common with chronic obstructions. Sequelae of long-standing calculi include acute sialadenitis, ductal strictures, ductal dilatation, and acinar atrophy. Fistulae, sinus tract, or ulceration may occur over the stone in chronic cases.

Pathological Features

Sialoliths range from white to yellowish white, with a smooth or rough surface and may be friable. Sialoliths frequently exhibit concentric laminations on cut sections (Figs 4.4A and B). Microscopically, the ductal epithelium of the affected salivary gland is usually compressed and commonly shows squamous, oncocytic, or mucous cell metaplasia.

Long-standing obstruction with retention of secretions leads to chronic obstructive sialadenitis. Histologic changes include periductal and lobular chronic inflammatory cell infiltrates, occasional acute inflammation, ductal dilatation,

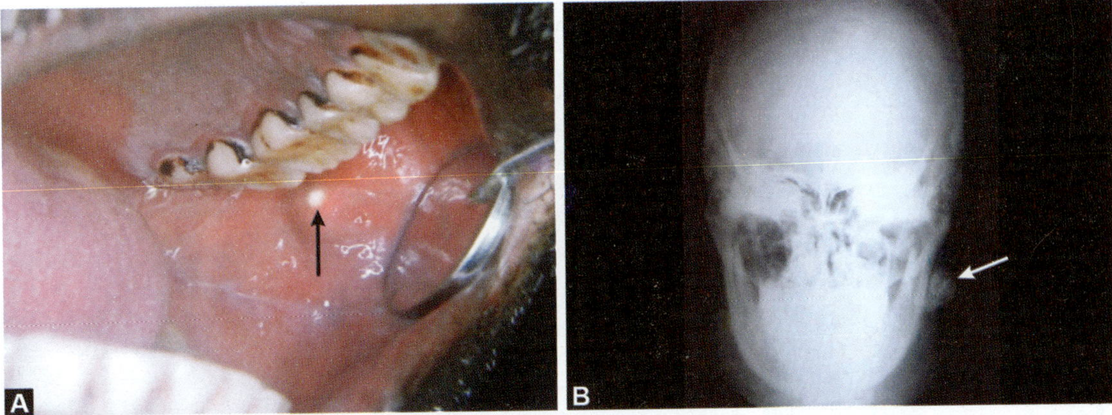

Figures 4.3A and B: Sialolith of parotid duct. The sialolith is seen as a small, round yellowish spot on the buccal mucosa (A). The anteroposterior view of the skull shows a large irregular radiopaque shadow (B) (*Courtesy:* Dr S Karthiga Kannan, Sree Mookambika Institute of Dental Sciences, Kanyakumari District)

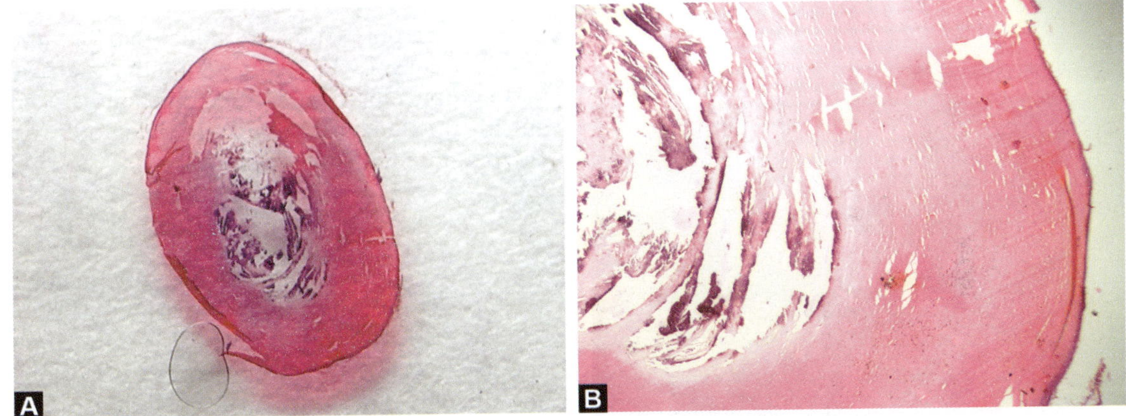

Figures 4.4A and B: Sialolith of the submandibular gland showing a central nidus surrounded by concentric calcifications

and parenchymal atrophy with scarring. Calculi may occur secondarily in association with neoplasms such as acinic cell carcinoma and mucoepidermoid carcinoma.

Diagnosis

Palpation along the pathway of the duct may confirm the presence of a stone. Radiographic examination is often necessary since the stone may not be accessible to bimanual palpation. Poorly calcified sialoliths will not be visible radiographically. An occlusal view is the recommended view for radiography of submandibular glands (Figs 4.5A to C) and in the case of sialolith present in the posterior part of the submandibular duct and gland a lateral oblique could be used (Fig. 4.6).

Parotid calculi can be more difficult to visualize due to the superimposition of other anatomic structures. An anteroposterior view of the skull is

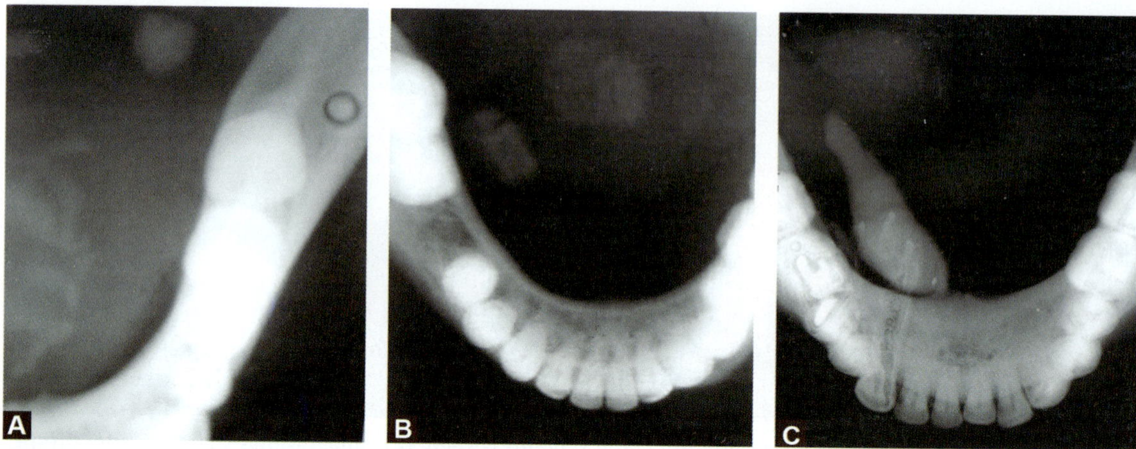

Figures 4.5A to C: Sialolith of submandibular duct. Mandibular occlusal view shows sialolith in the submandibular duct as a radiopaque mass. (*Courtesy:* Dr S Karthiga Kannan, Sree Mookambika Institute of Dental Sciences, Kanyakumari District)

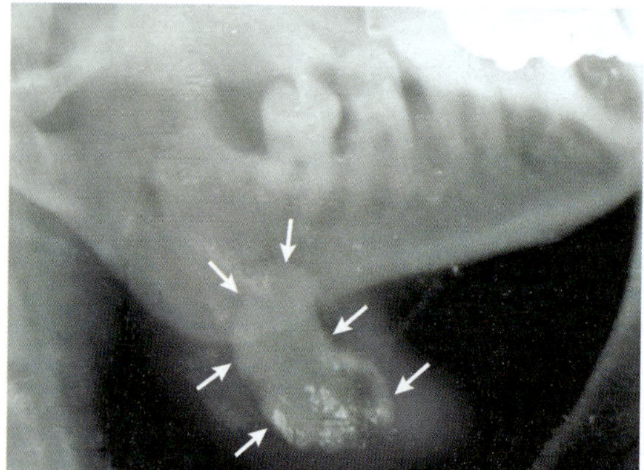

Figure 4.6: Sialolith of the submandibular gland is seen as a large, irregular radiopaque mass in the mandibular lateral radiograph. *Courtesy:* Dr S Karthiga kannan, Sree Mookambika Institute of Dental Sciences, kanyakumari District

useful for visualization of parotid calculi (see Figs 4.3A and B). One can also place an occlusal film intraorally adjacent to the duct. CT may be used for the detection of sialoliths and has 10 times the sensitivity of plain-film radiography for detecting calcifications.

Calcified phleboliths are stones that lie within a blood vessel, they can be easily mistaken radiographically for sialoliths. Phleboliths occur outside the ductal structure, and sialography can aid to differentiate these lesions.

Mucous Escape Reaction

Mucous escape reaction is pooling of mucous in a cavity within the connective tissue that is not lined by epithelium and is the most common non-neoplastic lesions of salivary glands. This lesion is described by various names like *mucous retention phenomena, mucous extravasation phenomenon, mucocele, ranula,* and *mucous retention cyst.* Early investigators believed that the lesion developed as a result of obstruction of the excretory duct of a salivary gland and the subsequent formation of an epithelium lined cyst. But, now it is generally accepted that these lesions arise due to traumatic severance of a duct with resultant pooling of mucous within the surrounding tissues.

Clinical Features

The mucous escape reaction may present in association with either a major or a minor salivary gland but is most frequently seen in association with the minor salivary glands. The most common cause is accidental biting of the lips and about 70% of extravasation mucoceles occur in the lower lip. More than two-thirds of mucous escape reactions occur in patients younger than 30 years, and males are more commonly affected than females.

The clinical presentation varies, depending on their depth within the soft tissues. Superficial lesions present as well circumscribed, soft and fluctuant, dome-shaped mucosal swellings. If the lesions are very close to the surface, the overlying epithelium may appear thinned, and appear translucent, bluish in color. They may vary in size from a few millimeters to more than a centimeter in diameter.

Lesions located deeper within the soft tissues are more nodular and lack the vesicular appearance of the superficial lesions. The surrounding mucosa is normal in color; however, like superficial lesions, they are usually well circumscribed and fluctuant when palpated (Figs 4.7A to D).

Mucous escape reaction commonly presents as a painless mucosal swelling that develops in a few days to a week and ruptures with apparent resolution, only to recur within few weeks to a month. Other lesions may persist for weeks or months and may occasionally increase in size, liberating a viscous, mucinous fluid, if ruptured. If the lesion becomes secondarily inflamed, mild symptoms may develop.

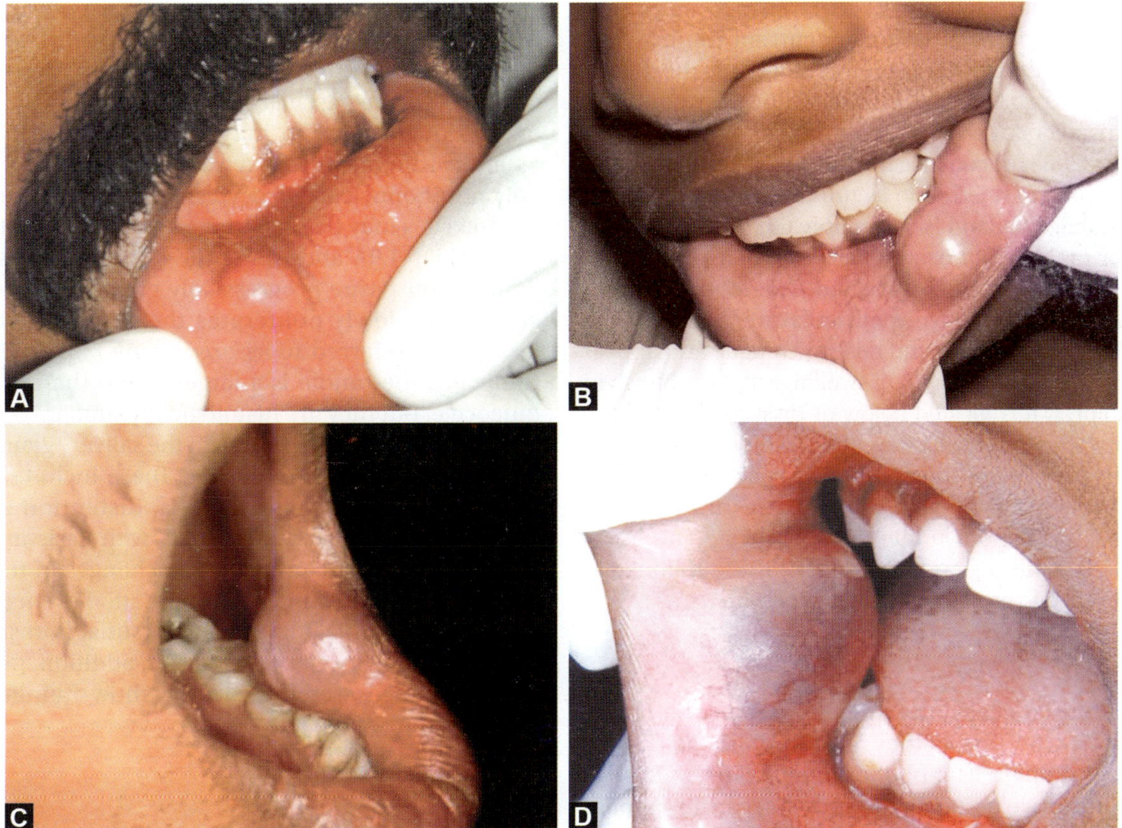

Figures 4.7A to D: Mucous escape reaction involving the labial (A to C) and buccal mucosa (D). (*Courtesy:* Dr S Karthiga Kannan, Sree Mookambika Institute of Dental Sciences, Kanyakumari District

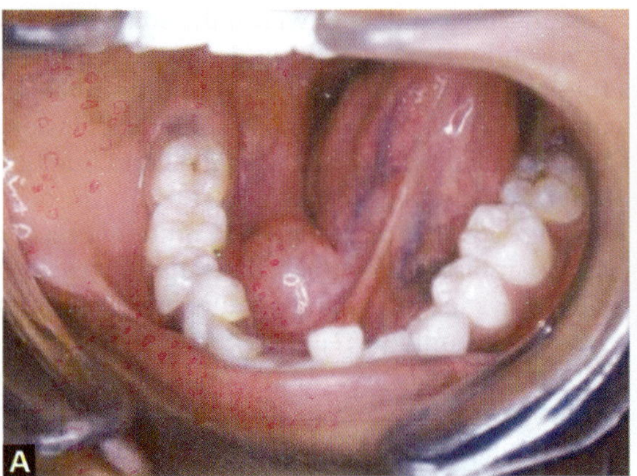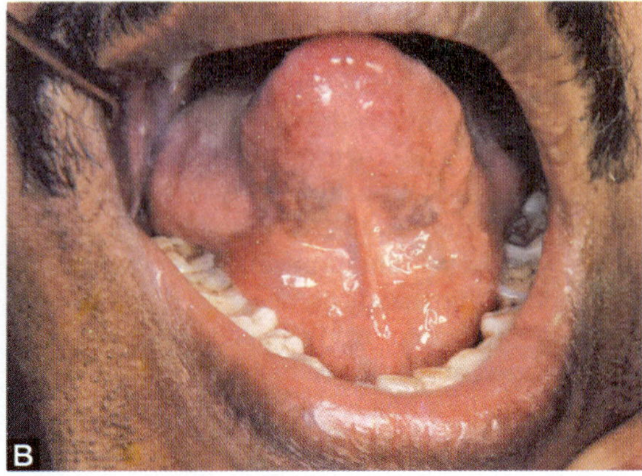

Figures 4.8A and B: Ranula presenting as a soft, fluctuant swelling in the floor of the mouth. (*Courtesy:* Dr S Karthiga Kannan, Sree Mookambika Institute of Dental Sciences, Kannyakumari District)

In superficial lesions, recurrent trauma may also result in extravasation of blood into the defect, which produces a reddish color that could be mistaken for a vascular lesion.

Large mucous escape reactions into the floor of mouth are referred to as *ranula* (Figs 4.8A and B). Sublingual gland is commonly the source of saliva for ranulas, but occasionally it may be associated with the submandibular gland. If the lesion is located above the mylohyoid musculature, it can fill the floor of the mouth and raise the tongue and appear as translucent, fluctuant swellings that are bluish in color. If it is located below or dissects through the mylohyoid musculature, the swelling is located in the area of the submandibular space and inferior border of the mandible. In rare cases, these lesions may dissect down into the suprahyoid and infra-mylohyoid regions of the neck. These lesions are referred to as *plunging or cervical ranulas.*

Histopathology

Microscopically, the mucous escape reaction is not a true cyst as they lack an epithelial lining. They appear as a pool of mucous in the fibrous connective tissue. In the early stages, they appear as well-defined cavity within the soft tissue that is filled with an eosinophilic material that stains positive for mucin. Within the material, an admixture of acute and chronic inflammatory cells and foamy histiocytes may be found. The tissue surrounding the cavity consists of compressed fibrovascular connective tissue, which on low magnification may be misinterpreted as an epithelial lining. A variable number of polymorphonuclear leukocytes, lymphocytes, and plasma cells may be seen in the surrounding soft tissue (Figs 4.9A and B). As the lesion matures, granulation tissue progressively grows into the cavity and slowly obliterates the defect. Such lesions are referred to as *organizing mucocele.* Clinically, the ranula is a larger lesion than the mucocele, but they are histologically similar.

Changes may also be seen in the salivary gland adjacent to the primary lesion. These include a generalized chronic sialadenitis, distention of intralobular and interlobular ducts, with stasis and inspissation of mucous, atrophic changes of the individual acinar elements, proliferation of small ducts; and variable degrees of interstitial fibrosis within the salivary gland lobules. In addition, the overlying mucosal epithelium may show thinning and flattening of the rete ridges.

Mucous Retention Cyst

Unlike the mucous escape reaction, the mucous retention cyst is a true cyst that is lined by epithelium. It is also known by various names like, *retention mucocele* and *oral sialocyst*. An

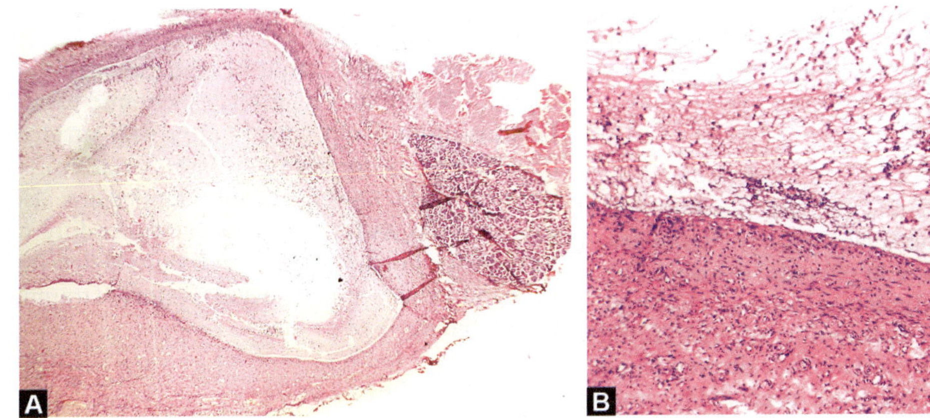

Figures 4.9A and B: Mucous escape phenomenon. The cystic cavity is lined by granulation tissue and is filled with mucin and inflammatory cells. Acini of the minor salivary gland can be seen adjacent to the cyst

obstruction within the duct may cause retention of saliva within the duct that causes dilatation of the duct without rupture. Hence, a retention cyst forms with an epithelial lining of compressed ductal epithelium.

Clinical Features

Usually presents as a slow growing, painless, often fluctuant mucosal swelling that may persist from months to years. The cysts varies in size, and like the mucous escape reaction, superficial lesions are more vesicular and bluish, whereas deep lesions are nodular and the same color as the overlying soft tissue.

Histopathology

Mucous retention cyst is a true cyst. Typically, the lining epithelium consists of a uniform, thin layer of non-keratinizing stratified squamous epithelium, and occasional mucous secreting cells can be seen within the epithelial lining of the cyst. The lumen of the cyst may be filled with an eosinophilic material that stains positive for mucin. Careful histologic examination is particularly important to exclude low-grade mucoepidermoid carcinoma because both the mucous retention cyst and the low-grade mucoepidermoid carcinoma may have mucous cells in the epithelial lining. However, mucous retention cysts show no piling up of cells in the wall of the cyst, nor do they show any proliferation or infiltration of islands of epithelium into the connective tissue that surrounds the lumen of the cyst.

Treatment and Prognosis

Mucous retention cysts usually require conservative surgical excision. Cysts distal to major salivary gland may be removed while sparing the gland. Cysts located within a major salivary gland or in association with a minor salivary gland usually require sacrifice of the gland.

Salivary Duct Cyst

Salivary duct cysts, or sialocysts, usually arise in the parotid gland. Similar in pathogenesis and histology to mucus retention cysts of minor salivary gland origin, salivary duct cysts represent true cysts with epithelial linings. Though these cysts develop as a consequence of duct obstruction, the cause of obstruction is typically not detectable.

Clinical Features

Commonly presents in the fifth decade of life as a slowly enlarging, painless, mass.

Pathologic Features

They are generally unilocular, rarely multicystic or show ectasia of the adjacent ducts. Metaplasia of the epithelial lining to cuboidal or columnar, squamous, mucous (goblet), and clear cells may be seen. Focal epithelial proliferations into the cyst lumen may occur and must be distinguished from cystadenoma, low-grade mucoepidermoid carcinoma and a unicystic acinic cell carcinoma.

Treatment and Prognosis

These cysts are treated by complete but conservative surgical excision. They should not recur if completely excised.

Necrotizing Sialometaplasia

Necrotizing sialometaplasia is a benign, necrotizing, self-limiting, reactive inflammatory disorder of the salivary tissue. Clinically, this lesion mimics a malignancy, and failure to recognize this lesion has resulted in unnecessary radical surgery.

Etiology

It is widely accepted that necrotizing sialometaplasia is initiated by a local ischemic event. Lesions often occur shortly after oral surgical procedures, restorative dentistry, or administration of local anesthesia although lesions also may develop weeks after a dental procedure or trauma. It is not uncommon for lesions to develop in an individual with no obvious history of trauma or oral habit.

Clinical Features

Most patients are older than 40 years of age. The lesion is two to three times more common in men than women. Necrotizing sialometaplasia has a rapid onset. Lesions initially present as a tender erythematous nodule. Once the mucosa breaks down, a deep ulceration with a yellowish base forms. Even though lesions can be large and deep, patients often describe only a moderate degree of dull pain.

Lesions occur predominately on the palate; however, lesions can occur anywhere salivary gland tissue exists, including the lips and the retromolar pad region (Figs 4.10A and B).

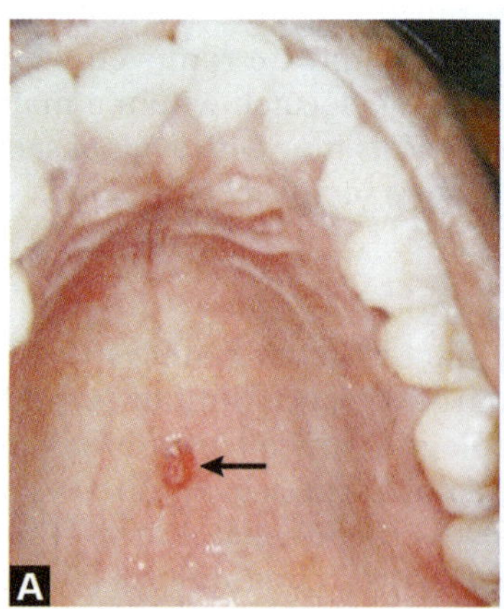
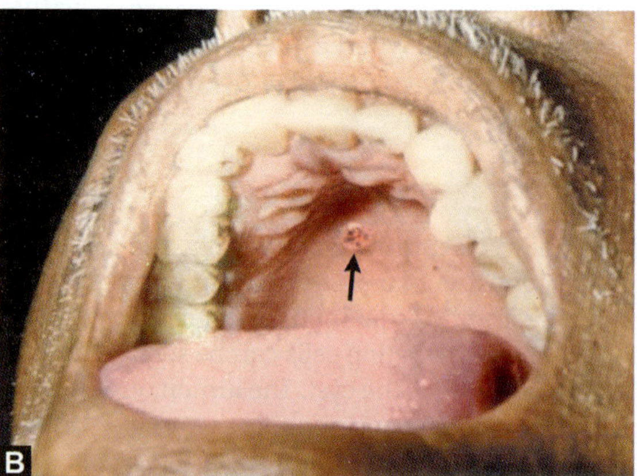

Figures 4.10A and B: Necrotizing sialometaplasia presenting as a round to oval ulcer on the palate (*Courtesy:* Dr S Karthiga Kannan, Sree Mookambika Institute of Dental Sciences, Kanyakumari District)

Pathological Features

Histologically, necrotizing sialometaplasia is characterized by various degrees of lobular necrosis and sialadenitis intermixed with squamous metaplasia of excretory ducts and acini. Careful examination will reveal that there are no malignant cells and that the lobular architecture is preserved even though necrosis is present.

Extremely early lesions may demonstrate lobules with complete or partial necrosis with minimal or almost no inflammation with occasional, mucin pools within areas of necrosis and granulation tissue. As this process evolves, areas of lobular necrosis is associated with acute and chronic inflammation and histiocytes involving the areas of necrosis. Older lesions have well-developed squamous metaplasia and usually have a greater degree of inflammation, edema, and fibrosis; foci of necrosis may not be present at this stage, since they may have already healed (Figs 4.11A to C).

In addition to the specimen, a complete clinical history should be provided to the pathologist to aid in distinguishing this lesion from squamous cell carcinoma. The uniformity and bland cytologic appearance of the squamous cells arranged in a lobular fashion and the location of residual ductal lumina in one or more of these squamous nests strongly support a benign metaplastic process. Also, the lack of incorporated mucous cells in the squamous epithelium can help to distinguish it from mucoepidermoid carcinoma.

Radiation Induced Sialadenitis

The salivary glands are often within the field of external-beam radiation that is used for treatment of head and neck tumors. Doses greater than 50 Gy

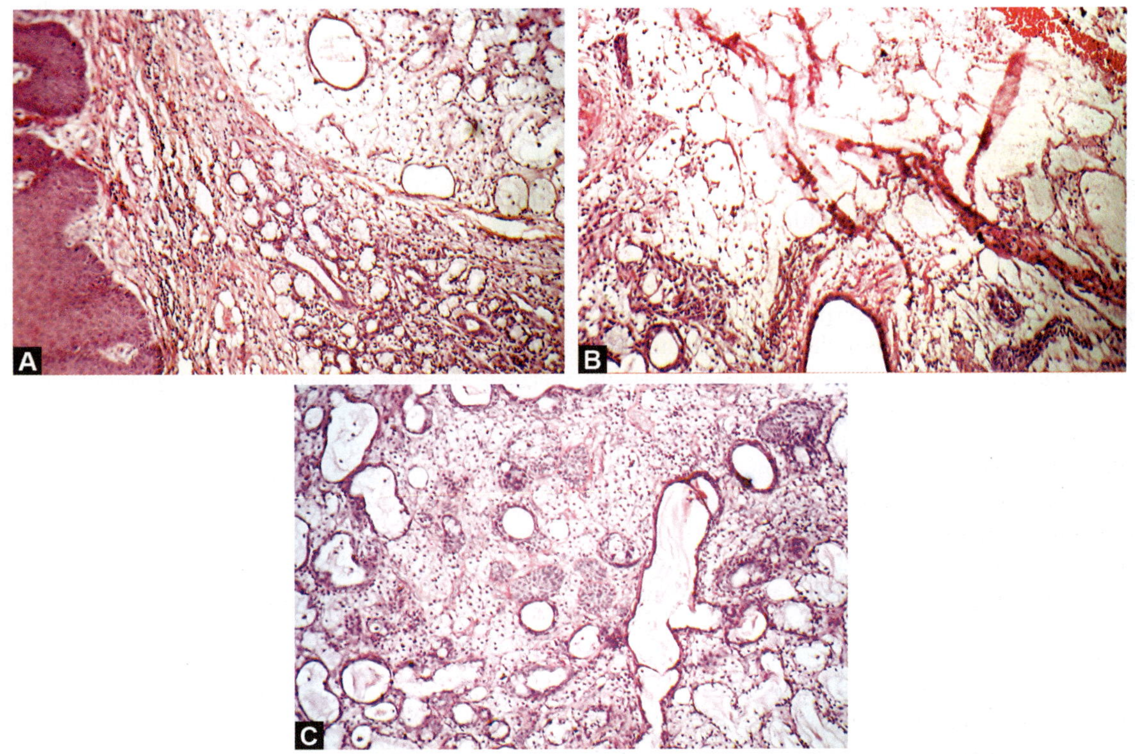

Figures 4.11A to C: Necrotizing sialometaplasia
(*Courtesy:* Dr I Ponniah, Tamil Nadu Government, Dental College and Hospital, Chennai)

results in permanent salivary gland damage and symptoms of oral dryness. Radioactive iodine (used for internal radiation therapy especially for thyroid) is taken up not only by thyroid tissue but also by the oncocytes in salivary gland tissue. Radioactive iodine can cause permanent salivary gland damage and fibrosis resulting in salivary gland hypofunction.

> Parotid gland is more affected than others due to the high radiosensitivity of the parotid gland, in contrast to the relative radioresistance of the other major salivary gland, the submandibular gland.

Numerous studies have demonstrated the destruction of serous cells with sparing of mucous cells. The high radiosensitivity of serous cells may be due to the presence of heavy metal ions like Fe, Cu, Zn and Mn in serous granules. There is a much higher prevalence of serous cells in the parotid gland as compared with the submandibular gland.

> The acute damage to the salivary gland is marked by elevation of serum and urinary amylase (the source of which is from the parotid gland).

Clinical Features

Radiation induced damage to the salivary glands which results in salivary hypofunction and consequent xerostomia which leads to various secondary effects like impairment of taste, mastication, swallowing, speech and sleep patterns. Furthermore, a reduction in saliva leads to diminished protection of the oral cavity against injuries to both hard and soft tissues, alters microbial flora to a more pathogenic type, precipitates a dry ulcerated painful mucosa and affects the wearing of oral prostheses.

Acute effects on salivary function can be recognized within a week of beginning treatments at doses of approximately 2 Gy daily and patients will often complain of oral dryness by the end of the second week. Various studies have revealed an over 50% reduction in parotid gland function within a few days following low irradiation doses of 2.5 to 10 Gy to the head and neck region. Eventually, the hypofunction exceeds 90% and the residual secreted whole-saliva obtains mucous-like properties.

Mucositis is a very common consequence of treatment and can become severe enough to alter the radiation therapy regimen. Typically, at doses > 50 Gy, salivary dysfunction is severe and permanent. Difficulty in speaking, dysphagia, and increased dental caries are common complaints that dramatically affect the quality of life for patients with radiation-induced salivary gland dysfunction. Saliva is minimal, and the saliva that is present tends to be thick and ropy.

Radiation caries is the term commonly used to describe the rapidly advancing caries, which characteristically occur at the incisal or cervical aspect of the teeth. The other oral complications include candidiasis and sialadenitis.

Pneumoparotid

Pneumoparotid is the reflux forcing of air through the parotid orifice and into the ducts. It usually occurs in wind instrument players, glass blowers, or any individual who increases intraoral pressure by forcefully blowing up the cheeks consciously or as a neurotic habit. The orifice of the parotid duct has a redundant papillary fold of buccal tissue which discourages such air reflux. Nevertheless, significant increase in the intraoral pressure distorts the musculature surrounding the orifice and favors the entrance of air into the duct.

Pneumoparotid presents either as unilateral or bilateral painless parotid swellings. The extraoral swelling is accompanied by a sense of fullness and follows the anatomic outline of the parotid gland. Palpation of the painless swelling shows a classic crackling sensation associated with tissue emphysema. When the gland is manually palpated, frothy bubbly saliva expells from the intraoral parotid orifice. This unique feature represents the mixture of air and saliva within the limited confines of the ductal system. Infection is an inevitable sequela of continued forced reflux. Consequently, chronic parotitis may be superimposed on the pneumoparotid and which may result in painful glandular enlargements with suppuration. Usually, the pneumoparotid regresses spontaneously.

Sialography shows a markedly dilated Stensen's duct due to longterm forced influx of air into the parotid system. Radiolucencies within the dye may be seen which result from pockets of air previously forced into the duct and trapped by the dye injection. In case of superimposed chronic infection sialography may show ductal dilatations and strictures (sausaging) associated with the chronic infection.

Because infection is a possibility, therapy should be aimed at cessation of the auto-insufflation. However, in case of an unintentional habit, conscious effort to stop may be difficult. Psychobehavioral or psychiatric care is indicated for those patients whose condition emanates from an emotional disturbance. The surgical rerouting of the parotid duct into the tonsillar fossa has been advocated. Surgical removal of the gland is only indicated in those situations in which infection has become a nonretractable problem.

Anesthetic Mumps

Bilateral and at times unilateral parotid sialadenopathy may be seen in association with general anesthesia during the intra-anesthetic or post-anesthetic periods. The exact mechanism for development of this anesthesia "mumps" is not fully understood, but it may represent a form of pneumoparotid.

Straining, coughing, and sneezing of the patient during a difficult anesthesia or postanesthesia period may increase the positive pressure in the oral cavity. Simultaneously, agents such as succinylcholine used as a muscle relaxant during the anesthetic procedure causes a loss of muscle tone around the parotid duct orifice. Hence, the flaccid musculature facilitates the retrograde passage of air into the parotid gland when the positive pressure in the oral cavity is significantly increased.

It is also possible that activation of a pharyngeal reflex causes a parasympathetic nerve stimulation that leads to vasodilation and hyperemia in the parotid glands. Tracheal intubation associated with coughing and straining against the endotracheal tube, serves as the stimulus for the pharyngeal reflex. Besides the endotracheal tube, endoscopy, bronchoscopy, and rigid esophagoscopy have all been implicated in the onset of bilateral parotid swelling.

Palpation reveals crepitations, a sign of tissue emphysema, which confirms the existence of an air distended parotid gland. The parotid swellings linked to a general anesthetic procedure are usually noted in the recovery room, often during extubation. Because the problem is only cosmetic and transient in nature, no treatment other than reassurance is indicated.

ALLERGIC AND IMMUNOLOGIC DISORDERS

Allergic Sialadenitis

Drugs and other allergens have occasionally been reported to cause salivary gland enlargement. Some of these reported cases may not be true hypersensitivity reactions, instead may represent secondary infections resulting from medications that reduce salivary flow. Drugs that have salivary gland enlargement as a potential side effect include phenobarbital, phenothiazine, ethambutol, sulfisoxazole, iodine compounds, isoproterenol, and heavy metals.

True allergic reactions are accompanied by angio-edema, skin rash, pruritus, or other signs of allergy.

Allergic sialadenitis is self-limiting. Avoiding the allergen, maintaining hydration, and monitoring for secondary infection are recommended.

Sjögren's Syndrome

Sjögren's syndrome (SS) is an autoimmune disease characterized by the progressive lymphocytic infiltration and destruction of exocrine glands, particularly the salivary and lacrimal glands. The characteristic symptoms are xerostomia and xerophthalmia, due to destruction of glandular epithelium with resultant decreased saliva and tear production.

Classification

The disease occurs in primary and secondary forms. *Primary Sjögren's syndrome* refers to the occurrence of xerostomia and xerophthalmia in the absence of another connective tissue disease and this was previously referred to as *Mikulicz's disease* or *sicca syndrome*. *Secondary Sjögren's syndrome* occurs in association with another connective tissue disease, such as rheumatoid arthritis, systemic lupus erythematosus, scleroderma, polymyositis, or polyarteritis. The revised European-American classification criteria is presented in Tables 4.1 and 4.2.

Table 4.1: Revised international classification criteria for Sjögren's syndrome

1. Ocular symptoms: A positive response to at least one of the following questions:
   - Have you had daily, persistent, troublesome dry eyes for more than 3 months?
   - Do you have a recurrent sensation of sand or gravel in the eyes?
   - Do you use tear substitutes more than 3 times a day?
2. Oral symptoms: A positive response to at least one of the following questions:
   - Have you had a daily feeling of dry mouth for more than 3 months?
   - Have you had recurrently or persistently swollen salivary glands as an adult?
   - Do you frequently drink liquids to aid in swallowing dry food?
3. Ocular signs: The objective evidence of ocular involvement is defined as a positive result for at least one of the following two tests:
   - Schirmer's test, performed without anesthesia (<5 mm in 5 minutes)
   - Rose bengal score or other ocular dye score (>4 according to van Bijsterveld's scoring system)
4. Histopathology: In minor salivary glands (obtained through normal-appearing mucosa) focal lymphocytic sialadenitis, evaluated by an expert histopathologist, with a focus score >1, defined as a number of lymphocytic foci (which are adjacent to normal-appearing mucous acini and contain more than 50 lymphocytes) per 4 mm^2 of glandular tissue.
5. Salivary gland involvement: Objective evidence of salivary gland involvement is defined by a positive result for at least one of the following diagnostic tests:
   - Unstimulated whole salivary flow (<1.5 ml in 15 minutes)
   - Parotid sialography showing the presence of diffuse sialectasias (punctate, cavitary or destructive pattern), without evidence of obstruction in the major ducts
   - Salivary scintigraphy showing delayed uptake, reduced concentration and/or delayed excretion of tracer
6. Autoantibodies: Presence in the serum of the following autoantibodies:
   - Antibodies to Ro(SSA) or,
   - La(SSB) antigens, or both

Table 4.2: Revised rules for classification

For primary SS

In patients without any potentially associated disease, primary SS may be defined as follows:
- The presence of any 4 of the 6 items in the Revised International classification criteria is indicative of primary SS, as long as either item IV (Histopathology) or VI (Serology) is positive.
- The presence of any 3 of the 4 objective criteria items (that is, items III, IV, V, VI).

For secondary SS

In patients with a potentially associated disease (for instance, another well defined connective tissue disease), the presence of item I or item II plus any 2 from among items III, IV, and V may be considered as indicative of secondary SS.

Exclusion criteria
- Past head and neck radiation treatment
- Hepatitis C infection
- Acquired immunodeficiency syndrome (AIDS)
- Pre-existing lymphoma
- Sarcoidosis
- Graft versus host disease
- Use of anticholinergic drugs (since a time shorter than 4-fold the half life of the drug)

Pathogenesis

Salivary glands are considered as a site of latent viral infections and hence, the putative role of various viruses in the etiopathogenesis of SS is hypothesised. These viruses include Epstein Barr virus, cytomegalovirus, hepatitis C virus, and lymphotropic viruses. These viruses are proposed to trigger the autoimmune process.

A possible relationship between Sjögren's syndrome and *Helicobacter pylori* infection has been suspected. In both these conditions there is an increased risk of developing mucosa-associated lymphoid tissue lymphoma. It has been suggested that infection with *H. pylori* might trigger a widespread clonal B-cell disorder observed in Sjögren's syndrome.

Immunohistochemical analysis of lymphocytic infiltrates in Sjögren's syndrome shows a predominance of T cells with fewer B cells and macrophages. The majority of T cells in the lymphocytic infiltrates are CD4+ T helper cells with a CD4/CD8 ratio well over two. Most of these T cells may contribute significantly to B cell hyperactivity.

The B cells make up roughly 20% of the infiltrating cell population in affected glands. The B cells produce immunoglobulins with autoantibody activity for IgG (rheumatoid factor), Ro/SS-A and La/SS-B. Production of IgG predominates in Sjögren's syndrome whereas synthesis of IgA is more abundant in normal salivary glands. A large number of autoantibodies have been reported in both primary and secondary Sjögren's syndrome, reflecting both B cell activation and a loss of immune tolerance in the B cell compartment.

Clinical Features

Sjögren's syndrome is most commonly encountered in post-menopausal women and up to 90% of patients with SS are females. The average age at diagnosis is 50 years; and is uncommon in patients under the age of 20. Among the major glands, the parotid gland is involved in 85% of cases and the remaining affect the submandibular gland and rarely the sublingual glands.

The principal clinical symptoms are due to dryness of the eyes and mouth, resulting in keratoconjunctivitis and difficulty with speaking and swallowing of food. Many patients present with firm, diffuse enlargement of the salivary glands, which is usually but not always bilateral. Induration of the glands without enlargement may be evident early in the course of the disease. These changes are usually painless or associated with slight tenderness.

The salivary and lacrimal glands are primarily affected, but other exocrine tissues, including the thyroid, lungs, and kidney, may also be involved. SS patients also frequently experience arthralgias, myalgias, peripheral neuropathies, and rashes.

Mucous secretions of the upper and lower respiratory tract may decrease in patients with SS, producing dryness of the nose, throat, and trachea; xerotrachea may result in a chronic dry cough. Diminished secretions of the exocrine glands of the skin may lead to dry skin, and vaginal dryness may cause pruritus, irritation, and dyspareunia.

Oral Manifestations

Virtually all patients complain of dry mouth and the need to sip liquids throughout the day. Oral dryness causes difficulty with chewing, swallowing, and speaking without additional fluids. Patients often have dry cracked lips and angular cheilitis. Some patients may not complain of oral dryness, but of an unpleasant taste, difficulty eating dry food, soreness, or difficulties in controlling dentures.

In the early stages of SS, the mouth may appear moist, but as the disease progresses, the usual pooling of saliva in the floor of the mouth becomes absent, the saliva that is present tends to be thick and ropy and lines of contact between frothy saliva and the oral soft tissues are seen. In advanced disease, the oral mucosa appears dry and glazed and tends to form fine wrinkles. Extreme dryness of the mouth, causing the tongue to stick to the palate, may lead to a 'clicking' quality in the speech of patients with SS. The surface of the tongue becomes red and lobulated, with partial or complete depapillation.

In patients with SS and severe salivary hypofunction, the mean number and proportion of

Streptococcus mutans and *Lactobacillus* organisms and the frequency of *Candida* organisms are reported to be increased. This leads to increased susceptibility to mucocutaneous candidiasis. Decreased salivary flow also results in increased dental caries and erosion of the enamel structure.

Ocular Manifestations

Dry eye is the most prominent ocular manifestation of SS. Symptoms of dry eye may include sensations of itching, burning, grittiness, soreness, and dryness, despite the eyes having a normal appearance. Diminished secretion of tears may lead to chronic irritation and destruction of corneal and bulbar conjunctival epithelium (keratoconjunctivitis sicca).

Ocular complaints may include photosensitivity, erythema, eye fatigue, decreased visual acuity, a discharge in the eyes, and the sensation of a film across the visual field. Because of decreased tear film and an abnormal mucous component, thick, rope-like secretions may accumulate along the inner canthus. Small superficial erosions of the corneal epithelium may result from desiccation; in severe cases, slitlamp examination may reveal filamentary keratitis, marked by mucous filaments that adhere to damaged areas of the corneal surface.

Diagnostic Criteria

Although minor salivary gland biopsy traditionally has been considered the 'gold standard' for the diagnosis of SS, newer criteria permit classification of SS without necessarily performing this procedure. The revised International classification criteria is presented in Tables 4.1 and 4.2 and the workup towards diagnosis is presented in Table 4.3.

Diagnostic Methods

The Schirmer test for the eye quantitatively measures tear formation by placement of filter paper in the lower conjunctival sac at the junction of the middle and lateral third of the lower eyelid margin (Fig. 4.12). The extent of wetting is measured by a ruler and the possible scores range

Table 4.3. Workup for Sjögren syndrome
1. Ocular
• Schirmer test
• Slitlamp examination with vital dye
• Tear breakup time
2. Oral
• Dental examination
• Estimate of salivary flow
• Salivary scintigram
• Minor salivary gland biopsy
3. Systemic
• Complete history and physical examination
• Complete blood cell count; ESR; liver enzymes; blood urea nitrogen/creatinine; Antinuclear antibody (ANA); Rheumatoid factor (RF), anti-SS-A/SS-B; total IgG, IgM and IgA; thyroid-stimulating hormone; and urine analysis
• Chest radiograph
4. Others (as indicated)
• Salivary gland sonography/magnetic resonance imaging
• Lymph node or bone marrow biopsy
• Additional laboratory testing
• Organ-specific antibodies (thyroid, liver, and neurologic)
• Viral (hepatitis B and C, EBV, and HIV)

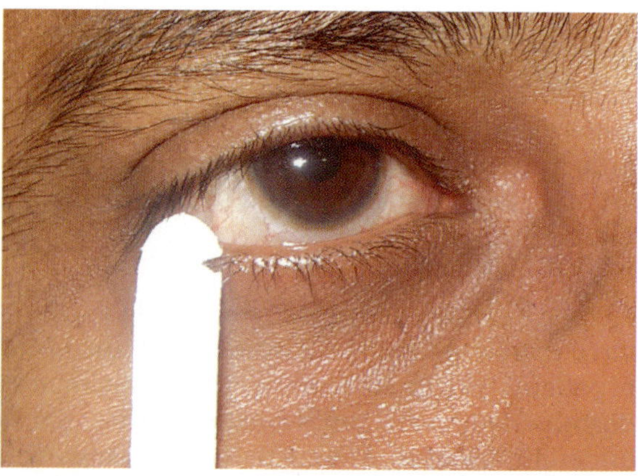

Figure 4.12: Schirmer test

from 0 to 35 mm, with lower scores indicating greater abnormality in tear production. The test could be done with or without an anesthetic agent.

A Schirmer test without anesthesia score of ≤ 5 mm in at least one eye is one of the required criteria for dry eye, according to the revised international classification criteria for Sjögren's syndrome. (see Table 4.1).

Rose bengal scoring involves placement of 25 ml of rose bengal solution in the inferior fornix of each eye and having the patient blink twice. Slitlamp examination detects destroyed conjunctival epithelium caused by desiccation. The rose bengal score is obtained by the sum of scores assigned to damage found in 3 regions of the eye.

The assessment of ocular surface damage can be done using a vital dye staining with 2% unpreserved sodium fluorescein and then 5% lissamine green dye. The corneal, temporal, and nasal regions of the conjunctiva are scored individually from 0-5 (for fluorescien) and 0-5 (for lissamine green) using the Oxford grading scheme. The Oxford score is derived by adding the scores for corneal fluorescein and nasal plus temporal conjunctival lissamine green staining. Total Oxford score could range from 0-15. The van Bijsterveld score (VB) was assessed using lissamine green staining of the cornea (0-3) and conjunctiva (0-3). Total VB score could range from 0-9. For all staining tests, higher scores indicate worse ocular surface damage.

Tear film stability is assessed using fluorescein tear film breakup time (TBUT). Five microliters of 2% sodium fluorescein is instilled into the inferior fornix and the patient is asked to blink several times. Using the cobalt blue filter and slitlamp biomicroscopy, the duration of time required for the first area of tear film breakup after a complete blink is determined. If the TBUT is less than 10 seconds, the test is repeated for a total of 3 values and the average is calculated.

Sialometry measures unstimulated salivary flow into a calibrated tube for 15 minutes. While being simple and noninvasive, sialometry alone does not distinguish between causes of xerostomia.

Other tests used to evaluate salivary gland involvement include parotid sialography and salivary gland scintigraphy. A typical sialographic feature of the affected parotid is the formation of punctate cavitary defects filled with radiopaque contrast medium, described as a 'fruit-laden, branchless tree'. This characteristic appearance is believed to be due to leakage of the contrast material through the weakened salivary gland ducts. Scintigraphic findings in patients with SS include decreased uptake and release of technetium Tc 99m pertechnetate. The extent of decreased uptake, parallels the degree of xerostomia and salivary flow rate.

The minor salivary gland biopsy specimen finding is considered to be the best sole diagnostic criterion for the salivary component of SS (Fig. 4.13). The grading system for quantifying the changes seen in the minor glands in SS, are as follows:

1. The number of infiltrating mononuclear cells are determined with an aggregate of 50 or more cells being termed as focus.
2. The total number of foci and the surface area of the specimen are measured.
3. The number of foci per 4 mm^2 is calculated. This constitutes the focus score. The range is from 0 to 12, with 12 denoting confluent infiltrates.
4. A focus score of 1 is considered positive for SS in some criteria although others require the score to be > 1.

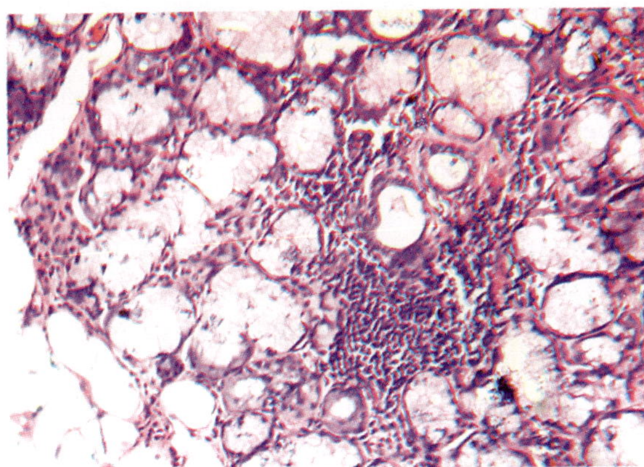

Figure 4.13: Sjögren's syndrome. (*Courtesy:* Dr I Ponniah, Tamil Nadu Government Dental College and Hospital, Chennai)

Serologic and laboratory findings associated with SS include diffuse hypergammaglobulinemia, which is found in approximately 80% of patients with the disease. Elevated levels of several autoantibodies are found including rheumatoid factors, antinuclear antibodies, and antibodies to the extractable cellular antigens Ro/SS-A and La/SS-B. Anti-Ro/SS-A is not specific for SS and occurs in other autoimmune disorders, particularly SLE. However, patients with SLE who have anti-La/SS-B antibodies usually have SS.

Histopathology

The microscopic hallmark of SS is focal lymphocytic infiltrates, located mainly around the glandular ducts (Fig. 4.13). These pathologic findings include lymphocyte infiltration of the salivary and lacrimal glands and other exocrine glands of the respiratory and gastrointestinal tracts and vagina. The infiltrate contains T cells, B cells, and plasma cells, with a predominance of activated CD4+ helper T cells. These T cells produce interleukins and tumor necrosis factor. Eventually, the infiltrate extends to occupy the acinar epithelium, leading to glandular dysfunction that manifests as dry eyes and dry mouth, and enlargement of the major salivary glands.

Early in disease, focal aggregates of lymphocytes are seen in parenchymal lobules with associated acinar involution. A focus score of greater than one focus (~50 lymphocytes) per 4 mm^2 is considered to be diagnostic of the disease. As the inflammation progresses, partial and then total parenchymal loss becomes evident, and the lymphocytic infiltrate dominates.

In later stages, epithelial and myoepithelial duct cells proliferate predominantly in the major glands and show metaplastic changes, producing the epimyoepithelial islands. Interlobular septa are typically preserved; thus, the affected gland maintains a lobular architecture.

Malignant Transformation

Patients with SS have almost 40 times higher risk for developing non-Hodgkin's lymphoma. The salivary gland enlargement in SS may progress from a benign sialadenitis with polyclonal lymphocytic infiltration to an oligoclonal infiltration and then progress to monoclonal lymphoid malignancy. Progressive unilateral swelling in an enlarged parotid gland in a patient with SS, especially in older females, is suggestive of lymphoma. The developing malignancy is usually a low-grade, monocytoid B-cell lymphoma.

METABOLIC DISORDERS

Sialadenosis

Principal regulation of major salivary gland function is via the autonomic nervous system. Dysregulation of autonomic control may lead to a benign form of salivary gland enlargement called sialadenosis. Various conditions that could dysregulate the autonomic control include obesity, starvation, anorexia nervosa, bulimia, starch ingestion, alcoholism, diabetes mellitus, celiac and liver disease, acromegaly, catecholamine excess, and heavy metal intoxication.

Clinical Features

Clinically, sialadenosis presents as painless, recurrent, bilateral swelling of the parotid glands (Figs 4.14A and B). The peak incidence is in the fifth and sixth decades. The clinical differential diagnosis includes other causes of bilateral salivary gland enlargement, such as sarcoidosis, Sjögren's syndrome, tuberculosis, malignant lymphoma, sialadenitis, gout, and Graves' disease.

Pathologic Features

Microscopically, glands appear essentially normal aside from increased acinar diameter and cytoplasmic changes. As a result of cellular hypertrophy, the diameter of acini may be two to three times the expected diameter. Individual acinar cells are swollen and appear basophilic (granular form) or translucent (honeycombed or vacuolated pattern). Inflammation is not a feature of sialadenosis. If the disease persists, there is

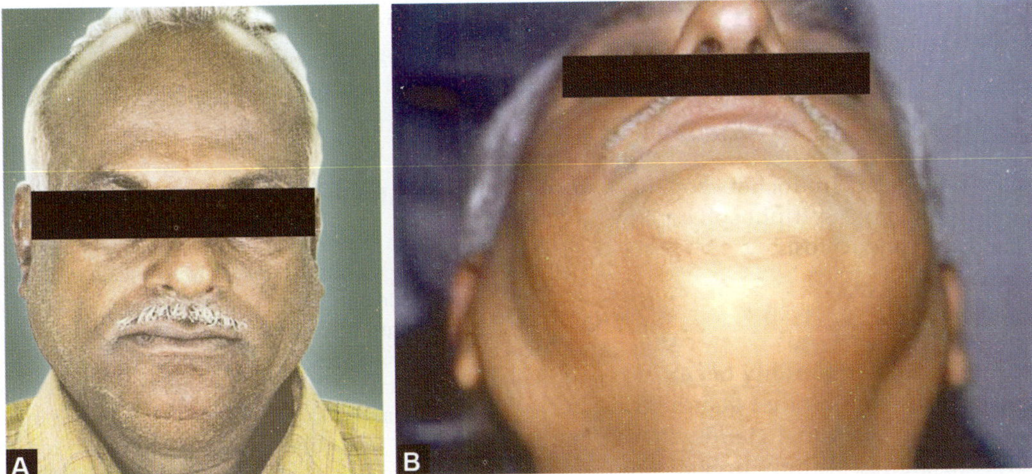

Figures 4.14A and B: Sialadenosis of parotid glands

eventual atrophy of the parenchyma with fatty replacement.

Iodide "Mumps"

Iodide "mumps" can develop after any imaging procedure that uses iodine-based contrast medium. Patients usually exhibit painless bilateral parotid or submandibular gland swellings that are rapid in onset (5 minutes to several days) and gradually disappear in a week. Usually either parotid or submandibular salivary gland is involved bilaterally, but occasionally all salivary glands can be enlarged and sometimes only one gland may be swollen.

Increased plasma iodide levels may result from an inadequately functioning kidney and/or the intravenous introduction of large amounts of iodide-containing compounds, the contrast dyes especially high-osmolar contrast dyes. In addition, iodine-contaning expectorants and agents increasing serum iodide levels, such as thiouracil, have also been implicated. Deiodination of contrast media occurs in the plasma.

Although the iodide is chiefly excreted by the kidney, salivary glands also have the ability to concentrate iodide and clear it from plasma. Salivary iodide concentration seems to occur in the salivary duct system. Extremely high plasma iodide levels can lead to inflammation of the ductal epithelium which in turn may lead to obstruction with glandular swelling.

Many patients with iodide manifestations have immediate reactions that probably are allergic in origin. Urticaria with pruritus, bronchospasms, and angioneurotic edema often accompany their salivary gland swellings. Patients with delayed swellings likely reflect a toxic gland reaction.

Preventive treatment is used in patients with allergic histories or histories of reaction to contrast media. Prednisolone and antihistamines may be administered. In addition, the low osmolar non-ionic dyes should be chosen. If a gland swelling develops, anti-inflammatory agents, anti-histamines, and steroids are accepted therapeutic modalities.

AGING

Oncocytosis

Greek word "onkousthai" means to swell. The term oncocyte was first applied by Hamperl in 1931 for the swollen, eosinophillic epithelial cells with granular cytoplasm. Focal replacement of normal glandular cells by these oncocytes is called oncocytosis. Foci of oncocytic metaplasia can be seen in ductal epithelium.

Etiology

Oncoytosis is thought to be an age-related phenomena, but it had also been ascribed as metaplastic, hyperplastic, developmental, or transformational process. It is presently thought to be a functional defect (mitochondropathy), since low levels of adenosine triphosphate have been associated with oncocytosis.

Clinical Features

Oncocytosis most commonly occur in parotid gland. It is also seen in other glandular tissues, i.e. bronchial and lacrimal glands, thyroid and parathyroid gland, kidney, breast, pancreas, pituitary gland, testicle, liver, stomach, and esophagus. Clinically, oncocytosis is asymptomatic. If there is diffuse or florid involvement of the glands it may present clinically as a swelling mimicking benign neoplasm.

Pathologic Features

Histologically, oncocytosis is made up of solitary or scattered foci of swollen, acidophilic epithelial cells, with granular cytoplasm and a centrally placed pyknotic nuclei. The cells may retain acinar pattern and may form sheets, trabeculae, or duct-like pattern. The lobular architecture of the gland is generally intact. Sometimes, oncocytes appear clear due to the intracytoplasmic glycogen. Oncocytes stain positive with phosphotungstic acid hematoxylin.

Ultrastructurally, the cytoplasm of the oncocyte is packed with large, pleomorphic mitochondria containing filamentous, tubular, and vesicular cristae. Accumulation of mitochondria is thought to compensate for an uncoupling of oxidative metabolism secondary to cellular aging. The oncocytic mitochondria in human salivary glands, lack the structural irregularity that has been reported for these organelles occurring in oncocytes in other organs.

Prognosis

Though focal or diffuse oncocytosis are non-neoplastic, rarely they have potential for neoplastic growth.

BIBLIOGRAPHY

1. Ahola SJ. Unexplained parotid enlargement: a clue to occult bulimia. Conn Med 1982;46:185-6.
2. Alcade RE, Ueyama Y, Lim DJ, Matsumura T. Pneumoparotid: report of a case. J Oral Maxillofac Surg 1998;56:676-80.
3. Anastassov GE, Haiavy J, Solodnik P, et al. Submandibular gland mucocele: Diagnosis and management. Oral Surg Oral Med Oral Pathol Oral Radiol Endod 2000;89(2):159-63.
4. Atkinson JC. Sjogren's syndrome: Oral and dental considerations. J Am Dent Assoc 1993;124:74-86.
5. Azuma M, Tamatani T, Fukui K, et al. Proteolytic enzymes in salivary extravasation mucoceles. J Oral Pathol Med 1995;24(7):299-302.
6. Banerjee AR, Soames JV, Birchall JP, et al. Ectopic salivary gland tissue in the palantine and lingual tonsil. Int J Pediatr Otorhinolaryngol 1993;27(2):159-62.
7. Barnes L, Brandwein M, Som PM. Surgical Pathology of the Head and Neck. 2nd edn. Marcel Dekker Inc: New York, 2001.
8. Baurmash HD. Mucoceles and ranulas. J Oral Maxillofac Surg 2003;61:369-78.
9. Bhide VN, Warshawsky RJ. Agenesis of the parotid gland: Association with ipsilateral accessory parotid tissue. AJR Am J Roentgenol 1998;170(6):1670-1.
10. Blitzer A. Inflammatory and obstructive disorders of salivary glands. J Dent Res 1987;66:675-81.
11. Bottrill ID, Chawla OP, Ramsay AD. Salivary gland choristoma of the middle ear. J Laryngol Otol 1992;106(7):630-2.
12. Bradley PJ. Benign salivary gland disease. Hosp Med 2001;62:392-5.
13. Brodie H, Chole R. Recurrent pneumosialadenitis. Otolaryngol Head Neck Surg 1988;98:350-3.
14. Bron AJ. The Doyne Lecture. Reflections on the tears. Eye 1997;11:583-602.
15. Burstein LS, et al. The crystal chemistry of submandibular and parotid salivary gland stones. J Oral Pathol 1979;8:284.

16. Cawson RA, Odell EW. Neoplastic and non-neoplastic diseases of salivary glands. In: Cawson's essentials of oral pathology and oral medicine, 7th edn. Churchill Livingstone. 2002;18:255-74.

17. Chilla R, Arglebe C. Function of the salivary glands and sialochemistry in sialadenosis. Acta Otorhinolaryngol Belg 1983;37:158-64.

18. Coleman H, Altini M, Nayler S, Richards A. Sialadenosis: A presenting sign in bulimia. Head Neck 1998;20:758-62.

19. Daniels TE, Fox PS. Salivary and oral components of Sjögren's syndrome. Rheum Dis Clin N Am 1992;18:571-89.

20. David M, Karga J. Pneumoparotid. Clin Pediatr 1988;27:506-9.

21. DiGiuseppe JA, Corio RL, Westra WH. Lymphoid infiltrates of the salivary glands: Pathology, biology, and clinical significance. Curr Opin Oncol 1996;8:232-37.

22. Dutta SK, Dukehart M, Narang A, Latham PS. Functional and structural changes in parotid glands of alcoholic cirrhotic patients. Gastroenterology 1988;16(4):215-8.

23. Ellis GL, Auclair PL, Gnepp DR. Surgical pathology of the salivary glands. 1st edn. WB Saunders: Philadelphia, Saunders, 1991.

24. Fox PC. Saliva and salivary gland alterations in HIV infection. J Am Dent Assoc 1991;122(12): 46-8.

25. Fox RI, Kang HI. Pathogenesis of Sjögren's syndrome. Rheum Dis Clin N Am 1992;18: 517-38.

26. Fox RI, Stern M, Michelson P. Update of Sjogren's syndrome. Curr Opin Rheumatol 2000;12: 391-8.

27. Gelbier MJ, Winter GB. Absence of salivary glands in children with rampant dental caries: A report of seven cases. Int J Paediatr Dent 1995;5:253-7.

28. Gnepp DR, Brandenwein MS, Henley JD. Salivary and lacrimal glands. In: Gnepp DR (Ed). Diagnostic surgical pathology of the head and neck. WB Saunders, Philadelphia, 2001.

29. Gnepp DR. Diagnostic Surgical Pathology of the Head and Neck. WB Saunders: Philadelphia, 2001.

30. Goguen LA, April MM, Karmody CS, Carter BL. Self-induced pneumoparotitis. Arch Otolaryngol Head Neck Surg 1995;121(12):1426-9.

31. Griesen O. Pneumatocele. J Laryngol Otol 1968; 82:477-80.

32. Grisius MM, Fox PC. Salivary gland diseases. In: Greenberg MS, Glick M (Eds). Burket's Oral Medicine Diagnosis and Treatment. BC Decker Inc, Ontario, 2003.

33. Harris MD, McKeever P, Robertson JM. Congenitals of the salivary gland: A case report and review. Histopathology 1990;17(2):155-7.

34. Hinni ML, Beatty CW. Salivary gland choristoma of the middle ear: Report of a case and review of the literature. Ear Nose Throat J 1996;75:422-4.

35. Jonsson R, Moen K, Verstrheim D, Szodoray P. Current issues in Sjogren's syndrome. Oral Dis 2002;8:130-40.

36. Kassan SS, Moutsopoulos HM. Clinical manifestations and early diagnosis of Sjogren. Arch Intern Med 2004;164:1275-84.

37. Kirsch CM, Shinn J, Porzio R, Trefelner E, Kagawa FT, Wehner JH, et al. Pneumoparotid due to spirometry. Chest 1999;116:1475-8.

38. Kubo S, Abe K, Ureshino T, Oka M. Aplasia of the submandibular gland. A case report. J Craniomaxillofac Surg 1990;18(3):119–21.

39. Lemp MA. Evaluation and differential diagnosis of keratoconjunctivitis sicca. J Rheumatol Suppl 2000; 61:11-4.

40. Lundeberg D. Non-neoplastic disorders of the parotid gland. West J Med 1983;138:589-95.

41. Mandel L, Kaynar A, Wazen J. Pneumoparotid: A case report. Oral Surg Oral Med Oral Pathol 1991;72:22-4.

42. Mandel L, Kayner A. Bulimia and parotid swelling: A review and case report. J Oral Maxillofac Surg 1992;50:1122-5.

43. Mandel L, Surattanont F. Bilateral parotid swelling: A review. Oral Surg Oral Med Oral Pathol Oral Radiol Endod 2002;93:221-37.

44. Martin-Granizo R, Herrera M, Garcia-Gonzalez D, Mas A. Pneumoparotid in childhood: Report of two cases. J Oral Maxillofac Surg 1999;57:1468-71.

45. Matsuda C, Matsui Y, Ohno K, Michi K. Salivary gland aplasia with cleft lip and palate: A case report and review of the literature. Oral Surg Oral Med Oral Pathol 1999;87(5):594-9.

46. McQuone SJ. Acute viral and bacterial infections of the salivary glands. Otolaryngol Clin North Am 1999;32:793-811.

47. Milunsky JM, Lee VW, Siegal BS, Milunsky A. Agenesis or hypoplasia of major salivary and lacrimal glands. Am J Med Genet 1991;41(2):269–70.

48. Neville BW, Damm DD, Allen CM, Bouquot JE. Oral and Maxillofacial Pathology, 2nd edn. WB Saunders Co., 2002.

49. Nordgarden H, Johannessen S, Storhaug K, Jensen JL. Salivary gland involvement in hypohidrotic ectodermal dysplasia. Oral Dis 1998;4(2):152–4.

50. Peel RL. Diseases of salivary gland. In: Surgical Pathology of the head and neck. Barnes L (Ed), Marcel Decker Inc, New York, 2001;1.

51. Pflugfelder SC, Tseng SC, Sanabria O, Kell H, Garcia CG, Felix C, Feuer W, Reis BL: Evaluation of subjective assessments and objective diagnostic tests for diagnosing tear-film disorders known to cause ocular irritation. Cornea 1998;17:38-56.

52. Powenell PH, Brown OE, Pransky SM, Manning SC. Congenital abnormalities of the submandibular duct. Int J Pediatr Otorhinolaryngol 1992;24(2):161–9.

53. Praetorius F, Hammarstrom L. A new concept of the pathogenesis of oral mucous cysts based on a study of 200 cases. J Dent Assoc S Afr 1992;47(5):226-31.

54. Rajendran R, Sivapathasundharam B. Diseases of salivary gland. In: Shafer's textbook of oral pathology, 5th edn. Elsevier, 2005.

55. Riad M, Barton JR, Wilson JA, Freeman CPL, Maran AGD. Parotid salivary secretory pattern in bulimia nervosa. Acta Otolaryngol (Stockh) 1991;111:392-5.

56. Rice DH. Non-inflammatory, non-neoplastic disorders of the salivary gland. Otolarynglogy Clinics of North America 1999;32(5):835-42.

57. Rice DH. Salivary gland disorders: Neoplastic and Non-neoplastic. Medical Clinics of North America 1999;83(1):197-218.

58. Rupp R. Pneumoparotid. Arch Otolaryngol 1963;77:665-8.

59. Schiodt M, Dodd CL, Greenspan D, Daniels TE, Cherroff D, Hollander H, et al. Natural history of HIV-associated salivary gland disease. Oral Surg Oral Med Oral Pathol 1992;74:326-31.

60. Schiodt M, Greenspan D, Daniels TE, et al. Parotid gland enlargement and xerostomia associated with labial sialadenitis in HIV-infected patients. J Autoimmun 1989;2(4):415-25.

61. Schiodt M, Greenspan D, Levy JA, et al. Does HIV cause salivary gland disease? AIDS 1989;3(12):819-22.

62. Schiodt M. HIV-associated salivary gland disease: A review. Oral Surg Oral Med Oral Pathol 1992;73:164-7.

63. Schubert MM, Izutsu KT. Iatrogenic causes of salivary gland dysfunction. J Dent Res 1987;66:680-7.

64. Schubert MM, Sullivan KM, Morton TH, Izutsu KT, Peterson DE, Flournoy N, et al. Oral manifestation of chronic graft-vs-host disease. Arch Intern Med 1984;144:1591-5.

65. Seifert G, Miehlke A, Haubrich J, Chillar R. Disease of the salivary glands. Stuttgart: George Thieme; 1986.

66. Shira RB. Anterior lingual mandibular salivary gland defect: Evaluation of 24 cases. Oral Surg Oral Med Oral Pathol 1991;71:131-6.

67. Sittel C, Jungehulsing M, Fischbach R. High-resolution magnetic resonance imaging of recurrent pneumoparotitis. Ann Otol Rhinol Laryngol 1999;108:816-8.

68. Stene T, Pederson KN. Aberrant salivary gland tissue in the anterior mandible. J Oral Surg 1977;44:75.

69. Strubel G, Rzepka-Glinder V. Structure and composition of sialoliths. J Clin Chem Clin Biochem 1989;27:244.

70. Terry JH, Loree TR, Thomas MD, Marti JR. Major salivary gland lymphoepithelial lesions and the acquired immunodeficiency syndrome. Am J Surg 1991;162:324-9.

71. Van Bijsterveld OP. Diagnostic tests in the sicca syndrome. Arch Ophthalmol 1969;82:10-4.

72. Vitali C, Bombardieri S, Jonsson R, Moutsopoulos HM, Alexander EL, Carsons SE, et al. Classification criteria for Sjögren's syndrome: A revised version of the European criteria proposed by the American-European Consensus Group. Ann Rheum Dis 2002;61:554-8.

73. Wang S, Zou Z, Wu Q, Sun K, Ma X, Zhu X. Chronic suppurative parotitis: A proposed classification. Chin Med J (Engl). 1996;109(7):555-60.

74. Zhao YF, Jia Y, Chen XM, Zhang WF. Clinical review of 580 ranulas. Oral Surg Oral Med Oral Pathol Oral Radiol Endod 2004;98:281-7.

5

Physiology and Functional Disorders of Salivary Glands

B Sivapathasundharam, AR Raghu, R Rajendran

PHYSIOLOGY OF SALIVARY GLANDS

Production of Saliva

The production of saliva is an active process occurring in two phases: *Primary secretion,* occurs in the acinar cells, which results in a product similar in composition and osmolality of plasma. *Ductal modification,* is the second stage which commences, as the primary secretion passes through the striated ducts, resulting in the production of hypotonic salivary fluid with decreased sodium and increased potassium in the end product (Fig. 5.1).

Primary Secretion

Primary saliva is believed to be formed by an active transport of ions chiefly the bicarbonate and chloride ions. Water, sodium and potassium ions follow down the osmotic and electrochemical gradient. The fluid component is derived from the interstitial fluid through passage across the basement membrane. The primary saliva taken from the lumen of an intercalated duct is isotonic (see Fig. 5.1).

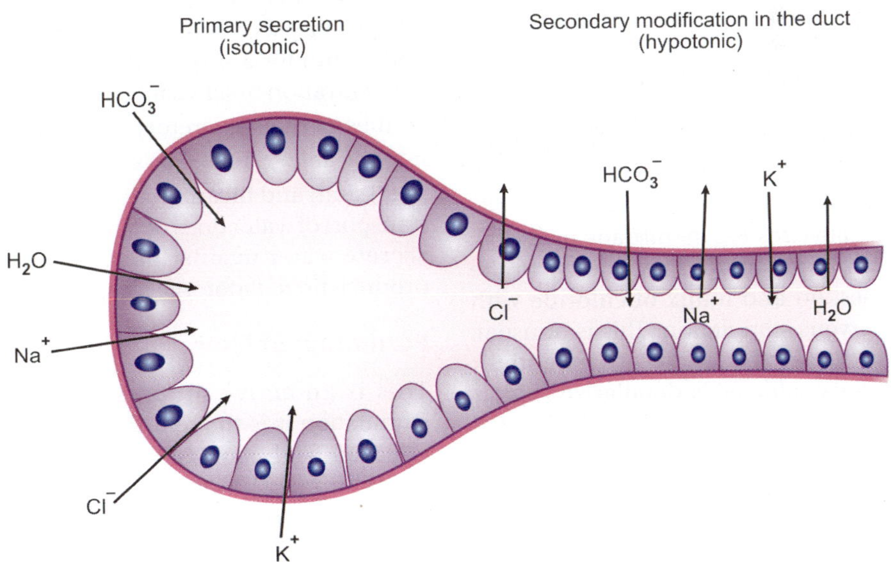

Figure 5.1: Two stage hypothesis of saliva production

Secondary Modification

Striated ducts reabsorb sodium ions from the primary secretion and secrete potassium ions. Chloride ions tend to follow the electrochemical gradient established by sodium reabsorption. Water is however impermeable at tight junctions of striated duct cells. So the water does not follow electrolytes and thus secondary saliva is hypotonic (see Fig 5.1).

The degree of modification of saliva relies heavily on the salivary flow rates. At fast flow rates, there is less time for secondary modification and saliva composition approach that of the primary saliva, yet it is hypotonic with respect to plasma. At slow rates, secondary modification results in low electrolytes and is increasingly hypotonic and potassium rich. In general, saliva is composed of 99.5% water in addition to proteins, glycoproteins, and electrolytes. Saliva is high in potassium (7x plasma), bicarbonate (3x plasma), calcium, phosphorous, chloride, thiocyanate, and urea. Saliva is low in sodium (1/10 x plasma). The normal pH of saliva is 5.6 to 7 at standard flow rate.

Fluid Dynamics

Water of the saliva enters at the level of terminal secretory units. The ductal reabsorption of Na^+ exceeds that of K^+ and HCO_3^- producing a hypotonic fluid. The salivary ducts rely heavily on the Na/K/2Cl co-transporter. The duct cells maintain a negative resting membrane potential, and these cells hyperpolarize secondary to the efflux of potassium and influx of chloride with autonomic nervous stimulation. This is unusual, and is referred to as the "secretory potential", because most excitable cells depolarize (rather than hyperpolarize) with stimulation. The striated and excretory ducts are impermeable to water and active transport of water does not occur against the osmotic gradient.

Salivary Secretion

Primary saliva produced by the acini consists of water, ions, small molecules and the secretory product of the secretory end piece. This fluid is derived from the interstitial fluid which in turn is an exchange product from the surrounding blood capillaries. This fluid passes through the basement membrane supporting the acini and is discharged either by the acinar cells or inter cellular spaces. The primary saliva is a protein containing isotonic fluid with increased sodium and decreased potassium.

Sodium ion and chloride ion concentration in primary saliva is approximately equal to those in plasma. Potassium concentration is lower when compared to that of sodium but more in saliva compared to that in plasma. Concentration of these electrolytes varies with flow rates. With increased flow sodium ions and chloride ions increase while potassium ions decrease. It is believed that striated ducts reabsorb sodium ion from the primary secretion and secretes the potassium ion and bicarbonates. Chloride tends to follow the electrochemical gradient established by the sodium reabsorption. So, at increased flow rates sodium reabsorption becomes less efficient and primary secretion is in contact with the ductal epithelium for a shorter time and hence sodium concentration of saliva increases. Microperfusion studies of main excretory duct have shown that it too is able to reabsorb sodium ion and secrete potassium and bicarbonate ions. Since the active transport of water does not occur the ducts cannot secrete water against the osmotic gradient to produce final hypotonic saliva.

Formation of Fluid

This is an active process. After appropriate stimulation it is thought that free calcium ion is released from storage within the endoplasmic reticulum (ER). Free cytoplasmic calcium ion concentration can increase 5 to 10 times in seconds after stimulation and this brings about significant compensatory changes that include the opening of two membrane ion channels for the passage of potassium ions and chloride ions, with chloride channels confined to the luminal surface of the cell and potassium channel confined to the baso-lateral surface.

When potassium ion is released, a compensatory uptake of sodium ions and chloride ions occur. Chloride ions exit the cells through the channel at the luminal surface and it is speculated that to maintain electrical neutrality, sodium ions enter the lumen through the para cellular pathway. The result of this ionic relocation is a flux of water into lumen via osmotic coupling of sodium chloride and water. As a result, it is proposed that the saliva production is a transcellular event.

Nervous Control

Physiologic activity of salivary gland is mediated through the autonomic nervous system (ANS). The release of neurotransmitter substance from the vesicles in the nerve terminal close to the parenchymal cells stimulates these to discharge their secretory granules. This process is referred to as stimulus secretion coupling. Neurotransmitter substances then interact with specific receptor located in the plasma membrane of the acinar cells. Norepinephrine, the sympathetic transmitter interacts with both alpha and beta adrenergic receptors where as acetylcholine interacts primarily with cholinergic receptors.

Stimulation of alpha adrenergic receptors or cholinergic receptors is mainly involved in water and electrolyte secretion. Receptor for peptide transmitter "substance P" stimulates secretion by elevating blood flow by acting on the feed arterioles. In addition vasoactive intestinal peptide (VIP) is present at the nerve endings of salivary glands which are also shown to induce secretion by salivary glands. Receptor stimulation results in the intracellular concentration of secondary messenger. In case of alpha adrenergic, cholinergic and substance P receptors, the membrane permeability of calcium is increased and there is a marked increase in the calcium influx. In addition there is increased release of calcium ion from intracellular stores from ER. Increased calcium concentration causes potassium efflux, water and electrolyte concentration and low levels of exocytosis (Fig. 5.2).

Stimulation of beta adrenergic receptors activates the plasma membrane enzyme adenylate cyclase which catalyzes formation of cyclic AMP from ATP. The increased cytoplasmic concentration of cyclic AMP from ATP activates cyclic AMP dependent protein kinase, an enzyme that phosphorylates other protein which inturn may be involved in exocytosis. Cyclic AMP also increases intracellular calcium concentration.

Salivation is entirely under the nervous control. Salivary flow rate from minor salivary gland is independent of the stimulation constituting seven to eight percent of total salivary output.

The physiologic control of saliva is mediated through the activity of autonomic nervous system (Fig. 5.3). Normally **parasympathetic stimulation** promotes continuous secretion of moderate amount of saliva. It keeps mucous membrane moist, lubricates the movement of tongue and lips during speech. Stimulation of parasympathetic nervous system results in abundant watery secretion with a decrease in amylase in saliva and increase in serum amylase. Acetylcholine is the active transmitter binding at muscarinic receptors in salivary glands.

In case of the parotid gland, parasympathetic fibers originate from glossopharyngeal nerve travel via lesser superficial petrosal nerve to synapse in otic ganglion, then to auriculo temporal nerve and finally the salivary gland. Parasympathetic fibers are secretomotor. They reach the gland through auriculotemporal nerve.

In case of submandibular and sublingual gland, parasympathetic fibers originate in seventh cranial nerve travel via the chordatympani to the submandibular ganglion, then release acetyl-choline in close proximity to the glands with no true postganglionic synapses.

Stimulation by the sympathetic nervous system results in a scant, viscous saliva rich in organic

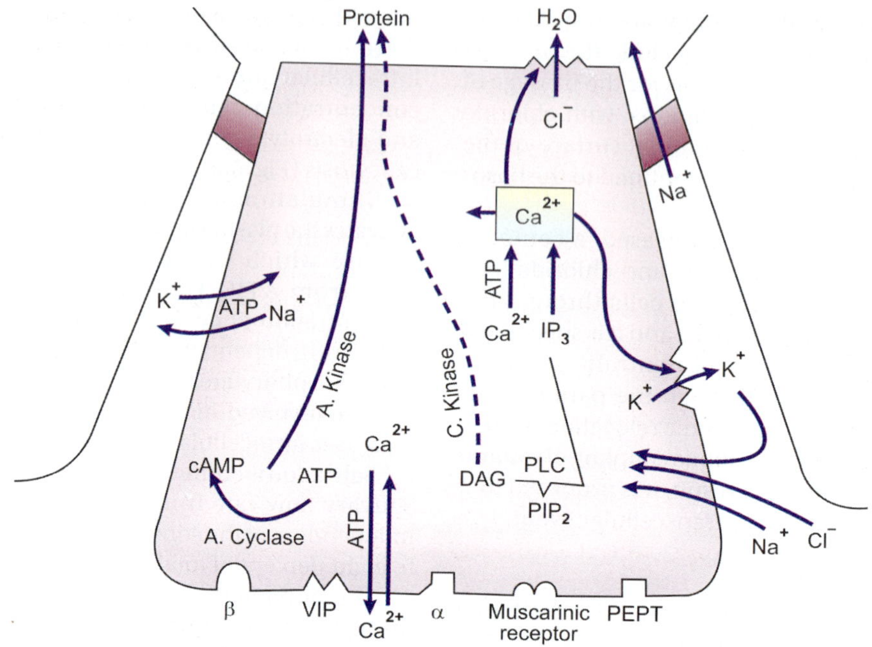

Figure 5.2: Intracellular events in production of saliva

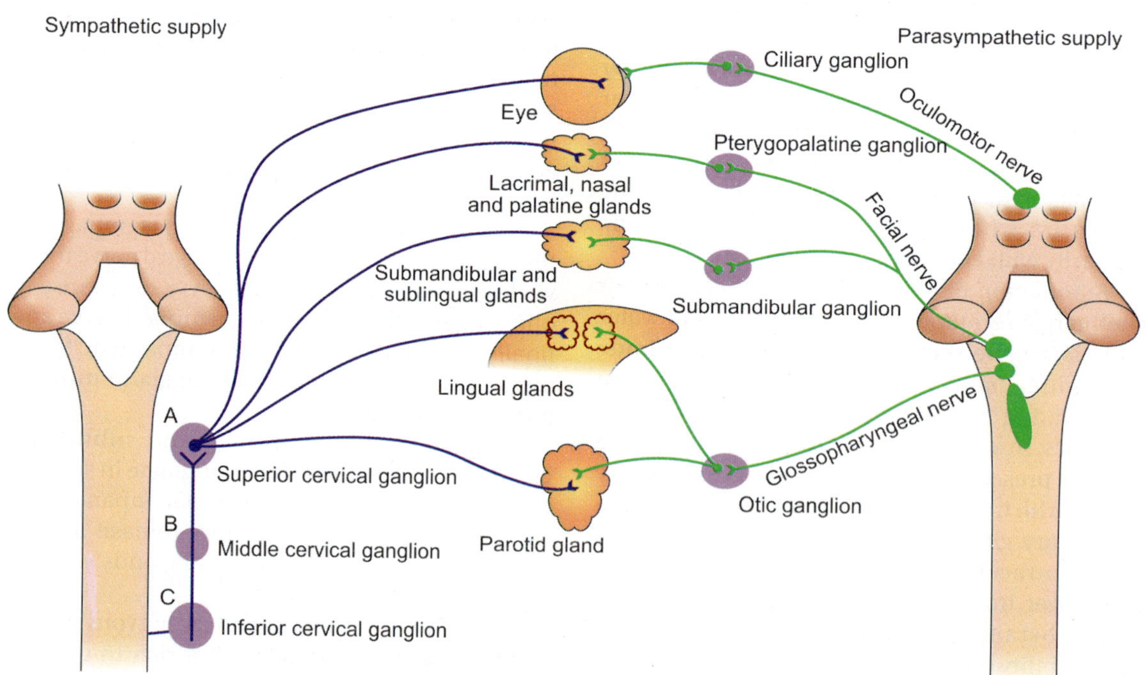

Figure 5.3: Sympathetic and parasympathetic supply to major and minor salivary glands

and inorganic solutes with an increase in amylase in the saliva and no change of amylase in the serum. Sympathetic stimulation dominates during stress resulting in dryness of mouth. Sympathetic nerves are vasomotor and are derived from the plexus around the external carotid artery. It contains postganglionic fibers from the superior cervical ganglion without any relay and supplies the vasomotor fibers to the two glands. For all of the salivary glands, these fibers originate in the superior cervical ganglion then travel with arteries to reach the glands, external carotid artery in the case of the parotid, lingual artery in the case of the submandibular, and facial artery in the case of the sublingual gland.

It was once thought that the sympathetic nervous system antagonizes the parasympathetic nervous system with respect to salivary output, but this is not true.

Nerve Supply

Two patterns of innervations are established. In the first described as epilemmal, axons remain in the connective tissue separated from the secretory cells by a basement membrane. When such axons come close to a secretory cell, they lose their Schwann cell covering and in the adjacent exoplasm, many vesicles containing transmitter substances exist. Presumably some neurotransmitters substances are released when a nerve impulse passes and diffuses some 100 to 200 nm across the basement membrane before influencing the secretory cell. The second described as hypolemmal, axons that penetrate the basement membrane lose their Schwann cell covering and run between the secretory cells separated from them by a gap of only 10 to 20 nm. With this type of innervation, a single axon may quickly affect several secretory cells or the single cell several times.

Autonomic Innervation

The parasympathetic nervous system is the primary instigator of salivary secretion. Interruption of parasympathetic innervation to the salivary glands results in atrophy, while interruption of sympathetic innervation results in no significant change in the glands.

Stimulation by the parasympathetic nervous system results in an abundant, watery saliva with a decrease in amylase in saliva and an increase in amylase in the serum. Acetylcholine is the active neurotransmitter, binding at muscarinic receptors in the salivary glands.

Stimulation by the sympathetic nervous system results in a scant, viscous saliva rich in organic and inorganic solutes with an increase in levels of amylase in the saliva and no change in the amylase levels in the serum.

Salivary Flow

The average volume of saliva secreted in a 24-hour period is 1 to 1.5 liters (approximately 1 cc/minute), most of which is secreted during meals. The basal salivary flow rate is about 0.001-0.2 ml/min/gland. With stimulation, salivary flow rate increases to about 0.2 to 5.0 ml/min (Table 5.1). Salivary flow rate from the minor salivary glands is however, independent of stimulation, constituting five to eight percent of total salivary output.

In the unstimulated state the relative contribution of the major salivary glands is as follows. Submandibular gland contributing about 69%, parotid gland about 26% and sublingual gland produce 5% of saliva (Table 5.2).

In the stimulated state the relative contribution of the major salivary glands is more in parotid which contributes about 69%, while submandibular gland and sublingual gland contribute to about 26 and 5% respectively.

Though the sublingual glands and minor salivary glands contribute only about 10% of all saliva, together they produce the majority of mucous and are critical in maintaining the mucin layer over the oral mucosa.

Ptyalism, or drooling, may be secondary to salivary hypersecretion. This is caused either by excessive salivary flow, or a salivary flow rate which

Table 5.1: Salivary flow rate			
Saliva	*Resting flow rate (ml/min)*	*Stimulated flow rate (ml/min)*	*pH*
Whole	0.2–0.4	2–5	6.7–7.4
Parotid	0.04	1–2	6.0–7.8
Submandibular	0.1	0.8	

Table 5.2: Nature and quantity of salivary secretion			
		Contribution of saliva (%)	
Gland	*Secretion*	*Unstimulated state*	*Stimulated state*
Parotid	Watery	26	69
Submandibular	Moderately viscous	69	26
Sublingual	Viscous	05	05
Minor		05	05

surpasses the ability to swallow the saliva. Possible surgical treatments for Ptyalism are tympanic neurectomies (eliminating parasympathetic innervation to the parotid gland) or parotid duct rerouting.

Eighty to ninety percent of salivary gland stones occur in the submandibular gland, and of those, 85% occur in Wharton's duct. Complete ductal obstruction generally results in atrophy of the gland, while partial obstruction usually results in glandular mucocele.

Effects of Aging

Acinar cells do degenerate with age. However, total salivary flow rates have been found to be independent of age. Xerostomia, or the subjective complaint of dry mouth, must be distinguished from the objective finding of decreased salivary flow. Xerostomia in the elderly is generally either secondary to medications or to systemic disease.

The submandibular glands are more sensitive to metabolic and physiologic changes. Thus, it is salivary flow in the unstimulated state which is more greatly affected by such changes.

Saliva

Saliva includes the combined secretion of all the major and minor salivary glands. Although the major production of salivary fluid is by the salivary glands *per se*, smaller amounts of other fluids are derived from the gingival sulcus, tonsillar crypts and general transudation from the epithelial lining of the oral cavity. Salivary glands produce about 1200 ml of saliva per day. The elemental role of this fluid to proper oral hygiene can be best demonstrated in those patients suffering from xerostomia.

Composition of Saliva

In addition to water which makes up about 99% of saliva, it contains both the organic and inorganic components. The solute portion of saliva which consists of electrolytes or inorganic ions plus proteins or other organic components, account for less than one percent. Human saliva is normally hypotonic with respect to plasma. The osmolarity of saliva varies according to the flow rate, being increased at higher flow rates.

Functions of Saliva

Saliva has numerous function related to both metabolic and non-metabolic activities.

Protection: Saliva keeps the mouth moist because of the glycoprotein content in it and thus protects the lining mucosa by forming a barrier against noxious stimuli, microbial toxins and abrasives. In fact, the mucin layer on the oral mucosa is thought to be the most important nonimmune defense mechanism in the oral cavity. Salivary fluid may help in lavage because of its fluid consistency and thereby provide a mechanical action that flushes away the non adherent bacterial and cellular debris from the mouth.

Lubrication: Saliva lubricates food, thereby assists in mastication and facilitates swallowing. Saliva importantly moistens dry food and cools the hot food. By coating the interior of the mouth, saliva helps in the free movement of tongue during speech and mastication.

Taste: Saliva provides a medium for dissolved foods to stimulate the taste buds. Saliva also contains a protein called *gusten*, which is necessary for growth and maturation of taste buds.

Formation of salivary pellicle: Because of the calcium binding proteins present in saliva, there is formation on the tooth of a protective film called salivary pellicle.

Buffering: Saliva has a high concentration of negatively charged phosphate and bicarbonate ions. It protects the oral cavity by two means. Firstly, the buffering property of saliva prevents the colonization of many potential pathogenic bacteria, denying them the optimal conditions for growth. Secondly, buffering prevents the demineralization of teeth from of the acids produced by the plaque microorganism.

Digestion: Saliva is important for digestion of cooked starch which begins in the mouth by salivary α amylase. Alpha-amylase, contained in saliva, breaks 1 to 4 glycoside bonds and continues to act in esophagus and stomach. Amylase digestion can continue in the stomach for approximately half an hour, until it is arrested by the excessive acidity of the gastric contents. Amylase is readily inactivated at pH less than 4.0. Lingual lipase is another digestive enzyme elaborated in saliva which helps in the breakdown of fat. Although not a very significant enzyme for the digestion of fat,

it is important in patients with cystic fibrosis in whom there is deficiency of pancreatic lipase. Saliva produces R protein, which binds to Vitamin B_{12}. It keeps it in an absorbable form during its passage through stomach and small intestine.

Antimicrobial: Saliva minimizes the risk of bacterial infection. Certain of the high molecular weight salivary glycoproteins aggregate specific strains of the oral microorganisms and prevent their adherence to oral tissues thus facilitating clearance from the mouth by swallowing. Secretion of peroxidase by acinar cells and thiocyanate by ductal system has bacteriostatic action. Peroxidase breaks down salivary thiocyanate which, in turn, oxidizes the enzymes involved in bacterial glycolysis. Another important bactericidal enzyme present in saliva is lysozyme or muramidase, that hydrolyzes the polysaccharide of bacterial cell wall resulting in cell lysis. Lysozyme agglutinates bacteria and activates autolysins.

Saliva also performs immunologic function, as noted by the presence of salivary immunoglobulin (IgA). IgA is synthesized by plasma cells in the connective tissue surrounding the secreory acini of the salivary glands and both dimeric and monomeric forms are released into the connective tissue. A secretory glycoprotein is synthesized by the salivary gland cells and inserted into the basal plasma membrane, where it serves as a receptor for dimeric IgA. When the dimeric IgA binds to the receptor, the secretory IgA complex thus formed is internalized by receptor mediated endocytosis and carried through the acinar cell to the apical plasma membrane, where it is released into the lumen as secretory IgA (sIgA). Secretory component also increases the resistance of IgA to denaturation and proteolysis. Small amounts of IgA and IgM can also be present and they primarily inhibit the adherence of microorganism to oral tissues.

Another important antimicrobial substance found in saliva is lactoferrin. Lactoferrin is an iron binding protein which binds to free iron and deprives bacteria of the essential element. Lactoferrin enhances the inhibitory effect of antibodies on the microorganism.

Maintenance of tooth integrity and tissue repair:
Saliva is saturated with calcium and phosphate ions. Calcium and phosphate in the saliva are essential for the mineralization of newly erupted teeth and for repair of precarious lesions of the enamel in erupted teeth. Bleeding time in the oral cavity is shorter and wound healing is faster possibly because of EGF secreted by submandibular salivary gland. Salivary gland produces various biologically active substances. For example, parotid gland produces a hormone called *parotin* which is said to promote the growth of mesenchymal tissue.

Diagnostic Application of Saliva

As a diagnostic fluid, saliva offers distinctive advantages over serum because it can be collected non-invasively by individuals with modest training. Furthermore, saliva may provide a cost-effective approach for the screening of large populations. Gland-specific saliva can be used for diagnosis of pathology specific to one of the major salivary glands. Whole saliva, however, is most frequently used for diagnosis of systemic diseases, since it is readily collected and contains serum constituents. These constituents are derived from the local vasculature of the salivary glands and also reach the oral cavity *via* the flow of gingival fluid. Analysis of saliva may be useful for the diagnosis of hereditary disorders, autoimmune diseases, malignant and infectious diseases, and endocrine disorders, as well as in the assessment of therapeutic levels of drugs and the monitoring of illicit drug use.

However, salivary flow rate may play a more important role in oral hygiene than any of these factors. The intraoral complications of salivary hypofunction include candidiasis, oral lichen planus (usually painful), burning mouth syndrome (normal appearing oral mucosa with a subjective sensation of burning), recurrent aphthous ulcers, and dental caries.

The best way to evaluate salivary function is to measure the salivary flow rate in stimulated (e.g. by using a parasympathomimetic such as pilocarpine) and unstimulated states. Xerostomia is not a reliable indicator of salivary hypofunction.

The cephalic phase response refers to the effects that the sensory stimuli have on the physiologic response to food. This is neuronally mediated via the parasympathetic nervous system. There is a hierarchy of sensory stimuli such that swallowing is more than mastication, which is more than taste, which is more than smell, which is more than sight and which is more than thought. Stimulation results in an increase in total salivary flow from 0.3 cc/min to more than 1 cc/min. In addition, the magnitude of salivary response is directly related to a subject's state of hunger.

DYSFUNCTION OF SALIVARY GLANDS

This could be a reflection of gross anatomical alterations of the glandular tissue or may be the result of a systemic change, manifested as deficient functional ability of the gland. The mucosal tissue, and oral mucosa not an exception, are frequent sites of complications arising from mucositis, xerostomia, osteonecrosis and local infection, which could all be linked ultimately to manifestations of salivary gland dysfunction. Because of the decrease in salivary secretion a number of essential functions are impaired that may result in difficulties with chewing, swallowing, and speech, oral mucosal inflammation, dental caries, and changes in taste perception.

FUNCTIONAL DISORDERS OF SALIVARY GLANDS

1. Sialorrhea (increase in salivary flow)
2. Xerostomia (dry mouth)
3. Sodium retention dysfunction syndrome
4. Dysfunctions in systemic diseases.

Sialorrhea (Drooling, Ptyalism or Excessive Salivation)

A common problem in neurologically impaired children (those with associated retardation or cerebral palsy) and in adults who have Parkinson's disease who had a stroke. Sialorrhea is most commonly caused by poor oral and facial muscle control. Contributing factors include hypersecretion of saliva, dental malocclusion, postural problems and an inability to recognize salivary spill (Hockstein NG et al 2004). It is a normal phenomenon in children prior to the development of oral neuromuscular control at age between 18 and 24 months. Sialorrhea causes a range of physical and psychosocial complications, including perioral soreness, dehydration, halitosis, and social stigmatization that can be quite discomforting for the patient. The flow of saliva is enhanced by sympathetic innervation, which promotes contraction of muscle fibers around the salivary ducts.

Etiology (Table 5.3)

Sialorrhea is usually caused by neuromuscular dysfunction, hypersecretion, sensory or anatomic (motor) dysfunction. In children, mental retardation and cerebral palsy are commonly implicated. In adults, Parkinson's disease is the most common cause. Pseudobulbar palsy, bulbar palsy, and stroke are less common causes. Hypersecretion commonly

Table 5.3: Etiological factors of sialorrhea

1. Neuromuscular/Sensory dysfunction
   - Mental retardation
   - Cerebral palsy
   - Parkinson's disease
   - Stroke
2. Hypersecretion
   - Inflammation (Teething, dental caries, mucosal infections, rabies)
   - Drug-side effects. (Tranquilizers and anti-convulsants)
   - Gastroesophageal reflux
   - Toxin exposure (Mercury vapor)
3. Anatomic
   - Macroglossia
   - Oral incompetence
   - Dental malocclusion
   - Orthodontic problems
   - Head and neck surgical defects (e.g. **Andy Gump** deformity)

Courtesy: Hockstein NG et al. American Family Physician, Vol 69 (11); 2004.

is caused by inflammation, such as associated with teething, dental caries, and oral infections. Other causes of hypersecretion include side effects from medications (i.e tranquilizers, anti-convulsants), gastro-esophageal reflex, toxin exposure (i.e. mercury vapor), and rabies. Sensory dysfunction may decrease a person's ability to recognize drooling and anatomic or motor dysfunction may impede the ability to manage increased secretions.

Anatomic abnormalities are usually not the sole cause of drooling but commonly exacerbate other causative conditions. Macroglossia and oral incompetence may predispose patients to salivary spill. Unfortunately, these conditions are difficult to be remedied. Malocclusion and other orthodontic problems may compound oral incompetence; orthodontic correction can reduce sialorrhea.

Surgical defects following head and neck resection and reconstruction also may cause sialorrhea. The most notable example of these anatomic defects is *Andy Gump* deformity, which is caused by the loss of the anterior mandibular arch (without adequate reconstruction).

Xerostomia (Dry Mouth)

Xerostomia is the symptom of oral dryness resulting from decreased salivary flow, particularly when it is reduced by 50%. Although the underlying mechanisms are different, each etiology results in a variable decrease of salivary function, which leads to the subjective complaint of dry mouth. Surprisingly few patients do not complaint of dry mouth, but admit that they have difficulty in taking dry food substances. It may or may not be associated with decreased salivary gland function. Xerostomia is a common complaint found often among older adults affecting approximately 20% of the elderly. However, it does not appear to be related to age itself but may be a complication of taking medications, to which the elderly are commonly used to. Oral dryness may be acute and transient in case of emotional disturbances and acute anxiety state. Table 5.4 lists the common causes of xerostomia

Table 5.4: Common causes of xerostomia

1. Iatrogenic
- Drugs
    - Antihypertensives
    - Antidepressants
    - Analgesics,
    - Tranquilizers,
    - Diuretics
    - Antihistamines
- Radiation to the salivary gland
- Complication of chemotherapy

2. Immune
- Graft versus host disease
- Sjögren's syndrome
- Sarcoidosis
- Primary biliary cirrhosis

3. Infectious causes
- HIV disease
- Hepatitis 'C' virus infection
- Mumps

4. Other causes
- Mouth breathing
- Excessive smoking
- Dehydration – Excessive sweating, vomiting, polyuria, hemorrhage, and fluid restriction
- Cystic fibrosis
- Diabetes mellitus
- Amyloidosis
- Hemochromatosis
- Wegener's granulomatosis
- Aplasia of salivary glands
- Endocrine disorders
- Stress, anxiety, depression
- Nutritional deficiencies
- Nerve damage—Trauma to head and neck area from surgery or wounds

Complications Associated with Xerostomia

Xerostomia is often a contributing factor for both minor and serious health problems. It can affect nutrition rather considerably resulting in associated deficiency manifestations, a constant sore throat, burning sensation of the oral mucosa, difficulty of speaking and swallowing, hoarseness of voice and/or dry nasal passages. It contributes to the occurrence of periodontal decay with resultant tooth loss in adults. If left untreated, xerostomia decreases the oral pH and significantly increases the development of plaque and dental caries. Oral candidosis is one of the most common oral infections seen in association with xerostomia.

Clinical Presentation

The patients often complain of problems with eating, speaking, swallowing, and wearing dentures. Dry and crumbly foods, such as cereals and crackers, may be particularly difficult to chew and swallow. Denture wearers may have problems with denture retention, denture sores and stickiness of the tongue to the palate. Patients with xerostomia often complain of taste disorders (dysguesia), a painful tongue (glossodynia), and persistent thirst, especially at night. It can lead to increased tendency for dental caries, parotid gland enlargement, inflammation and fissuring of the lips (cheilitis), inflammation and ulcers of the tongue and buccal mucosa, oral candidiasis, salivary gland infection (sialadenitis), halitosis, and cracking and fissuring of the oral mucosa.

Diagnosis and Evaluation of Xerostomia

Diagnosis of xerostomia may be based on evidence obtained from the patients history, an examination of the oral cavity and/or sialometry; a simple procedure that measures the flow rate of saliva. In women the **lipstick** sign where the lipstick adheres to the front teeth may be a useful indicator of xerostomia.

Several clinical tests can be utilized to ascertain the function of salivary glands. In sialometry, collection devices are placed over the parotid gland or the submandibular/sublingual duct orifices and saliva is stimulated with citric acid. The normal salivary flow rate for unstimulated saliva from the parotid gland is 0.4 to 1.5 ml/min/gland. The normal flow rate for unstimulated, 'resting' whole saliva is 0.3 to 0.5 ml/min; for stimulated saliva, 1 to 2 ml/min. Values less than 0.1 ml/min are typically considered xerostomic. Although reduced flow rate may not always be associated with complaints of dryness.

Sialography is an imaging technique that may be useful in identifying salivary gland stones and masses. It involves the injection of a radiopaque media in to the salivary glands. Salivary scintigraphy can be useful in assessing salivary gland function. Technetium 99m sodium pertechnate is injected intravenously to ascertain the rate and density of uptake and the time of excretion in the mouth. Minor salivary gland biopsy is often used in the diagnosis of Sjögren's syndrome, HIV-salivary gland disease, sarcoidosis, amyloidosis and graft versus-host disease. Biopsy of major salivary gland is resorted to in cases of suspected malignancies.

Sodium Retention Dysfunction Syndrome

The normal proportional relationship between salivary flow and sodium concentration is absent in a number of persons. Not only are smaller flow rates measured but also the sodium concentration is relatively low and fluctuates around a steady state of 2.5 mmol/L while most other substances are slightly raised. In some cases, the saliva has a milky appearance. These indications of sodium retention dysfunction syndrome are fairly typical and may be found at all ages, although they are more prevalent in later life. Prominent clinical signs are the sensation of a dry mouth and incidental unilateral painless swelling of the parotid gland for a few hours, e.g. during breakfast with some exceptions, the dysfunction persists through life. Risk factors can be listed in subgroups such as both hyper and hypotension, Cardiac failure, local and systemic edema from other causes, and dehydration. A sudden onset of sodium retention is seen after arteriovenous shunt in hemodialysis. This phenomenon is not related to the time at which dialysis was actually performed. Increased sodium reabsorption may be due to hormonal effects on the sodium/potassium exchange rate or even to elongation of the striated duct. The reduced flow with sodium retention and low bicarbonate values accompanying the sodium retention dysfunction syndrome may

have a profound impact in the oral environment. This kind of gland dysfunction is in fact a common finding in periodontal disease, superficial glossitis, glossodynia, and taste disorders.

Dysfunctions in Systemic Diseases

Collagen vascular diseases such as rheumatoid arthritis, systemic lupus erythematosus, and systemic sclerosis, associated with Sjögren's syndrome can cause decreased salivary flow, alteration in salivary protein secretion, and changes in ductal electrolyte reabsorption.

Salivary gland enlargement and protein alteration occurs in endocrine disorders including diabetes mellitus. Hypertension leads to decrease in salivary sodium levels. Patients with alcoholic cirrhosis have low salivary flow rate and lower levels of electrolytes and proteins. In cystic fibrosis there is abnormal chloride regulation in exocrine glands including mucous salivary glands, which results in increased protein, sodium, chloride, calcium, and urea concentrations.

BIBLIOGRAPHY

1. Bailey CM, Wadsworth PV. Treatment of the drooling child by submandibular duct transposition. J Laryngol Otol 1985;99(11):1111-7.
2. Barnes L, Brandwein M, Som PM. Surgical Pathology of the Head and Neck. 2nd edn. Marcel Dekker Inc. New York, 2001.
3. Baum BJ. Principles of saliva secretion. Ann N Y Acad Sci 1993;694:17-23.
4. Borg M, Hirst F. The role of radiation therapy in the management of sialorrhea. Int J Radiat Oncol Biol Phys 1998;41:1113-9.
5. Dirix P, Nuyts S, Bogaert WV. Radiation-induced xerostomia in patients with head and neck cancer: a literature review. Cancer 2006;107(11):2525-34.
6. Domaracki LS, Sisson LA. Decreasing drooling with oral stimulation in children with multiple disabilities. Am J Occup Ther 1990;44:680-4.
7. Dutta SK, Dukehart M, Narang A, Latham PS. Functional and structural changes in parotid glands of alcoholic cirrhotic patients. Gastroenterology 1988;16(4):215-8.
8. Fox PC, Busch KA, Baum BJ. Subjective reports of xerostomia and objective measures of salivary gland performance. J Am Dent Assoc 1987;115:581-4.

9. Grisius MM, Fox PC. Salivary gland diseases. In: Burket's Oral Medicine Diagnosis and Treatment. Greenberg MS, Glick M (Eds) BC Decker Inc, Ontario, 2003.

10. Nederfors T. Xerostomia: Prevalence and pharmacotherapy. With special reference to beta-adrenoceptor antagonists. Swed Dent J Suppl 1996;116:1-70.

11. Neville BW, Damm DD, Allen CM, Bouquot JE. Oral and Maxillofacial Pathology, 2nd edn. WB Saunders Co., 2002.

12. O'Connell AC. Natural history and prevention of radiation injury. Adv Dent Res 2000;14:57-61.

13. Rajendran R, Sivapathasundharam B. Diseases of salivary gland. In: Shafer's textbook of oral pathology, 5th edn. Elsevier, 2005.

14. Schubert MM, Izutsu KT. Iatrogenic causes of salivary gland dysfunction. J Dent Res 1987;66:680-7.

15. Sreebny LM, Yu A, Green A, Valdini A. Xerostomia in diabetes mellitus. Diabetes Care 1992;15:900-4.

16. Valdez IH, Fox PC. Diagnosis and management of salivary dysfunction. Crit Rev Oral Biol Med 1993;4:271-7.

17. Valdez IH, Fox PC. Diagnosis and management of salivary dysfunction. Crit Rev Oral Biol Med 1993;4:271-7.

18. Vissink A, Jansma J, Spijkervet FKL, Burlage FR, Coppes RP. Oral sequelae of head and neck radiotherapy. Crit Rev Oral Biol Med 2003;14(3):199-212.

19. Wasserman T. Radioprotective effects of amifostine. Semin Oncol 1999;26(Suppl 7):89-94.

6

Histogenesis and Molecular Pathogenesis of Salivary Gland Tumors

G Sriram, Geetha Prakash

INTRODUCTION

Tumors of the salivary glands represent 2 to 4% of head and neck neoplasms. They are broadly categorized into malignant epithelial tumors, benign epithelial tumors, soft tissue tumors and hematolymphoid tumors. Seventy percent of salivary gland tumors originate in the parotid gland, 8% arise in the submandibular gland and 22% in the minor salivary glands. Seventy-five percent of parotid tumors are benign, a little more than 50% tumors of the submandibular and 60 to 80% of minor salivary gland tumors are malignant. Pleomorphic adenomas are the most common benign tumors comprising 85% of all salivary gland neoplasms.

One of the major problems in classification and histogenesis is that most of the salivary gland tumors arise from or differentiate toward the same cell lines, luminal (intercalated and acinar) and abluminal (basal and myoepithelial). To add to our woes, each of these cells can undergo a variety of metaplastic changes (e.g. oncocytic, sebaceous, squamous and chondroid), thus confounding the origin of the cell.

The advent of immunohistochemistry and molecular genetics have dramatically changed our understanding of the etiology, histogenesis, prognosis and treatment protocols of neoplasms. Immunohistochemistry has helped us to delineate the luminal and abluminal cells, and hence the extent of participation of these cells in any particular neoplasm. A word of caution here is that immunohistochemistry requires expert interpretation as one has to know to deal with background staining and strong and weak positive results. It can be misleading and totally alter a diagnosis if the interpretation is incorrect. The immunophenotypic profile of the normal cells of the salivary gland is tabulated in Table 6.1.

ETIOLOGY

Viruses

Epstein-Barr virus (EBV) is shown to be strongly associated with lymphoepithelial carcinomas, especially among Asians. EBV has not been shown in any other salivary gland carcinomas or neighboring normal gland. SV40 sequences have been demonstrated in pleomorphic adenomas but there is no convincing association between human salivary gland tumors and other viruses, including polyoma virus and papilloma virus.

Radiation

Long-term follow-up studies of the survivors of the atomic bomb explosions in Hiroshima and Nagasaki show an increased relative risk of 3.5 for benign, and 11 for malignant salivary gland neoplasms. The risk was directly related to the level of exposure to ionizing radiation. There was a high frequency of both mucoepidermoid carcinomas and Warthin's tumors in these individuals.

Therapeutic radiation, particularly of the head and neck region, has been linked with a significantly increased risk of developing salivary gland cancers. There appears to be a risk from iodine 131 used in the treatment of thyroid disease, as the isotope is also concentrated in the salivary glands.

Table 6.1: Immunophenotypic profile of luminal and abluminal cells of normal salivary gland

Marker	Luminal Cells		Abluminal Cells	
	Acinar	Ductal	Myoepithelial	Basal
Pancytokeratin	-/+	+	+ (often weak)	+
Low molecular weight cytokeratins	+	+	+	+
High molecular weight cytokeratins	-	-	+	+
Amylase	+	-	-	-
EMA	+ (luminal)	+ (luminal)	-	-
CEA	+ (luminal)	+ (luminal)	-	-
S100	-	-/+	-/+	-
Myoid markers (Actin, Myosin, Calponin)	-	-	+	-
Desmin	-	-	-	-
GFAP	-	-	+/-	-

Abbreviations: EMA: Epithelial membrane antigen; CEA: Carcinoembryonic antigen; GFAP: Glial fibrillary acidic protein

There is evidence that exposure to routine dental radiographs and ultraviolet radiation is associated with an increased risk of salivary gland carcinoma.

Occupation

Increased incidences of salivary gland carcinomas have been reported among workers in a variety of industries which include rubber, asbestos, arsenic, plumbing, automobile and cosmetics.

Lifestyle and Nutrition

No association between tobacco use and alcohol consumption and salivary gland cancers could be demonstrated. However, there is a strong association between smoking and Warthin's tumor.

Hormones

Estrogen receptors were reported to be found in nearly 80% of normal glands in males and females and four out of eight salivary tumors in women had estrogen receptor levels similar to those of hormonally dependent breast carcinomas. Estrogen receptors have been reported in a minority of cases of acinic cell carcinoma, mucoepidermoid carcinoma and salivary duct carcinoma, but were not detected in adenoid cystic carcinoma. In some studies, estrogen receptors have been reported to be present in pleomorphic adenomas but in others, estrogen receptors were absent.

Progesterone receptors have been reported in normal salivary glands. They have been detected in a minority of pleomorphic adenomas but high levels of expression were reported in recurrent pleomorphic adenomas and this could be used as a prognostic factor.

Androgen receptors are reported to be present in over 90% of salivary duct carcinomas, carcinoma ex-pleomorphic adenoma and basal cell adenocarcinoma.

HISTOGENESIS

Over the last four decades a variety of histogenetic concepts for salivary gland tumors have evolved. These concepts were based on histologic observation of fetal salivary gland and the cellular differentiation in specific segments of the ductal system.

Hypotheses of the earlier times were based on *unicellular theory of origin* which proposed that the neoplasms arise from their adult differentiated counterparts of the salivary gland unit. For instance, mucoepidermoid carcinomas and squamous cell carcinomas would arise from excretory duct cells, oncocytic tumors from striated duct cells, acinic cell carcinomas from acinar cells and all adenomas and other adenocarcinomas from the intercalated duct cells. But this unicellular theory of origin was rejected on the fact that induction of neoplasm would require dedifferentiation of already specialized cells such as acinar and striated duct cells.

Eversole in 1971 proposed the bicellular theory of origin of salivary gland tumors which is termed as the *semipleuripotential bicellular theory*. Eversole had postulated the bicellular theory based on his observations in the embryonic development of palatal minor salivary glands. Eversole observed existence of reserve cells during embryogenesis of palatal salivary glands. The palatal minor salivary glands develop as downgrowths of bilayered ducts, and it was assumed that the inner or luminal layer derived from the outer or basal layer. These basal cells were considered as reserve cells that function as stem cells, particularly for generation of duct luminal and acinar cells. It was further assumed that with development and maturation of the salivary glands, the reserve cells remained confined to the basal cell layer of excretory and intercalated ducts. The reserve cells associated with intercalated duct cells was presumed to be responsible for replacement of intercalated ducts, striated ducts and acinar cells. Similarly, the reserve cells associated with the excretory duct give rise to the columnar and squamous cells of the excretory duct. But, this theory was not initially accepted due to lack of specific evidence.

In 1977, Regezi and Batsakis adopted the reserve cell hypothesis and proposed that the differentiated cell types in mature salivary glands are incapable of undergoing neoplastic alteration. The role of repair and replenishment could be assumed only by uncommitted stem (reserve) cells (Batsakis, 1990), and by inference, such cells were solely at risk for neoplastic induction. Henceforth, the semipleuripotential bicellular theory became most accepted theory.

On the other hand, there are evidences accumulating against the semipleuripotential bicellular theory. Both *in vitro* and *in vivo* studies have shown that mitotic figures are more frequently seen in luminal than basal cells, acinar cells divide, and that luminal epithelial cells with mitotic figures are present at all levels of the ductal system. Under certain circumstances like duct obstruction and chronic sialadenitis, luminal cells in the excretory duct can undergo squamous, goblet and ciliated cell metaplasia. Similarly, the acinar cells are capable of dedifferentiation to duct like cells and squamous metaplasia. These data suggest that any of the cells found in the normal salivary ductal system could probably serve as a precursor for neoplasia (Table 6.2). This *multicellular histogenetic concept* is proposed by Dardick et al, 1991.

HISTOGENESIS AND MOLECULAR GENETICS OF BENIGN SALIVARY GLAND TUMORS

Pleomorphic Adenoma

Histology of the tumor reveals epithelial cells, myoepithelial cells, mucinous, chondroid and even osseous foci intermingled with the epithelial elements. Myoepithelial cells seen in salivary, lacrimal and mammary glands support

Table 6.2: Cells of origin of salivary gland tumors

Cells of origin	Salivary gland tumors
Intercalated duct cell	Pleomorphic adenoma
Myoepithelial cell	Pleomorphic adenoma Basal cell adenoma
Striated duct cell	Oxyphilic adenoma (oncocytoma)
Heterotopic salivary tissue within lymph nodes	Adenolymphoma
Acinar epithelium Excretory duct cell	Acinic cell carcinoma Mucoepidermoid carcinoma squamous cell carcinoma

a morphological relationship of these organs. Myoepithelial cells secrete a substance resembling stromal mucins. The presence of a chondromyxoid stroma is practically pathognomonic of pleomorphic adenoma.

Histogenesis

Pathological alterations in glandular and ductal elements result in altered to completely different to physiological, morphological and immuno-histochemical features. For instance, presence of squamous cells in mucoepidermoid carcinomas; sebaceous cells derived from metaplastic changes in excretory duct can be observed in sebaceous adenoma, sebaceous lymphadenoma and sebaceous carcinoma; clear cells in pleomorphic adenoma, acinic cell carcinoma, mucoepidermoid carcinoma and epithelial-myoepithelial carcinoma: oncocytes which may be derived from mucous cells, serous cells, excretory cells and also myoepithelial cells can be seen in oncocytosis, Warthin's tumor, oncocytic adenocarcinoma and pleomorphic adenoma. These indicate the high potential for multidirectional differentiation of the cells of salivary gland.

Presence of both epithelial and mesenchymal elements had raised a lot of controversy regarding the histogenesis of the tumor. The various theories put forth to explain the histogenesis of pleomorphic adenoma are as follows:

1. The early German school suggests that it simultaneously arises from epithelial and mesenchymal components, corresponding to the concept of mixed tumor.
2. The French school suggest that the tumor is exclusively derived from epithelium and develops from mature salivary tissue, wheras the mesenchymal components are the result of stromal metaplasia occurring as a result of chemical influences, secreted by epithelial tumor cells.
3. The present and most accepted theory suggests that the tumor has a concomitant origin from epithelial and myoepithelial cells. This concept

is supported by various immunohistochemical and ultrastructural investigations. The ultra-structure of stromal cells reveals perinuclear tonofilaments, ectoplasmic actin micro-filaments and remnants of basement membrane indicating their origin from myoepithelial cells. The mesenchymal components are thought to be product of these myoepithelial cells (Flow chart 6.1).

Origin of Cartilage

Mcfarland states that the simultaneous presence of cartilage and epithelium is due to differentiation from embryonal and ectodermal cells isolated during the development of the face. Stein et al proposed that the cartilage arose from a precartilaginous substance included within the tumor at an early age of its evolution and that once stimulated this matrix proliferated and surrounded the neoplastic element. Another theory is that the cartilage represents the end result of a chemical transition of secretions produced by the epithelial tumor cells.

Pleomorphic adenomas show two types of mucin, an epithelial and a mesenchymal mucin. Mesenchymal mucin is believed to be produced by the myoepithelial cells. Epithelial mucin contains mainly neutral glycoproteins; whereas the mesenchymal mucin contains glyco-saminoglycans composed of hyaluronic acid, chondroitin sulfate. The chemical nature of the mesenchymal mucin is similar to that of cartilage, indicating that the mesenchymal mucin forms the precursor for cartilage found in the tumor.

Molecular Genetics

Cytogenetic studies of pleomorphic adenomas have shown that approximately 70% of the tumors are karyotypically abnormal. Four major cyto-genetic subgroups may be discerned:

1. Tumors with rearrangements involving 8q12 (39%)
2. Tumors with rearrangements of 12q13-15 (8%)
3. Tumors with sporadic, clonal changes not involving 8q12 or 12q13-15 (23%)

Flow chart 6.1: Cellular differentiation in pleomorphic adenoma

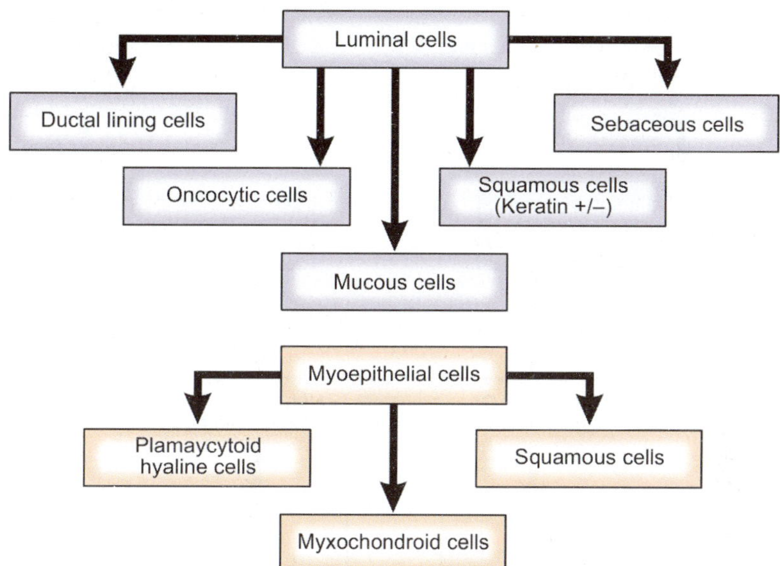

4. Tumors with an apparently normal karyotype (30%).

Whereas t(3;8)(p21;q12) and t(5;8) (p13;q12) are the most frequently observed translocations in the first subgroup, a t(9;12) (p24;q14-15) or an ins(9;12)(p24;q12q15) are the most frequent rearrangements seen in the second subgroup. Previous studies have also indicated that patients with karyotypically normal adenomas are significantly older than those with rearrangements of 8q12 and that adenomas with normal karyotypes are often more stroma rich than tumors with 8q12 abnormalities.

The target gene in pleomorphic adenomas with 8q12 abnormalities is *PLAG1*, a developmentally regulated zinc finger gene. The PLAG1 protein is a nuclear oncoprotein that functions as a DNA-binding transcription factor. Deregulation of *PLAG1* target genes, including *IGF2*, is likely to play a major role in the genesis of pleomorphic adenomas (Flow chart 6.2).

The target gene in adenomas with rearrangements of 12q14-15 is the high mobility group protein gene, *HMGA2*. *HMGA2* encodes an architectural transcription factor that promotes activation of gene expression by modulating the conformation of DNA. High-level expression of *HMGA2* resulting from gene amplification was recently suggested to be of importance for malignant transformation of pleomorphic adenomas (Flow chart 6.3).

Molecular studies of the *RAS* and *ERBB2* oncogenes have shown that mutation and activation of *RAS* frequently occur in pleomorphic adenomas, particularly in tumors with *PLAG1* activation, whereas amplification and/or overexpression of *ERBB2* seem to be rare. Similarly, TP53 alterations are infrequent in adenomas. In contrast, mutation and overexpression of TP53 are found in a relatively high proportion of carcinoma ex pleomorphic adenomas.

Studies using the human androgen receptor gene assay have demonstrated that the stromal and epithelial cells in pleomorphic adenomas are clonal and derived from the same progenitor cell. It was recently demonstrated that pleomorphic adenomas contain Simian virus 40 (SV40) DNA sequences and express the SV40 large T antigen, suggesting that this oncogenic virus may be involved in the genesis and/or progression of this tumor.

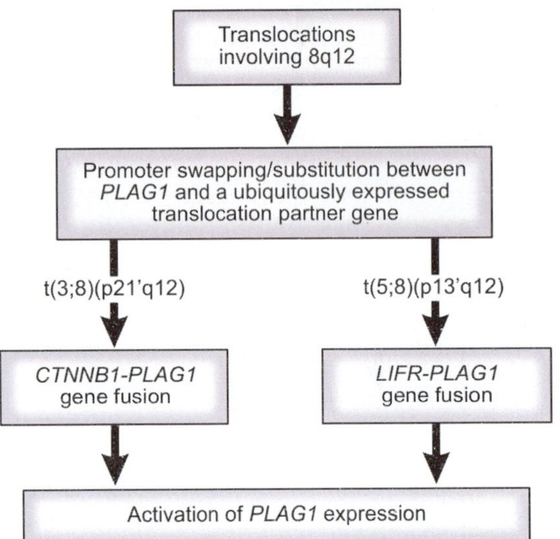

Flow chart 6.2: Cascade of events leading to activation of PLAG1 expression

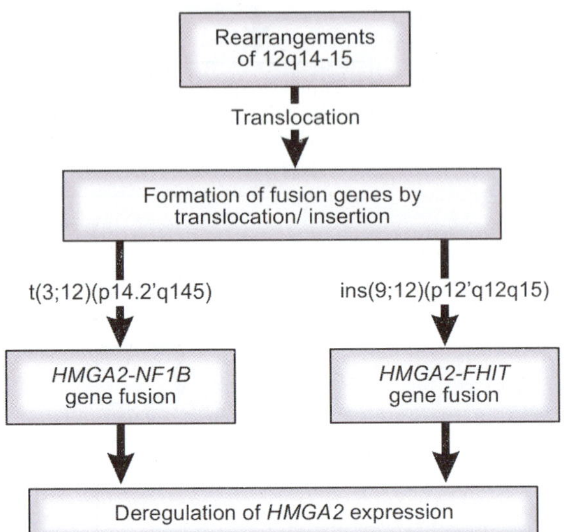

Flow chart 6.3: Cascade of events leading to activation of HMGA2 deregulation

Myoepithelioma

A benign tumor composed almost exclusively of neoplastic myoepithelial cells and their derivatives. Less than 5 to 10% ductal component is generally present. Immunoreactivity for pan cytokeratin and myoepithelial markers such as calponin, actin, S-100, GFAP, and CK 14 are positive. Ultrastructure shows hemidesmosomes (epithelial features) and myofilaments with focal densities, and pinocytotic vesicles (myoid features).

Ectomesenchymal chondromyxoid tumor of the anterior tongue is thought to be a peculiar variant of myoepithelioma that arises from undifferentiated ectomesenchyme of the tongue. Immunoreactivity for GFAP and cytokeratin is present, though inconsistently positive for actin and S100 protein.

Cytogenetic studies of myoepitheliomas have demonstrated various structural alterations of chromosomes 1, 9, 12, and 13 which include t(1;12)(q25;q12), del(9)(q22.1q22.3), del(13)(q12q22).

Warthin's Tumor (Adenolymphoma, Papillary Cystadenoma Lymphomatosum)

Etiology

Studies have shown a strong association between cigarette smoking and Warthin's tumor. The exact mechanisms are not clear but it is speculated that irritants in tobacco smoke cause metaplasia in the parotid. Increased incidence of this tumor in atomic bomb survivors has led to hypothesize the role of radiation exposure.

Histogenesis

A tumor characterized by bilayered oncocytic and basaloid epithelium forming cystic structures, separated by a lymphoid stroma is known by variety of names that reflect the diverse views concerning the histogenesis of this tumor.

Branchiogenic theory: This theory was proposed by Ssobolew in 1912. He contends that the tumor arises from the ectodermal portion of the branchial arches. This theory was proposed based on the fact that branchial cysts have similar relationship of epithelial and lymphoid tissue and they may be found in and around parotid gland. However, this theory was not accepted, as many investigators consider that branchial cysts do not arise from epithelial remnants of branchial arches, and there is no similarity in the staining characteristics or nuclear arrangement of the epithelium in branchial cysts and Warthin's tumor.

Eustachian tube theory: Based on the fact that the epithelial lining of tumor is similar to that of lining of Eustachian tube and both have subepithelial lymphoid tissue. Warthin proposed that the tumor arises from an aberrant anlagen of the Eustachian tube.

Orbital inclusion theory: The orbital inclusion gives rise to the orbital salivary glands in certain carnivore (cats, dogs). In human embryo, it appears as a vestigial rudiment. Orbital inclusion was thought to be source of origin for the tumor based on the close relationship of orbital inclusion to the parotid gland during development and the microscopic cystic dilation of the inclusion. However, this theory was not accepted as this structure lies medial to the masseter muscle as the embryo grows (whereas the tumor is commonly present in a posterior and superficial relationship to the body of parotid gland).

Oncocytic theory: This theory was proposed by Jaffe who states that the tumor arises from oncocytes in heterotopic salivary duct tissue in lymph nodes. However, this theory was not accepted for the following reasons. Oncocytes normally are seen in an aging salivary tissue, whereas the tumor arises in a young individuals. Secondly, it does not explain the almost exclusive occurrence of the tumor in parotid glands (oncocytes are present in all the salivary glands, pharynx, tongue, trachea, esophagus and pancreas).

Heterotopic salivary gland theory: This theory was proposed by Albrecht and Arzt. This theory was based on the following observations:

- Salivary gland tissue may be found in lymph nodes in and around the parotid gland.
- Proliferation of this salivary tissue, leading to formation of cysts with the lymph nodes may occur.
- During early stages of cyst formation, part of the lymph node is replaced by the tumor.
- Warthin's tumor exhibits subcapsular and medullary sinusoids.
- Warthin's tumor-like proliferation occurs outside the lymph nodes but they lack the lymphocytic component. This would suggest that the lymphocytic component is not secondary to epithelial proliferation.
- The tumor can arise in any lymph node that contains salivary gland inclusions.

Submandibular and sublingual salivary glands develop as compact mass, parotid gland on the other hand develops in loose arrangement containing aggregates of lymphoid tissue, and encapsulation occurs late in development. Thus, salivary tissue becomes included within lymph nodes which are both within and outside the capsule of parotid gland. Similarly, lymph nodes become entrapped within the parotid gland, due to late capsule formation. This explains the occurrence of the tumor in and around the parotid gland and the occasional multicentricity of the tumor. This theory is the most accepted theory till date.

Delayed hypersensitivity theory: Allegro stated that oxyphilic metaplasia of striated duct and papillomatous proliferation along with secretion leads to cyst formation. This leads to infiltration of the basement membrane by basophils and histiocytes which eventuate in a delayed hypersensitivity reaction and formation of a lymphoid stroma. Presence of Langerhan's cells, and distribution of IgA and IgG in the tumor that is similar to that seen in autoimmune thyroiditis support this hypothesis.

Other recent theories: Warthin's tumor develops as a benign epithelial neoplasm or proliferation that attracts a heavy lymphoid reaction, similar to that seen in certain other salivary neoplasms. More recently, it has been suggested that Warthin's tumor initially develops in a parotid lymph node as an adenomatous epithelial proliferation in reaction to as yet unidentified stimuli (probably including tobacco either as a direct stimulus or a promoter), followed by lymphocytic infiltration.

Molecular Genetics

Immunohistochemistry has shown that the oncocytic cells are immunoreactive for keratin, and ultrastructure shows mitochondria in these granular cells. The epithelial cells are immunoreactive for CEA, lactoferrin, and lysozyme. The lymphoid stroma is predominantly composed of B lymphocytes, but also shows a few T cells , mast cells, and S -100 protein positive dendritic cells.

Analysis of the X chromosome-linked human androgen receptor gene showed that Warthin, tumor is non-clonal, and thus likely to be non-neoplastic. This finding supports that Warthin's tumor resulted from the induction of cystic changes in branchial cleft epithelium by an inflammatory infiltrate, accompanied by oncocytic change in the epithelium. Mitochondrial DNA damage may account for the ultrastructural changes seen in the mitochondria, as well as the oncocytic change seen morphologically.

Oncocytic Lesions (Oncocytosis, Oncocytoma and Oncocytic Carcinoma)

Oncocytes are large cells with plentiful granular, markedly eosinophilic cytoplasm originally thought to be metaplastic products and not specifically of any stem cell derivation. Oncocytic cells are considered as somatic mutants, rather than as a new or specific cell lineage. They represent acini or intralobular ducts of normal or abnormal salivary tissue which have undergone cytoplasmic changes induced by unknown cause. Oncocytic transformation of the epithelial cells is not a degenerative process, but rather is considered as a re-differentiation of the epithelial cells which develop an increased but unbalanced metabolism.

Electron microscopy of oncocytes show the cytoplasm of oncocytes to be distended by mitochondria with atypical outlines and large numbers of cristae. PTAH (phosphotungstic acid hematoxylin) stains the mitochondria as deep blue cytoplasmic granules. These oncocytes are positive for anti-mitochondrial antibody. Unlike normal mitochondria, the mitochondria of oncocytic cells produce very minimal quantities of ATP. The cell compensates for this functional defect by increased number of mitochondria and increased surface area of the mitochondrial membrane. Hence, oncocytic transformation must be considered as an acquired disturbance of the mitochondrial enzyme organization, i.e. a form of mitochondriopathy. This functional defect is transferred to the offspring, as the oncocytes have the ability to divide.

Basal Cell Adenoma

A tumor composed of basaloid cells separated from the stroma by basement membrane, exhibits a monotonous solid, trabecular, tubular or membranous growth pattern. These tumors arise from neoplastic transformation of the reserve cells in the intercalated duct with histodifferentiation toward ductal and myoepithelial differentiation. Basal cell adenomas show differentiation of both epithelial and myoepithelial elements. Epithelial markers (CK, CEA, EMA) as well as myoepithelial markers (calponin, actin, GFAP, S-100, vimentin) can be variably demonstrated in the luminal and basal/myoepithelial cells respectively.

Canalicular Adenoma

Canalicular adenomas are characterized by bilayered strands of cells which abut and separate haphazardly, generally arranged in single file, canaliculi and pseudopapillary pattern. These tumors arise from neoplastic transformation of the reserve cells in the intercalated duct with histodifferentiation toward ductal cells with none to very minimal myoepithelial differentiation.

Immunohistochemistry and electron microscopy reveal luminal cell differentiation of the cells without myoepithelial participation. Immunoreactivity for cytokeratin, vimentin, infrequently for CEA and S-100 protein is present, while actin and GFAP are negative, thereby supporting the epithelial origin of the tumor cells.

Ductal Papillomas

Three distinct types of papillary tumors have been recognized, namely, sialadenoma papilliferum, inverted ductal papilloma, and intraductal papilloma based on their unique histopathologic features. Various theories have been put forward to explain the histogenesis of sialadenoma papilliferum. The possible cell of origin has been variously reported as the excretory duct reserve cell, intercalated duct cells or striated duct cells. Based on the location of the tumor, it seems probable that the salivary gland excretory duct cell is the possible cell of origin.

As most of the squamous papillomas of the oral mucosa are being associated with papilloma virus infection in the recent past, there is speculation if sialadenoma papilliferum may also be of viral origin. But till date, no strong evidence points in this direction.

Sebaceous Adenoma and Sebaceous Lymphadenoma

Sebaceous cells can occur normally in the oral mucosa, parotid gland and submandibular gland. Tumors are rare arising from these sebaceous differentiated cells. Other salivary gland tumors like pleomorphic adenoma, Warthin's tumor and mucoepidermoid carcinoma can show focal sebaceous differentiation. Fat stains are helpful in identifying sebaceous cells. No definite immuno-histochemical marker has been documented.

It has been postulated that sebaceous lymph-adenoma originates from ectopic salivary gland in parotid lymph node, but the tumor cells differentiate towards sebaceous cells instead of oncocytic epithelial cells. Some authors postulate that lymphoid stroma in sebaceous lymphadenoma is a tumor associated host reaction. In fact, this explanation has been given even for the lymphoid stroma in Warthin's tumor.

HISTOGENESIS OF MALIGNANT SALIVARY GLAND TUMORS

Acinic Cell Carcinoma

Acinic cell adenocarcinoma is a malignant epithelial neoplasm in which at least some of the tumor cells demonstrate serous acinar differentiation. The tumor is composed of cells arranged in varying patterns which include solid, microcystic, papillary-cystic, and follicular. These may contain acinar, intercalated ductal, vacuolated, clear, and nonspecific glandular cells. The acinar cells are polygonal and have abundant, pale, basophilic cytoplasm with purplish cytoplasmic granules, and eccentrically placed, basophilic to vesicular nuclei. The zymogen-type secretory granules are PAS positive, diastase resistant and mucicarmine positive.

Histogenesis

Most investigators consider that these tumors arise from neoplastic transformation of the reserve cells in the intercalated duct cells with histodifferentiation toward serous acinar cells. But proponents of multicellular theory have shown that normal serous acinar cells undergo mitotic division, and some acinic cell carcinomas could arise from transformation of these cells.

The varying patterns of differentiation seen in acinic cell carcinomas are attributed to the attempt of the terminal tubule or intercalated duct reserve cells to simulate the neoplastic equivalent of the normal phenotypic expression of lobules of acini. The complete expression of this differentiation of these neoplastic cells results in the classically defined acinic cell carcinomas (lobules of acini). Those acinic cell carcinomas with imperfect differentiation retain areas of tubular or solid epithelial masses.

Immunohistochemistry reveals differentiation towards acinar cells and ductal cells exhibiting positivity for low molecular weight cytokeratin, CEA and amylase.

Molecular Genetics

Molecular analysis of acinic cell carcinomas has shown that 84% of the tumors had LOH in at least one of the 20 loci on chromosomes 1,4,5,6 and 17. The most frequently altered regions were noted at chromosomes 4p, 5q, 6p and 17p regions, suggesting the presence of tumor suppressor genes associated with the oncogenesis of these tumors.

Mucoepidermoid Carcinoma

Tumor characterized by squamous cells occurring in association with mucin secreting elements and intermediate cells in variable combinations, forming cysts and solid islands. There is no definite myoepithelial component in the tumor. The tumor is composed of haphazardly dispersed mucin filled cysts and irregular tumor nests of mucus, epidermoid, intermediate, columnar and clear cells in variable combinations.

Histogenesis

Mucoepidermoid carcinomas (MECs) are thought to arise from the excretory duct cells. Excretory ducts are structures devoid of myoepithelial cells, hence MECs are derived from a single parent cell probably the basal cells of the excretory duct that undergoes luminal and myoepithelial differentiation. This hypothesis is strengthened by immunohistochemical observations. MECs stain for cytokeratin and may show a focal positivity to vimentin. They are also negative for glial fibrillary acidic protein and usually negative for S-100 protein and muscle-specific actin. These findings suggest that MECs are epithelial in origin, with at most limited myoepithelial differentiation.

It is hypothesized that the neoplastic basal cells of the excretory duct could be the parent cell that differentiates into mucous, intermediate, goblet, columnar, and clear cells. The intermediate cell, in turn, could differentiate into epidermoid and clear cells.

Molecular Genetics

Molecular studies of MECs have also reported infrequent genetic loss at chromosomes 9p21, 8q, 5p, 16q and 12p. Several MECs have been reported to possess t (11:19) (q21;p13) translocation. A specific chromosomal translocation has been recognized in MEC. t (11;19)(q21;p13), which fuses *MECT1* (mucoepidermoid carcinoma translocated-1) at 19p13 with *MAML2* (mastermindlike gene family) at 11q21, is found in up to 70% of cases. The fusion protein is expressed in all different cell types that constitute MEC. This genetic alteration disrupts the Notch signaling pathway. *MECT1–MAML2* fusion-positive patients have significantly less local recurrences, metastases and tumor-related deaths compared with fusion-negative patients. Median survival for fusion-positive patients exceeds 10 years, whereas that for fusion-negative patients is only 1.6 years. These findings suggest that *MECT1–MAML2* fusion may be a useful prognostic marker for MEC.

Adenoid Cystic Carcinoma

Adenoid cystic carcinoma (AdCC) is an invasive neoplasm composed of basaloid cells with a predominant myoepithelial/basal cell differentiation arranged in anastomosing cords, in masses and around cavities giving the tumor a cribriform appearance. Interspersed ductal structures associated with myxohyaline stroma are seen.

Histogenesis

Adenoid cystic carcinomas are thought to arise from the neoplastic transformation of reserve cells of the terminal duct system. These neoplastic cells differentiate along the lines of ductal or myoepithelial cells. This is supported by the presence of epithelial-type mucin in the true ducts and basement membrane-like material in the pseudocysts. In addition, immunohistochemistry shows that the cells lining the true ducts are positive for cytokeratins, carcinoembryonic antigen and epithelial membrane antigen, and may be positive for S-100 protein. The cells lining the pseudocysts, and the component tumor cells of the cribriform and solid patterns, are positive for muscle-specific actin, calponin and smooth muscle myosin heavy chains, and may or may not stain for S-100 and cytokeratins. Hence, the myoepithelial cells play a key role in the architectural pattern of the tumor.

Molecular Genetics

Molecular studies of AdCCs have reported alterations at chromosomes 6q, 9p and 17p12-13 regions. The t(6;9) (q21-24;p13-23) has been reported in several tumors and is considered to be a primary event in at least a subset of these tumors. A recent study has reported LOH in chromosome 6q23-25 in 76% of cases of AdCC and this alteration correlated with histologic grade and clinical behavior.

The gene expression profile of AdCC has reported the most overexpressed genes encode for basement membrane and extracellular matrix proteins of myoepithelial differentiation (e.g. laminin-b1, versican, biglycan and type IV collagen-a1). While the most underexpressed genes are those encoding for proteins of acinar-type differentiation (e.g. amylase, carbonic anhydrase and salivary proline-rich proteins).

Allelic loss of chromosomal arm 19q has been reported in adenoid cystic carcinoma. In addition, mutations in 14-3-36, CTNNB1 (b-catenin gene), AXIN1 (axis inhibition protein 1) and APC (adenomatosis polyposis coli tumor suppressor) genes have been found. Increased expression of PCNA with higher expression in submandibular derived malignancies has been noted. It has been postulated that cumulative mutations in the p53 and retinoblastoma genes are associated with transformation from cribriform and tubular areas to solid areas.

Overexpression of cyclin D1, p53 mutations, HER-2/neu, overexpression or loss of pRb expression is considered to be associated with transformation to dedifferentiated adenoid cystic carcinoma. Decreased expression of E cadherin is also seen in high grade tumors. Brain derived neurotropic factor (BDNF), a growth factor involved in neurogenesis has been found to be uniformly expressed by adenoid cystic carcinomas and is presumed to play a causative role in the predilection of these tumors for perineural invasion. Expression of c-kit, a transmembrane receptor tyrosine kinase, has recently been reported to be expressed in adenoid cystic carcinoma but not in polymorphous low grade adenocarcinoma.

Polymorphous Low Grade Adenocarcinoma (Terminal Duct Carcinoma, Lobular Carcinoma, Low Grade Papillary Adenocarcinoma)

Tumor characterized by diverse architectural patterns but unified by bland looking tumor cells. The tumor is composed of tumor cells arranged in solid sheets, trabeculae, ductular, tubular, glandular, papillary or papillary-cystic, and cribriform patterns. Myoepithelial cells are a minor component.

Histogenesis

Polymorphous low grade adenocarcinomas (PLGA) are thought to arise from the neoplastic transformation of reserve cells of the terminal duct system. These neoplastic cells differentiate mainly along the lines of ductal cells with a limited potential to differentiate along lines of myoepithelial cells. This is supported by immunohistochemical findings. Almost 90% of both luminal and nonluminal cells stain for EMA, cytokeratin and S-100 and are negative for calponin and smooth muscle myosin heavy chains. Hence in PLGA, myoepithelial differentiation is very minimal.

Molecular Genetics

Molecular studies have reported alterations at 8q12, 12q rearrangements, clonal t(6;9) (p21;p22) and a monosomy 22. Cytogenetic alterations in PLGA have frequently displayed chromosome 12 abnormalities affecting the q arm and the p arm.

Basal Cell Adenocarcinoma

Basal cell adenocarcinoma is an epithelial neoplasm that is cytologically and immuno-histochemically similar to basal cell adenoma but is infiltrative and has a potential for metastasis. Basal cell adenocarcinomas also show the same solid, membranous, trabecular and tubular patterns seen in their benign counterpart. Immunohistochemically there is reactivity for smooth muscle actin and vimentin. Tumors are positive for cytokeratin and often focally reactive for S-100 protein, EMA and CEA.

Molecular Genetics

Molecular studies have reported chromosomal gains at 9p21.1-pter, 18q21.1-q22.3, and 22q11.23-q13.31 as well as losses at 2q24.2 and 4q25-q27. A study of two familial cases and two sporadic basaloid tumors for alterations at the 16q12-13 regions showed high frequency (80%) of LOH in both sporadic and familial basaloid tumors and dermal cylindromas of the familial cases. The minimally deleted region contained the CYLD gene. This study indicates that these tumors share the same alterations as dermal cylindromas and implicates the CYLD gene in their development.

Salivary Duct Carcinoma

Salivary duct carcinoma is a rare highly aggressive malignant neoplasm composed of structures that resemble expanded salivary gland ducts and is considered as counterpart of invasive ductal carcinoma of the mammary gland. Immuno-histochemistry and electron microscopy confirm the luminal epithelial nature of the tumor cells. In confirmation the cells show immunoreactivity for cytokeratin, EMA, and CEA, but not myoepithelial markers.

Molecular Genetics

A high incidence of LOH has been reported at 6q, 16q, 17p and 17q regions. Mutations and overexpression of the TP53 gene and protein are frequent. Most cases express GCDFP-15 (BRST-2) and c-erbB-2. Rarely there may be positivity for progesterone receptor, androgen receptor or prostate specific antigen. A high expression of peroxisome proliferator-activated receptor gamma (PPAR) has been reported in a recent study. Seventy nine percent of the tumors are non-diploid and the mean S phase fraction is 11%.

The chromosomal locus 9q21 contains the CDKN2A/p16 tumor suppressor gene that has been implicated in a variety of tumor types, including SDC. More polymorphic genetic markers located at this particular region suggest that inactivation of CDKN2A/p16 gene is associated with progression of the tumor.

Myoepithelial Carcinoma

Myoepithelial carcinoma is a rare, malignant salivary gland neoplasm in which the tumor cells almost exclusively manifest myoepithelial differentiation. Cytologic abnormalities and infiltrative growth distinguish them from myoepithelioma. The cellular morphology is similar to that of benign myoepithelioma and includes the spindle cell, plasmacytoid, clear and epithelioid types. The tumor cells show immunoreactivity for cytokeratin, CK14, actin, calponin, S-100 protein, GFAP, EMA, and are negative for CEA and HMB-45.

Histogenesis

Myoepithelial carcinomas may arise *de novo*, but about half of cases develop in pre-existing pleomorphic adenomas, or from benign myoepitheliomas, particularly in recurrences. They can also arise as a result of progression of epithelial myoepithelial carcinoma to high grade myoepithelial carcinoma, characterized by overgrowth of the myoepithelial component with nuclear anaplasia. This phenomenon has also been reported as 'epithelialmyoepithelial carcinoma with myoepithelial anaplasia'.

Carcinoma Ex-Pleomorphic Adenoma

Carcinoma ex-pleomorphic adenoma is malignant transformation of a pre-existing pleomorphic adenoma. The malignant component is either a poorly differentiated adenocarcinoma, poly-morphous low grade adenocarcinoma, squamous cells carcinoma, mucoepidermoid carcinoma or any other type of salivary gland carcinoma, including malignant myoepithelioma.

Histogenesis

Sequential evolution can sometimes be traced in the development of carcinoma ex-pleomorphic adenoma, and these different phases have prognostic significance.

1. In the earliest phase, carcinoma cells with large atypical nuclei replace the neoplastic ductal luminal cells while retaining an intact layer of non-atypical myoepithelial cells of the pre-existing pleomorphic adenoma. This can be considered a form of 'carcinoma *in situ*', and there is no metastatic potential.
2. With time, the carcinoma cells may break out from the confines of the neoplastic myoepithelial sheath and invade into the surrounding stroma. If this process is still confined within the parent pleomorphic adenoma, the carcinoma is considered 'intracapsular'. The prognosis is excellent with complete excision. There has been no metastasis, except for a single case report with cervical lymph node metastasis.
3. If the invasion extends beyond the fibrous capsule of the parent pleomorphic adenoma, the carcinoma ex-pleomorphic adenoma is considered 'invasive'. However, it should be further categorized as being 'minimally invasive' or 'frankly invasive', although the optimal cut-off point to define minimally invasive carcinoma (tumor with minimal metastatic potential) is currently unsettled. In the current WHO classification, tumors with invasion of < 1.5 mm from the tumor capsule are considered minimally invasive.

Cell Types that Undergo Malignant Change in Pleomorphic Adenoma

In most cases, luminal epithelial cells undergo malignant change. In the other cases, the supervening carcinoma shows dual epithelial-myoepithelial differentiation or pure myoepithelial differentiation.

Molecular Genetics

Deletions of chromosome 5(q22-23, q32-33) and t(10;12) (p15;q14-15) with 12q breakpoint at the 5' of the HMGA2 and translocation of the entire gene to the 10 marker chromosome followed by deletion/amplification of the segment containing HMGA2 and MDM2 genes have been reported. Alterations at 12q13-15 with amplification and overexpression of CDK4, HMGA2 and MDM2 genes have also been reported. These genes may contribute to the malignant transformation of pleomorphic adenoma.

Alterations or rearrangements of chromosome 8q21 and 12q13-15 are frequent in carcinoma ex pleomorphic adenoma, similar to its benign counterpart. However, the carcinoma shows additional alterations in 17p.

Sialoblastoma

A tumor of newborns and infants also known as embryoma, congenital carcinoma or congenital basal cell adenoma is of low malignant potential. The tumor is composed of many islands and sheets of primitive basaloid cells separated by a fibrous or fibromyxomatous stroma. Most of the tumor cells are primitive looking and have large ovoid vesicular nuclei and moderate cytoplasm with indistinct cell borders. Immunohistochemical staining for cytokeratin has shown accentuation of the ductal structures with positivity for vimentin, actin and S-100 protein in the outermost layer of the ducts.

Histogenesis

This tumor arises from primitive cells recapitulating the embryonic salivary tissue, and occasional ductal formation confirms the epithelial nature of the tumor. The retained blastema cells rather than basal reserve cells give rise to the tumor. Dysembryogenic parotid changes have been described adjacent to the tumor, with proliferation of the terminal ductal epithelial bulbs.

*Clear Cell Carcinoma and
Hyalinizing Clear Cell Carcinoma*

Both these tumors are characterized by epithelial cells with clear cytoplasm and show their definite epithelial origin by positivity for cytokeratin. Both the tumors do not show any reactivity with myoepithelial markers such as actin, myosin or calponin. Ultrastructural studies show features of only duct differentiation and no myoepithelial differentiation.

TUMOR PROGRESSION IN SALIVARY GLAND TUMORS

Tumor progression is a multistep process, which often involves sequential accumulation of genetic changes. Salivary gland tumors can progress in one of the following ways:
1. Malignant transformation of benign salivary gland tumors. (e.g. Pleomorphic adenoma to carcinoma ex-pleomorphic adenoma; Basal cell adenoma to basal cell adenocarcinoma; Myoepithelioma to myoepithelial carcinoma, oncocytoma to oncocytic carcinoma)
2. Progression from low grade to high grade carcinoma. (e.g. Adenoid cystic carcinoma, mucoepidermoid carcinoma, epithelial-myo-epithelial carcinoma). Epithelial-myoepithelial carcinoma progress to myoepithelial carcinoma.
3. Dedifferentiation of a carcinoma to high grade carcinoma with loss of original line of differentiation.
4. Stromal invasion.

Dedifferentiation in Salivary Gland Tumors

Dedifferentiation refers to the transformation of a salivary gland carcinoma to a high grade carcinoma in which the original line of differentiation is no longer evident. Acinic cell carcinoma was the first salivary gland carcinoma to be reported to undergo dedifferentiation. The dedifferentiated component could be a form of high grade adenocarcinoma, poorly differentiated carcinoma or undifferentiated carcinoma. The other tumors that are reported to undergo dedifferentiation are mucoepidermoid carcinoma, adenoid cystic carcinoma, polymorphous low grade adenocarcinoma, myoepithelial carcinoma, epithelial-myoepithelial carcinoma, salivary duct carcinoma and hyalinizing clear cell carcinoma.

Some of the genetic changes that could mediate dedifferentiation are *p53* mutation, increased cyclin D1 expression, loss of expression of Rb protein, and c-erbB2 protein overexpression or gene amplification.

CONCLUSION

Histogenesis of many of the tumors both benign and malignant is still rather uncertain. Electron microscopy has an extremely limited role in the routine diagnosis of salivary gland tumors, except those of myoepithelial origin. Immunohisto-chemistry can clearly delineate the tumors as to their luminal, or abluminal differentiation and also indicate to a certain extent the cell of origin (Table 6.3). Immunohistochemistry however, requires expert interpretation and the pitfalls at the hands of a novice can prove to be more of a problem than help.

Molecular studies are still in their infancy as far as their application to salivary gland neoplasms is concerned. Though there is still a long way to go, the day is not too far when molecular genetics could pinpoint the cell of origin and help in distinguishing benign from malignant tumors and also aid in the prognosis and therapy of these neoplasms.

Table 6.3: Cell types and their immunoreactivity

Ductal cells	Oncocytic cells	Squamous nests	Basaloid cells	Spindle cells	Clear cells
Pleomorphic adenoma Warthin's tumor Adenosquamous myoepithelial Epithelial myoepithelial carcinoma Adenoid cystic carcinoma Salivary duct carcinoma Polymorphous low grade adenocarcinoma Clear cell carcinoma Hyalinizing clear cell carcinoma	Warthin's tumor Oncocytic tumor Oncocytic carcinoma Oncocytic cystadenoma	Squamous cell carcinoma Adenosquamous carcinoma Pleomorphic adenoma High grade mucoepidermoid carcinoma Warthin's tumor Pilomatrixoma	Basal cell adenoma Basal cell adenocarcinoma Adenoid cystic carcinoma Basaloid squamous carcinoma	Myoepithelioma Malignant myoepithelioma Salivary anlage tumor Pleomorphic adenoma Various benign and malignant mesenchymal tumors	Hyalinizing clear cell carcinoma Epithelial carcinoma Clear cell carcinoma Oncocytoma Sebaceous adenoma Metastatic clear cell carcinoma

Immunoreactivity

Ductal cells	Oncocytic cells	Squamous nests	Basaloid cells	Spindle cells	Clear cells
CK + EMA + CEA + S-100 +	PTAH + Mitochondrial antibody +	CK + CEA + EMA +	CK + CEA + EMA + Actin + Calponin + GFAP + S-100 + Vimentin +	Calponin + S-100 + GFAP + Actin + CK 14 +	CK + EMA + S-100 + Actin + Calponin+

BIBLIOGRAPHY

1. Auclair PL, Ellis GL, Gnepp DR, Wenig BM, Janney CG. Salivary gland neoplasms: General considerations. In: Ellis GL, Auclair PL, Gnepp DR, (Eds). Surgical pathology of the salivary glands. 1st edn. Philadelphia: WB Saunders Company; 1991. pp. 135-64.
2. Barnes L, Brandwein M, Som PM. Surgical Pathology of the Head and Neck. 2nd edn. Marcel Dekker Inc: New York, 2001.
3. Barnes L, Eveson JW, Reichart P, Sidransky D. World Health Organization Classification of Tumours. Pathology and Genetics of Head and Neck Tumours. Salivary glands. Lyon, IARC Press, 2005;5.
4. Batsakis JG, Luna MA, el-Naggar AK. Basaloid monomorphic adenomas. Ann Otol Rhinol Laryngol 1991;100:687-90.
5. Batsakis JG, Regezi JA, Luna MA, El-Naggar AK. Histogenesis of salivary gland neoplasms: A postulate with prognostic implications. J Laryngol Otol 1989;103:939-44.
6. Batsakis JG. Salivary gland neoplasia: An outcome of modified morphogenesis and cytodifferentiation. Oral Surg Oral Med Oral Pathol 1980;49:229-32.
7. Batsakis JG. Tumors of the Head and Neck: Clinical and Pathological Considerations, 2nd edn. Baltimore, MD: Williams and Wilkins, 1979.
8. Chan JK, Yip TT, Tsang WY, Poon YF, Wong CS, Ma VW. Specific association of Epstein-Barr virus with lymphoepithelial carcinoma among tumours and tumor like lesions of the salivary gland. Arch Pathol Lab Med 1994;118:994-7.
9. Chapnik J. The controversy of Warthin's tumor. Laryngoscope 1983;93:695-716.
10. Cheuk W, Chan JK, Ngan RK. Dedifferentiation in adenoid cystic carcinoma of salivary gland: An uncommon complication associated with an accelerated clinical course. Am J Surg Pathol 1999;23(4):465-72.
11. Cheuk W, Chan JKC. Advances in salivary gland pathology. Histopathol 2007;51:1-20.
12. Daa T, Kashima K, Kaku N, Suzuki M, Yokoyama S. Mutations in components of the Wnt signaling pathway in adenoid cystic carcinoma. Mod Pathol 2004;17(12):1475-82.
13. Dardick I, Burford-Mason AP. Current status of histogenetic and morphogenetic concepts of salivary gland tumorigenesis. Crit Rev Oral Biol Med 1993;4:639-77.
14. Dardick I, Byard RM, Carnegie JA. A review of the proliferative capacity of major salivary glands and the relationship to current concepts of neoplasia in salivary glands. Oral Surg Oral Med Oral Pathol 1990;69:53-67.
15. Dardick I, Dardick AM, Mackay AJ, Pastolero GC, Gullane PJ, Burford-Mason AP. Pathology of salivary glands, IV: Histogenetic concepts and cycling cells in human parotid and submandibular glands cultured in floating collagen gels. Oral Surg Oral Med Oral Pathol 1993;76:307-18.
16. Dardick I, Thomas MJ, van Nostrand AW. Myoepithelioma-new concepts of histology and classification: A light and electron microscopic study. Ultrastruct Pathol 1989;13:187-224.
17. Dardick I. Mounting evidence against current histogenetic concepts for salivary gland tumorigenesis. Eur J Morphol 1998;36:257-61.
18. DiGiuseppe JA, Corio RL, Westra WH. Lymphoid infiltrates of the salivary glands: Pathology, biology, and clinical significance. Curr Opin Oncol 1996;8:232-7.
19. Ellis GL, Auclair PL, Gnepp DR. Surgical pathology of the salivary glands. 1st edn. WB Saunders: Philadelphia, Saunders, 1991.
20. El-Naggar Ak, Callender D, Coombes MM, Hurr K, Luna MA, Batsakis JG. Molecular genetic alterations in carcinoma ex-pleomorphic adenoma: A putative progression model? Genes Chromosomes Cancer 2000;27:162-8.
21. Fonseca I, Felix A, Soares J. Dedifferentiation in salivary gland carcinomas. Am J Surg Pathol 2000;24:469-71.
22. Klijanienho J, Vielh P. Salivary gland tumours: Monographs in clinical cytology. Karger: Basel, 2000;15.
23. Kotwell C. Smoking as an etiologic factor in the development of Warthin's tumour of the parotid gland. Am J Surg 1992;164:646-7.
24. Mariette X, Loiseau P, Morinet F. Hepatitis C virus in saliva. Ann Intern Med 1995;122:556.
25. Meer S, Altini M. CK7+/CK20− immunoexpression profile is typical of salivary gland neoplasia. Histopathology 2007;51:26-32.

26. O'Connell AC. Natural history and prevention of radiation injury. Adv Dent Res 2000;14:57-61.

27. Ogata T, Hongfang Y, Kayano T, Hirai K. No significant role of Epstein-Barr virus in the tumorigenesis of Warthin's tumour. J Med Dent Sci 1997;44:45-52.

28. Pinkston JA, Cole P. Cigarette smoking and Warthin's tumor. Am J Epidemiol 1996;144: 183-7.

29. Rajendran R, Sivapathasundharam B. Diseases of salivary gland. In: Shafer's textbook of oral pathology, 5th edn. Elsevier, 2005.

30. Saku T, Hayashi Y, Takahara O, et al. Salivary gland tumours among atomic bomb survivors, 1950-1987. Cancer 1997;79:1465-75.

31. Santucci M, Gallo O, Calzolari A, Bondi R. Detection of Epstein-Barr viral genome in tumour cells of Warthin's tumour of parotid gland. Am J Clin Pathol 1993;100:662-5.

32. Savera AT, Gown AM, Zarbo RJ. Immunolocalization of three novel smooth muscle-specific proteins in salivary gland pleomorphic adenoma: Assessment of morphogenetic role of myoepithelium. Mod Pathol 1997;10:1093-1100.

33. Thompson AS, Bryant HC. Histogenesis of papillary cystadenoma lymphomatosum (Warthin's tumor) of the parotid salivary gland. Am J Pathol 1950;26:807-49.

34. Yu GY, Ussmuller J, Donath K. Histogenesis and development of membranous basal cell adenoma. Oral Surg Oral Med Oral Pathol Oral Radiol Endod 1998;86:446-51.

7

Benign Tumors of Salivary Glands

Einstein T Bertin A, B Sivapathasundharam

Salivary gland tumors are quite uncommon, but they elicit considerable medical interest because of their multifaceted clinical presentation, varied histologic appearance, and difficulties encountered in predicting their prognosis. They may arise from the major, or the minor salivary glands present in the oral mucosa and pharynx, the seromucous glands of the nasal passages, sinuses, larynx, the ectopic salivary gland tissue.

Nearly 90% of the salivary gland neoplasms are epithelial in origin and can be either benign or malignant in nature. This chapter discusses in detail the benign epithelial tumors of salivary glands. Even though the non-epithelial or mesenchymal tumours account for only 10% of salivary gland neoplasms, they are highly significant. The mesenchymal tumors are, in fact, the most common tumors in children. Considering this, we also discuss the mesenchymal neoplasms of salivary glands origin.

Benign epithelial tumors of salivary glands account for 60 to 65% of all epithelial salivary gland tumors. A vast majority of these tumors occur in the parotid glands. Nearly one fourth of the benign epithelial tumors involve the minor salivary glands.

Among the benign epithelial salivary gland tumors arising from parotid glands, pleomorphic adenomas predominate, accounting for 50 to 75%, followed by Warthin's tumor (5–15%). Pleomorphic adenomas again predominate in the submandibular salivary glands. Interestingly, Warthin's tumor is rare in this location.

In the minor salivary glands, pleomorphic adenomas account for nearly 40% of the cases. Palate is the most common location of minor salivary gland tumors, followed by the lips and buccal mucosa. Labial tumors are predominant in the upper lips, accounting for up to 90% of the tumors.

PLEOMORPHIC ADENOMA (MIXED TUMOR)

'Pleomorphic adenoma' or 'mixed tumor' is a benign neoplasm of salivary gland origin composed of epithelial (luminal) and myoepithelial (abluminal) cells with variable amounts of characteristic stroma. It is the most common neoplasm of both the major and minor salivary glands.

The term 'mixed tumor', more commonly used by pathologists in the United States, has emerged from the belief that this tumor possibly arises from cells of more than one germ layer. The co-existence of apparently epithelial and mesenchymal elements has given credence to this assumption. The same belief has given rise to various names such as branchioma, enclavoma, teratoma, myxochondrocarcinoma, cylindroma, myxochondrosarcoma, and chondromyxohemangioendotheliosarcoma.

Immunohistochemical studies and molecular analyzes have, however, proved convincingly that this neoplasm is a pure epithelial tumor with divergent differentiation rather than a collision of independent epithelial and mesenchymal elements. The term 'mixed tumor' does not refer to the fact it is an 'admixture' of both ductal and myoepithelial cells, because many other salivary gland tumors also show myoepithelial differentiation.

The term 'pleomorphic adenoma', more common among pathologists in Europe, Canada, and Asia and also used in the WHO classification system, is a reference to the varied microscopic appearance arising due to the confluence of cellular and stromal elements. This term also is inappropriate as there is no true pleomorphism of the tumor cells.

Clinical Presentation

Pleomorphic adenoma is the most common neoplasm of parotid, submandibular, and minor salivary glands. The most common minor salivary gland sites are the hard and soft palates, cheek, tongue, and floor of the mouth. They are exceedingly rare in the sublingual salivary gland, as this is seldom a site for salivary gland neoplasia. Rare cases have been reported possibly arising from ectopic salivary gland tissue present in lymph nodes, the mandible, or the maxilla.

This benign tumor commonly presents during the third through fifth decades of life. It is also the most common salivary gland tumor in children and adolescents. A slightly increased incidence in the female population and Caucasians has been documented.

Pleomorphic adenomas are asymptomatic, slow-growing, and discrete masses that grow to large sizes if left untreated. They are usually firm on palpation, except for predominantly myxoid lesions that are soft to palpation.

Tumors of parotid glands present as well-delineated, ovoid or irregular, movable masses over the angle of the mandible, below and in front of the ear arising from the lower pole of the superficial (lateral) lobe of parotid glands (Figs 7.1A to C). With continued growth, these tumors become more nodular and less movable. Recurrent lesions of parotid gland are less mobile than the original tumors and often present as multiple discrete nodules.

About 10% of parotid tumors appear in the deep lobe of the gland, extending between the ascending ramus of the mandible and the stylomandibular ligament in a dumb-bell shape into the parapharyngeal space. These deep-lobe tumors are often misdiagnosed owing to the oropharyngeal swelling caused by them, leading to peroral biopsy. There is seldom involvement of the facial nerve in spite of the grotesque sizes to which the parotid tumors grow. In rare cases, facial paralysis occurs due to extrinsic compression of facial nerve.

Tumors of the submandibular glands present as firm, discrete masses within the gland. Pleomorphic adenomas arising from the minor salivary

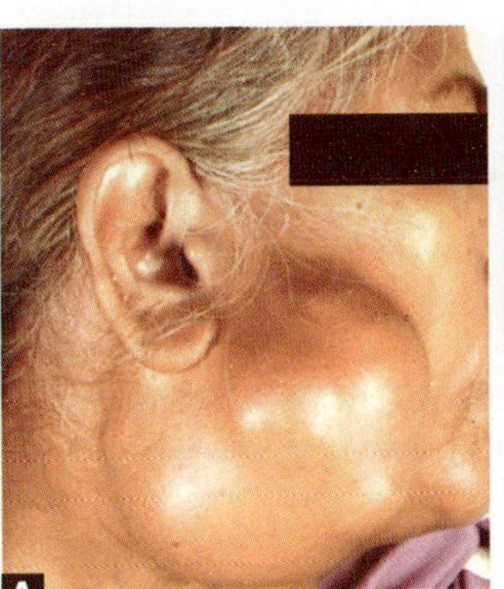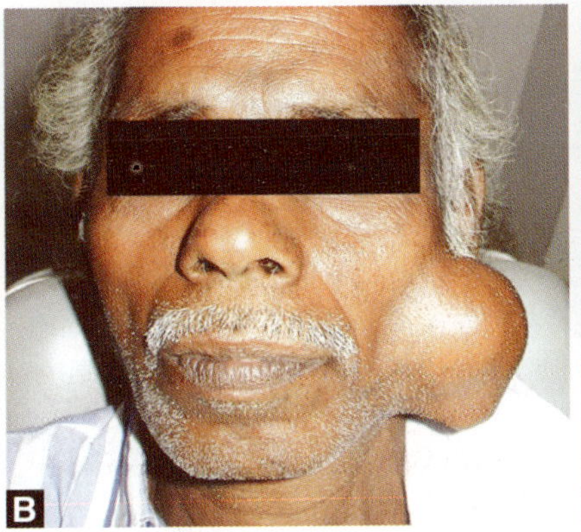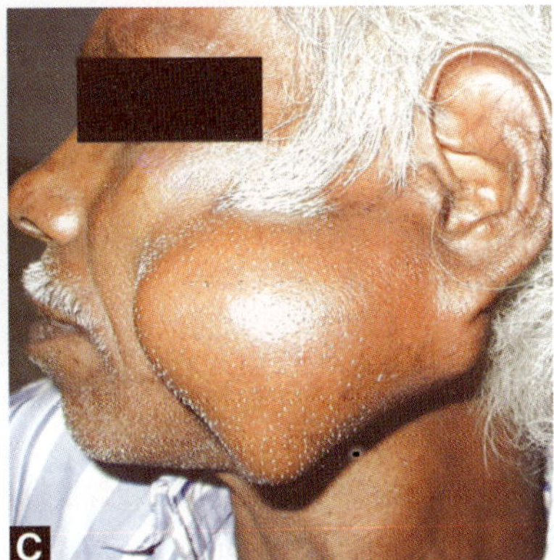

Figures 7.1A to C: Pleomorphic adenoma of parotid gland presenting as irregular masses over the angle of the mandible

glands present as firm submucosal masses. The overlying mucosa is not ulcerated, unless it has been traumatized. Palatal tumors are characteristically located lateral to the midline, with very limited mobility (Figs 7.2A to D). However, minor salivary gland tumors of other sites such as labial or buccal mucosa are mobile. Intraoral tumors are usually less than 3.0 cm in diameter when excised.

Macroscopic Features

Gross examination of the lesional tissue reveals a well-circumscribed, thinly encapsulated, solitary mass with a smooth or bosselated surface. Recurrent tumors are multicentric, with multiple nodules scattered over the field of previous operation. This multifocal recurrence is due to a surgical "shelling-out" procedure that leaves tiny pseudopod-like transcapsular processes of the tumor in the salivary gland or may result from rupture of a mucoid mixed tumor during removal, leading to seeding of the tumor bed. These recurrent nodules are usually myxoid in nature.

> Intraoral tumors such as in the palate lack a definite capsule. In such instances, the tumor buds are directly in contact with the adjacent salivary gland tissue.

Cut surface of the tumor is rubbery, fleshy, mucoid, or glistening depending on the content

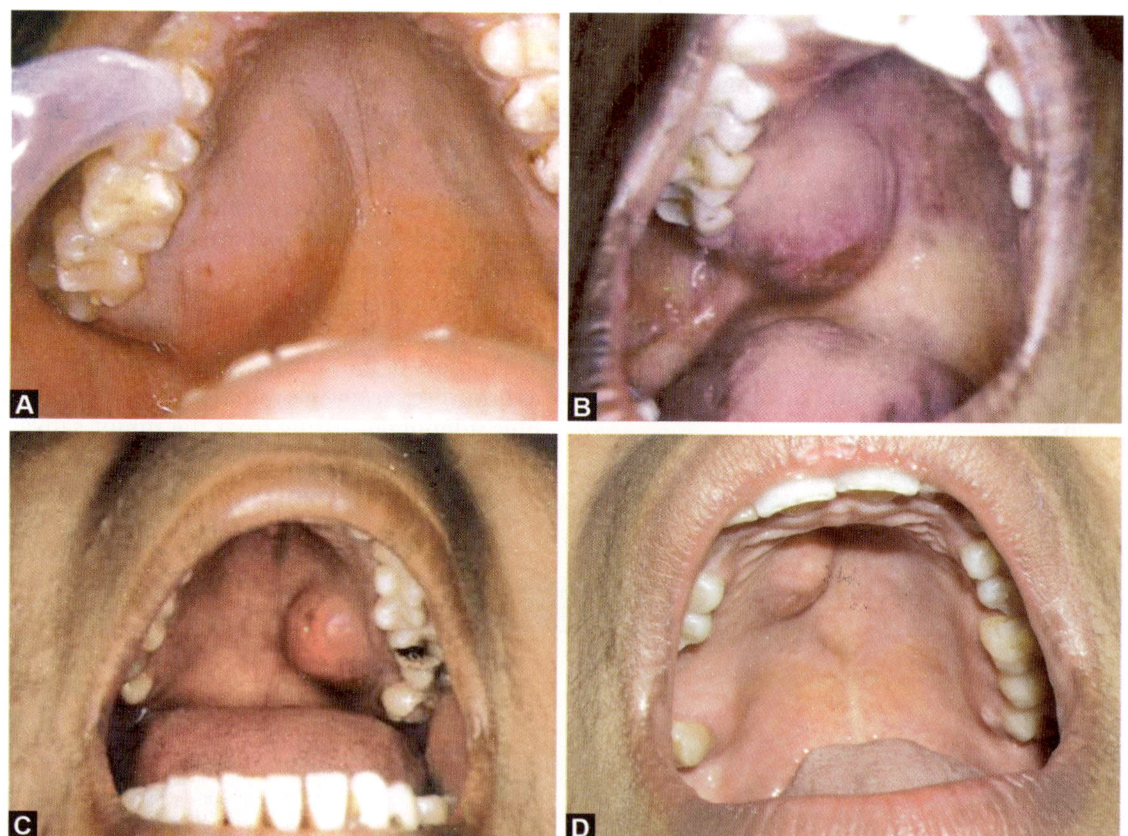

Figures 7.2A to D: Pleomorphic adenoma of minor salivary glands of the palate presenting as smooth, long standing, submucosal masses (*Courtesy:* Dr S Karthiga Kannan, Sree Mookambika Institute of Dental Sciences, Kanyakumari District)

and amount of stroma in the tumor. Cartilaginous tissue appears as firmer, translucent, and bluish areas. Predominantly myxoid tumors produce soft, somewhat gelatinous tissue. Areas of infarction or hemorrhage may be observed in large, long-standing tumors or may result from prior surgical manipulation, such as biopsy or fine needle aspiration.

Microscopic Features

Pleomorphic adenoma is well-encapsulated tumor characterized by extreme cytomorphologic and architectural diversity. It is usually well covered by a thin capsule, except in few areas where smooth contoured buds project through the fibrous capsule (Fig. 7.3A). In few occasions, tumor islands may appear outside the capsule away from the tumor. These are in fact outgrowths continuous with the main tumor and can be demonstrated by serial sectioning.

The morphologic diversity in pleomorphic adenomas is due to ductal and myoepithelial differentiation, production of variable quantities of mucopolysaccharide matrix, and chondroid osseous metaplasia. The tumor is essentially made of narrow tubular structures, enveloped by myoepithelial mantles, submerging in a chondromyxoid stroma. These myoepithelial mantles radiate centrifugally into sheets, clusters, and isolated cells, appearing to "melt" into the sea of stroma they produce (Figs 7.3A to P).

Epithelial Component

The epithelial component may present as anastomosing tubules, small cysts, ribbons, and small sheets, made of columnar, cuboidal, or flat cells. Rarely, metaplasia to squamous, sebaceous, oncocytic, or clear cells may occur. The ductal lumina are empty or contain eosinophilic colloid-like PAS positive, diastase resistant, and variably mucicarmine positive material.

Myoepithelial Component

Myoepithelial/modified myoepithelial cells appear as cuboidal, spindle, stellate, plasmacytoid, epitheloid, and clear cells. The spindle or cuboidal cells may surround the ductal cells in a single layer as seen in normal salivary gland tissue or form a thick mantle, or radiate outwards from the ducts. They also form non-descript sheets, trabeculae, or cribriform structures. In some occasions, they might form fibrous-like interlacing fascicles, or rarely even schwannoma-like palisading of nuclei.

Plasmacytoid cells are the most distinctive form of myoepithelial cells. They are oval shaped, with a homogeneous eosinophilic hyaline cytoplasm, round and eccentrically located nuclei, and peripheral margination of dense chromatin. Even though called as plasmacytoid cells because of the superficial resemblance to plasma cells, these cells show less coarse clumping of chromatin, lack a perinuclear Golgi zone, and are larger, compared to plasma cells. These plasmacytoid cells are usually arranged in aggregates or sheets without any particular orientation. Identification of plasmacytoid cells is of high diagnostic value especially in small biopsies as these cells are observed only in pleomorphic adenomas and myoepitheliomas.

The stellate shaped cells occur singly or form anastomosing strands, suspended in an abundant myxoid matrix. The squamous cells may occasionally form squamous nests sometimes with keratin pearl formation. They are observed usually in solid cellular zones of presumed myoepithelial cells or in myxoid areas rather than in relation to pre-existing ducts. Cystic squamous epithelium-lined structures filled with keratin are also observed (Figs 7.3J and K).

Stroma

Stroma can be scanty to abundant in pleomorphic adenomas. It is chiefly made of acidic mucosubstances, commonly heparan sulfate,

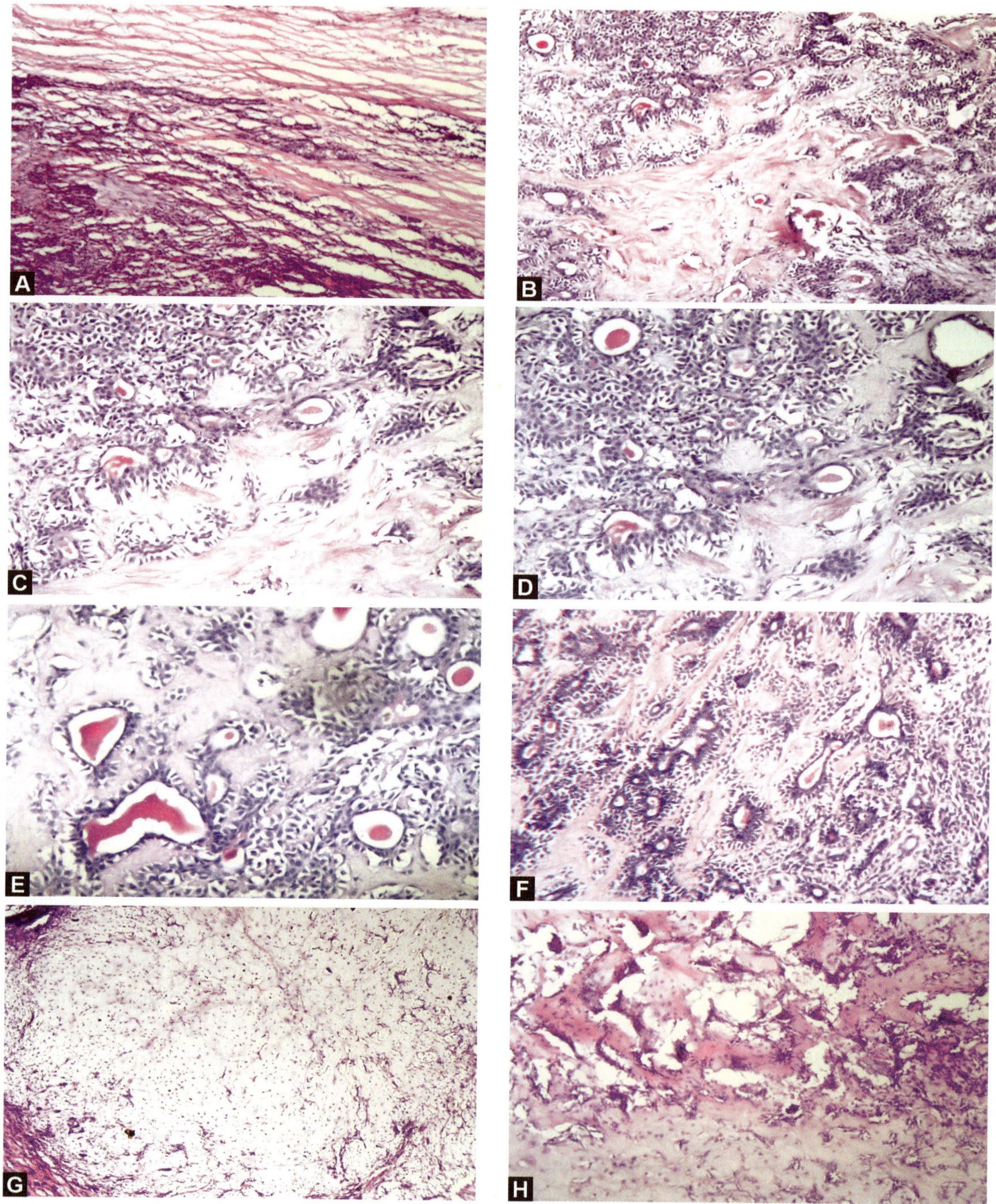

Figures 7.3A to H: Various histological patterns of pleomorphic adenoma: (A) The tumor is usually well covered by a thin capsule, except in few areas where smooth contoured buds project through the fibrous capsule; (B to F) Ductal structures are surrounded by myoepithelial cells and many of these ductal structures contain the eosinophilic material; (G Cartilaginous foci); (H) Osseous differentiation adjacent to a chondroid focus (Continued)

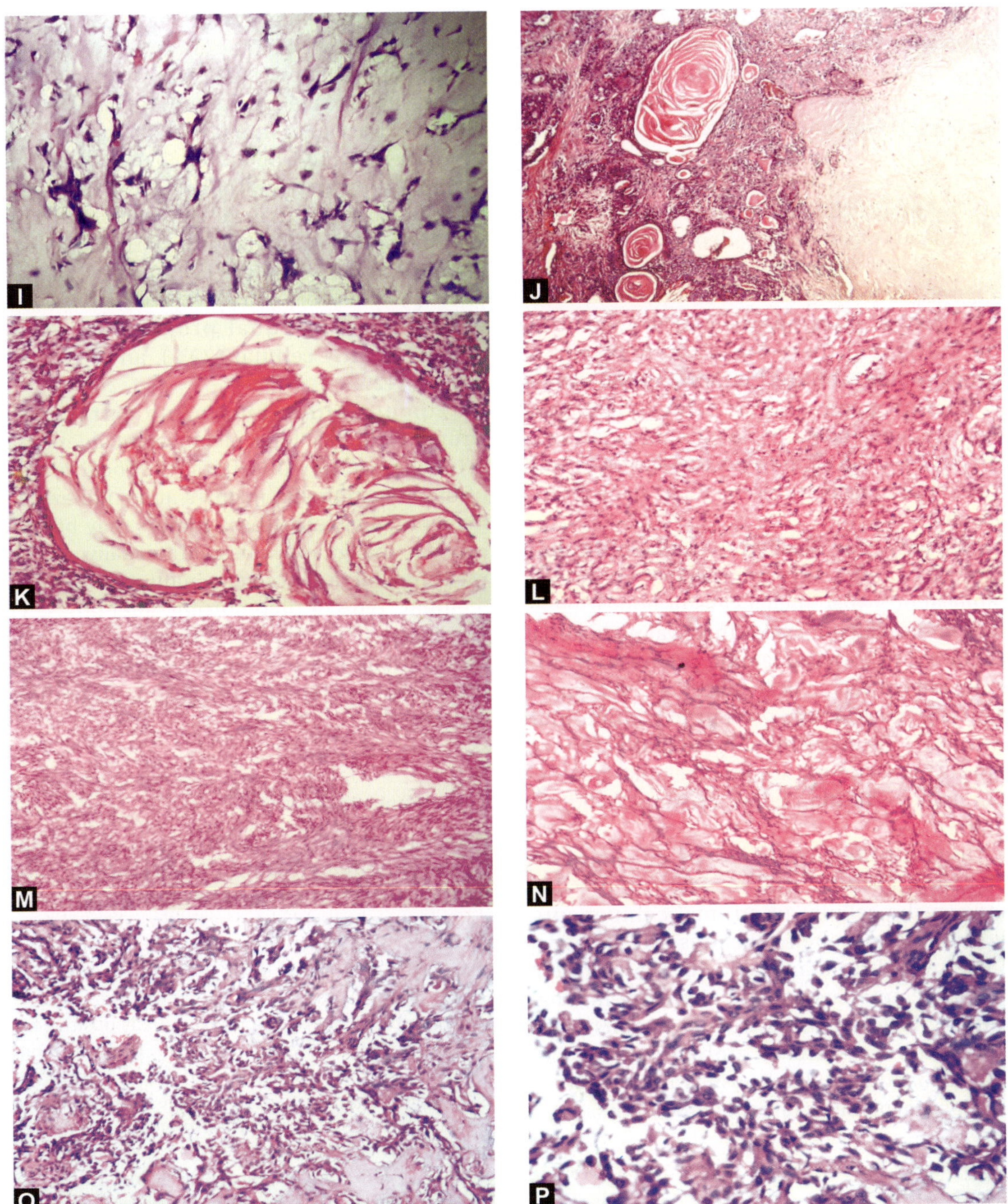

Figures 7.3I to P: Various histological patterns of pleomorphic adenoma: (I) Myxoid areas with separation of the spindle to stellate shaped myoepithelial cells; (J-K) Squamous differentiation with formation of multiple squamous epithelium lined cysts; (L) Cellular area with formation of occasional tubular structures; (M-N) Areas with a prominent spindle shaped myoepithelial component with nuclear palisading and hyalinized areas resembling neurilemmoma; (O-P) Acantholytic areas with plasmacytoid cells

produced by the modified myoepithelial cells (Positive for alcian blue and variably positive for PAS). Stroma may take the form of a mixture of chondroid (hyaline cartilage), myxoid, chondromyxoid, hyaline, and, very rarely, osseous and adipose tissues. Isolated or groups of stellate, oval or polygonal cells may be suspended in the matrix. Adipose differentiation is more common in cutaneous pleomorphic adenomas.

Chondroid stroma results from accumulation of myxohyaline material around individual cells, which further undergo vacuolar degeneration (Fig. 7.3G). But these areas rarely resemble mature hyaline cartilage. Chondromyxoid stroma in a salivary gland tumor is pathognomonic of pleomorphic adenoma. In pleomorphic adenomas with predominant chondromyxoid stroma, ductal structures can be best observed just beneath the capsule.

Homogeneous, fibrillary, or radiating hyaline material can be seen interspersed among the epithelial or myoepithelial cells or appearing as foci within cellular masses. This hyaline material is believed to be basal lamina produced by the myoepithelial cells. Focal collections of adipose tissue are occasionally present in pleomorphic adenomas. The occasional bone that is formed appears to result from stromal metaplasia rather than from ossification of pre-existing chondroid stroma.

Crystalloids composed of collagenous substance, tyrosine, and oxalate can develop between the cellular or stromal components. Tyrosine crystals often appear as "daisy-heads" in the myxoid stroma. Elastic fibers are present in variable amounts and are abundant in long-standing lesions. These fibers, demonstrated by van Gieson stain as globular masses or irregular bands, are of diagnostic value as they are uncommon in other salivary gland tumors.

Histologic Classification of Pleomorphic Adenomas

Seifert has subclassified pleomorphic adenoma into four types based on the relative proportion of stroma and cellular components, namely, type 1 with an extracellular stroma 30 to 50% of the tumor (30% of cases); type 2 with an extracellular stroma ~80% of the tumour (55% of cases); type 3 with an extracellular stroma of 20-30% of the tumor (9% of cases); and type 4 wherein the extracellular stroma is similar to type 3 but a focal monomorphic differentiation occurs in the epithelial component.

Foote and Frazell have categorized pleomorphic adenomas similarly into 4 types, namely, principally myxoid (36%), myxoid and cellular components in equal proportions (30%), predominantly cellular (22%), and extremely cellular (12%).

Tumors with scanty or no extracellular stroma or the 'cellular pleomorphic adenomas' are diagnosed by observing the focal melting of the myoepithelial mantles and solid areas of myoepithelial cells. These tumors may be more prone to malignant change. Minor salivary gland pleomorphic adenomas usually belong to the 'cellular' type of pleomorphic adenomas. The 'stroma-rich' or 'myxoid' tumors, on the other hand, recur more frequently because of the higher chance of spillage of mucoid stroma during surgery.

Immunohistochemistry

Immunohistochemistry helps to diagnose uncertain cases, by demonstrating the glandular and myoepithelial components. Inconspicuous ductal lamina can be highlighted by Epithelial membrane antigen (EMA) or Carcino embryonic antigen (CEA). Myoepithelial and modified myoepithelial cells are positive for CK and vimentin, but not EMA or CEA. Myoepithelial components are usually positive for S-100 protein and GFAP. However, in the luminal cells, S-100 positivity can be variably observed. The most reliable marker for neoplastic myoepithelium is calponin. Its expression is strongest in the cells at a juxtaluminal location.

Low proliferative index (Ki 67), rare immuno-reactivity for p53 protein, and weak bcl-2 staining are parameters that differentiate pleomorphic adenomas from adenoid cystic carcinomas.

Ultrastructural Studies

Electron microscopy has identified tonofilaments and actin microfilaments, linear densities of the plasma membrane, pinocytotic vesicles, and remnants of basement membrane within the cytoplasm of 'mesenchymal cells', confirming the myoepithelial origin of these cells.

Cytogenetic Abnormalities

Cytogenetic abnormalities involving the chromosome regions 12q13-15 have been reported in pleomorphic adenomas. Recurrent reciprocal translocation t(3;8)(p21;q12), putative pleomorphic adenoma gene (PLAG) 1 mapped to chromosome 8q12, HMGI-C, NFIB, and FHIT, have all been implicated in the genesis of these tumors. But these studies have not established any role in the diagnosis of pleomorphic adenomas.

Malignant Transformation

Pleomorphic adenomas can undergo malignant transformation to carcinoma ex-pleomorphic adenoma. These malignancies however can also arise de novo, without any pre-existing benign tumor.

Clinically, rapid growth of the tumor and facial nerve involvement in a pleomorphic adenoma are features suggestive of malignant transformation. High-risk factors include old age, submandibular location, larger size, and recurrence.

Histologically, high mitotic count, bizarre mitotic figures, coagulative necrosis, widespread cellular pleomorphism, tumor cell infiltration into parenchyma, vascular permeation, perineural extension and presence of an expansile nodule within the parent adenoma are features suggestive of a supervening malignancy.

It is important to remember that capsular invasion, hypercellularity and intravascular tumor plugs are not supportive of malignancy. When abnormal cytological features are confined within the capsule, the terms intracapsular carcinoma, carcinoma *in situ* or non-invasive carcinoma ex mixed tumor have been used.

Differential Diagnosis

Goblet or mucous cells formed rarely by the epithelium along with the squamous cells, results in areas resembling mucoepidermoid carcinoma. Extensive areas of epithelial differentiation in the form of tubules or trabeculae well-delineated from the characteristic stroma mimics mucoepidermoid carcinoma or adenoid cystic carcinoma. But these pleomorphic adenomas are identified by the absence of infiltration, limited cystic component, and presence of myxochondroid elements.

Cellular pleomorphic adenomas mimic monomorphic adenomas such as basal cell adenoma. A diagnosis of pleomorphic adenoma is arrived at in such cases if the epithelial pattern is similar to that seen in a typical pleomorphic adenoma and if there is some evidence of spindle or plasmacytoid differentiation, even in the absence of any appreciable myxochondroid stroma.

Pleomorphic adenomas of minor salivary glands resemble polymorphous low-grade adenocarcinomas (PLGA). But PLGA has perineural growth, infiltrates adjacent fibrous connective tissue, fat, and salivary parenchyma, and forms small tubular structures or single file cords of tumor cells at the periphery.

Myxoid or stroma-rich pleomorphic adenomas mimic mesenchymal neoplasms such as myxoma, myxoid lipoma, or myxoid neurofibroma. Careful search for typical epithelial areas, even if small in size, in sections from multiple blocks solves the diagnostic dilemma in such cases.

Other differential diagnoses include epithelial-myoepithelial carcinoma, carcinoma ex pleomorphic adenoma, acinic cell carcinoma, and mesenchymal tumors such as nerve sheath tumor.

Metastasizing Pleomorphic Adenoma

A rare and curious complication of surgical excision of pleomorphic adenomas is the iatrogenic spread of tumour cells through the vascular route resulting in distant metastasis. This 'metastasizing pleomorphic adenomas' characteristically retain the benign features of the primary tumor and commonly present in the bone (50%), lungs (30%), and lymph nodes (20%). In spite of the benign appearance of the tumor cells, up to 37%

of the patients die of the disease. A more rapidly progressive course is noted in an immuno-compromised host.

MYOEPITHELIOMA

Myoepithelioma is a benign tumor made, almost exclusively, of neoplastic myoepithelial cells and their derivatives. A minor epithelial component is, however, present and the characteristic chondro-myxoid stromas of pleomorphic adenoma are absent.

It is believed that pleomorphic adenoma, basal cell adenoma, and myoepithelioma are in a continuum. Myoepithelioma have been argued as representing an extreme form of basal cell adenoma without a ductal component, while basal cell adenoma can be viewed as pleomorphic adenoma 'without' the characteristic stroma. It is, however, prudent to accept that myoepitheliomas only represent one end of the spectrum of pleomorphic adenomas, because of the presence of occasional ductal elements. This has led to myoepitheliomas being alternatively referred to as 'mixed tumor with myoepithelial predominance'. Barnes et al have suggested that a tumor can be referred to as 'mixed tumor with a high content of myoepithelial cells if one or more ductal structures are noted in every 20 X magnification field or if more than one small cluster of ducts is present within the tumor. Such distinction between tumors is strictly academic, considering the benign nature of all these entities.

Clinical Features

Myoepitheliomas are rare neoplasms, with a preponderance to occur in the parotid and the minor salivary glands. Most common site for intraoral myoepitheliomas is the palate. Less commonly, myoepitheliomas are reported in the skin, breast, or soft tissue. The tumor presents as a slow growing, asymptomatic mass, in the third to fourth decade of life with no gender predilection.

Microscopic Features

The gross findings in myoepitheliomas are very similar to pleomorphic adenomas except that the myxoid or chondroid areas will be absent in myoepitheliomas. The neoplastic myoepithelial cells can be spindle shaped or plasmacytoid in appearance with rare epithelioid or clear cell differentiation. Of these cells, either the spindle or the plasmacytoid cell types predominate or a mixture of these two cell types may result. The spindle cell pattern is more common in parotid tumors and the plasmacytoid variant is more common in palatal tumors.

The most common variant of myoepithelioma, the *spindle-cell predominant tumor*, is highly cellular, made of elongated spindle cells, with a vesicular nuclei and eosinophilic cytoplasm. The tumor cells are arranged in a storiform, swirling pattern or exhibit a herringbone fascicular arrangement, with very little stroma.

In the *plasmacytoid variant*, the tumor cells are similar to the plasmacytoid cells seen in pleomorphic adenomas, loosely cohesive and accompanied by an abundant myxoid stroma, rich in hyaluronic acid and lacking mucin. These cells are oval shaped, with a homogeneous eosinophilic hyaline cytoplasm, round and eccentrically located nuclei, and peripheral margination of dense chromatin. Even though called as plasmacytoid cells because of the superficial resemblance to plasma cells, these cells show less coarse clumping of chromatin, lack a perinuclear Golgi zone, and are larger compared to plasma cells. These plasmacytoid cells are usually arranged in aggregates or sheets without any particular orientation or may be suspended in myxoid matrix in the form of isolated cells, cords, or aggregates. True chondroid differentiation is, however, absent.

Epithelioid cells are large, polygonal cells with eosinophilic cytoplasm and centrally placed bland nuclei. They often show a reticular, trabecular, or solid growth pattern. Clear cells are rich in glycogen and are present as focal areas or rarely as large sheets, leading to errors in diagnosis. Collagenous crystalloids may be observed in myoepitheliomas in the form of radially arranged and intercellular hyaline materials.

Immunohistochemistry

The tumor cells show positivity for pan-cytokeratin, vimentin, and myoepithelial markers such as muscle-specific actin, GFAP, S-100 protein, calponin, and CK14. S-100 is the most reliable, but lacks specificity. Some cells express EMA also, but only rarely CEA.

Ultrastructural Findings

Electron microscopy has identified epithelial (presence of desmosomes) and myoid (cytoplasmic microfilaments in the presence or absence of dense bodies, pinocytotic vesicles with basal lamina separating the tumor cells from the stroma) features.

Differential Diagnosis

Tumors that closely resemble myoepitheliomas are pleomorphic adenoma and basal cell adenoma. But absence of the characteristic chondromyxoid areas of pleomorphic adenomas and the ductal structures of basal cell adenomas help to overcome the diagnostic dilemma.

The spindle-cell variant of myoepithelioma mimics mesenchymal lesions such as benign fibrous histiocytoma, leiomyoma, and benign peripheral nerve sheath tumor. However, positive staining for immunoreactive cytokeratin, S-100 protein, and GFAP helps to confirm the myoepithelial nature of the tumor.

Predominance of clear cells in myoepitheliomas may mimic clear cell adenocarcinoma. But myoepitheliomas lack infiltrative areas and cellular atypia seen in clear cell adenocarcinomas.

Myoepitheliomas are differentiated from synovial carcinomas by the lack of nuclear abnormality, increased mitotic activity, and infiltrative areas. Further, myoepitheliomas do not show the nuclear abnormality that is observed in metastatic renal cell carcinoma.

Ectomesenchymal Chondromyxoid Tumor of the Tongue: A Variant of Myoepithelioma

Ectomesenchymal chondromyxoid tumor of the tongue is a benign tumor that presents as slow growing, painless nodule in the anterior dorsum of the tongue, commonly in the third decade of life. Even though this tumor has been postulated to arise from the undifferentiated ectomesenchyme of the tongue, the morphologic similarity and immunohistochemical profile strongly points out the possibility of this tumor being a peculiar variant of myoepithelioma.

Microscopically, this well-circumscribed tumor consists of lobular proliferation of ovoid, fusiform or stellate cells disposed in cords and a characteristic lattice pattern. The nuclei are round or multilobulated with occasional atypia. Abundant hyaline, myxoid or chondromyxoid matrix is present. The tumor cells are positive for GFAP and cytokeratin and inconsistently positive for actin and S-100 protein.

PAPILLARY CYSTADENOMA LYMPHOMATOSUM (WARTHIN'S TUMOR)

Papillary cystadenoma lymphomatosum (PCL) is a benign neoplasm of salivary gland origin characterized by distinctive clinical and histologic features, thus making it one of the most readily identifiable salivary gland neoplasms.

This tumor has been also referred to as cystic papillary adenoma, branchial cysts of the parotid, branchiogenic adenoma, oncocytome, adenolymphoma, lymphoglandular cystome, and Warthin's tumor (named after Warthin, who first coined the term papillary cystadenoma lymphomatosum). But papillary cystadenoma lymphomatosum is the most appropriate designation as it describes fully the histology of the tumor, namely, the glandular epithelium thrown into papillary folds, projecting into the lumen of cystic structures they form, and a prominent lymphoid stroma demarcated from the glandular epithelium. Among the other common terms in use today, Warthin's tumor is held synonymous with PCL, but the term adenolymphoma should be discouraged as it overstates the lymphoid component and even suggests a malignancy.

Clinical Features

The PCL is the second most common benign parotid salivary gland tumor. Most of the tumors occur in the parotid and paraparotid region, with very few examples in the submandibular gland and minor salivary glands of lower lip. The tail of the parotid gland is commonly involved even though few tumors develop from the deep lobe of the gland and from the lymph nodes in the superficial and medial portions of the gland (Fig. 7.4)

PCL accounts for 4 to 11 percent of all salivary gland tumors. A definite male preponderance has been reported. However of late, there has been a decline in men and increase in women, possibly due to a decline in smoking habit, an established risk factor of this tumor (eight times more risk), in men and increase of this habit among women. Besides smoking, radiation and EBV infection have also been correlated with this tumor. A high incidence has been reported in whites.

PCL is commonly reported in the sixth and seventh decades of life. It is usually multicentric, synchronous or metachronous, and unilateral or bilateral more often than any other salivary gland tumor. More than one tumor is reported in at least 12% of the cases. Bilateral occurrence is seen in 5 to 8% of cases. Frequently, the tumor is also associated with a second tumor, commonly pleomorphic adenoma, which may develop synchronously or metachronously.

PCL presents as a painless, doughy or sometimes fluctuant, well circumscribed ovoid or spherical mass of the lower portion of the parotid gland, next to the angle of the mandible and is usually 2 to 4 cms in size. In contrast to other monomorphic adenomas, PCL can present with a variety of symptoms such as pain, facial weakness, ipsilateral ear symptoms (ache, tinnitus), and deafness. Leakage of fluid into the surrounding tissues and retrograde infection from the oral cavity through the Stensen's duct might result in a sudden painful increase in size of the tumour associated with acute pain, a condition also referred to as papillary cystadenoma lymphomatosum syndrome. Rarely facial palsy might result in a tumor complicated by inflammation and fibrosis, which may be mistaken clinically or intraoperatively for carcinomas.

Macroscopic Features

The parotidectomy specimens of PCL should be observed thoroughly for separate tumor foci. The tumor is usually a well-circumscribed, spherical to ovoid lesion, measuring not more than 4 cms in size and covered by an intact, thin, tough capsule. The cut surface is light brown and lobular, with cystic structures and solid rubbery areas. The cystic structures, which might be single or multiple, contain clear, serous, mucous, brown tinged (chocolate color) fluid or caseous semi-solid debris (as seen in tuberculous lymphadenitis). Fine papillary projections of the tan-brown tumor are seen projecting into the cystic spaces. The solid areas appear grey-white and refer to the lymphoid component. Tiny white nodules can be seen on scraping the surface of these areas and represent the lymphoid follicles. The gross appearance is thus pathognomonic.

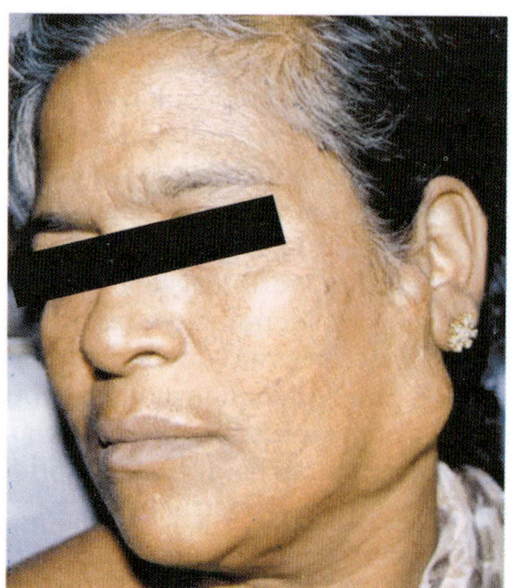

Figure 7.4: Warthin's tumor typically presents as swelling in the tail of the parotid

Microscopic Features

PCL is a well-encapsulated tumor, essentially composed of a bilayered oncocytic epithelium thrown into papillary folds, projecting into the lumen of irregular cystic structures they form, and a prominent lymphoid stroma demarcated from the glandular epithelium (Figs 7.5A to C).

The epithelium is made of two layers of cells, the inner or luminal layer of columnar cells supported by a discontinuous outer layer of triangular, basaloid cells. The ovoid nuclei of the luminal cells appear darkly stained and pyknotic and are centrally placed near the luminal space. The basaloid cells, present beneath and between the columnar cells, possess round to oval nuclei that are perpendicular to the long axis of the columnar cells and have small but conspicuous nucleoli. The bright eosinophilic granular cytoplasm of the cells of both these layers is due to the accumulation of mitochondria. The luminal cells are rarely ciliated, but often demonstrate a fuzzy luminal surface, attributed to the presence of microvilli. The epithelial layer can also show downward extension to form some loosely arranged or closely packed salivary glands.

The cystic lumen contains thick proteinaceous secretions, cellular debris, cholesterol crystals, and, at times, laminated bodies (resembling corpora amylacea).

The epithelial lining is separated from the underlying lymphoid stroma by a distinct layer of basement membrane. The lymphoid stroma

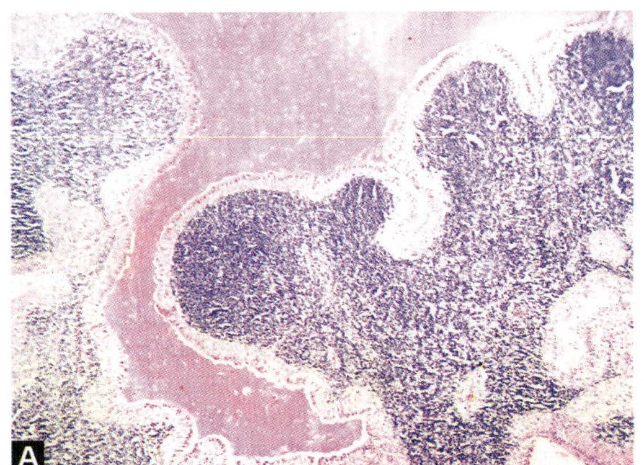

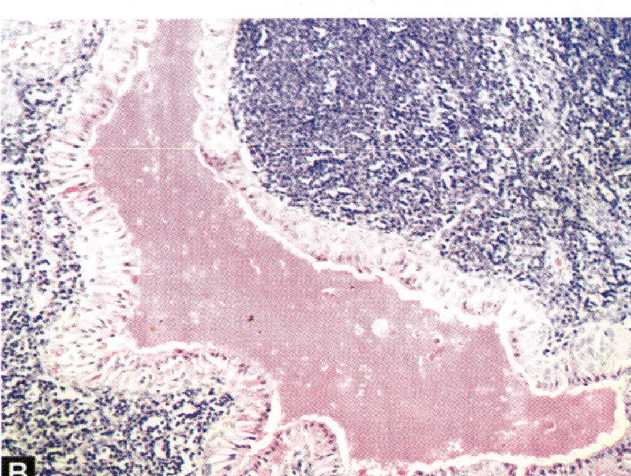

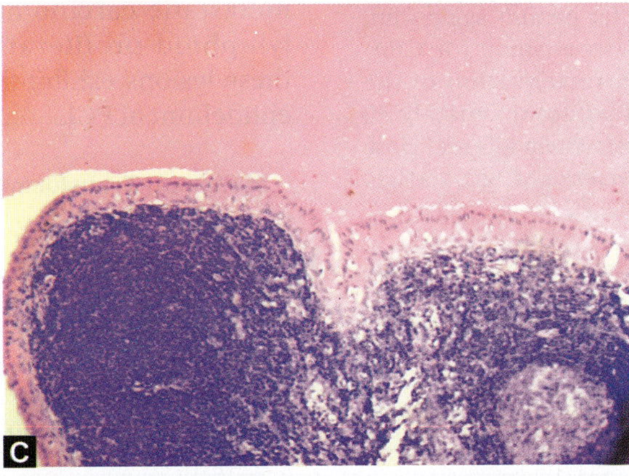

Figures 7.5A to C: Bilayered oncocytic epithelium is thrown into papillary folds, projecting into the lumen of irregular cystic structures they form. A prominent lymphoid stroma is seen

resembles a normal lymph node with lymphoid follicles and germinal centers and consists of small lymphocytes and few plasma cells, histiocytes, and mast cells. The ratio of B to T cells is 0.8:1. Rarely, a granulomatous reaction may ensue with Langhans-type giant cells.

The most frequent histologic variations observed in PCL include oncocytosis, squamous metaplasia, mucous cell prosoplasia, and rarely, inclusions of sebaceous glands. Oncocytosis is characterized by sheets and nests of disorganized oncocytic cells that show loss of papillary formation. The epithelial component might undergo metaplasia to form squamous or mucous cells, especially in response to inflammation or infarction.

Histologic Classification

Seifert has subclassified PCLs into four types based on the relative proportion of epithelial and lymphoid components: subtype 1 (classical PCL) is 50% epithelial (77% of cases); subtype 2 (stroma-poor) is 70 to 80% epithelial (14% of cases); subtype 3 (stroma-rich) is only 20 to 30% epithelial (2% of cases); and subtype 4 is characterized by extensive squamous metaplasia. Subtype 2 shows morphologic overlap with oncocytoma.

Immunohistochemistry

The luminal epithelial cells are reactive for IgA and the basal cells are reactive for peanut agglutinin. The epithelial cells are also positive for CEA. Immunohistochemical characterization of the immunoglobulins reveal that approximately 50 percent of the B lymphocytes contain IgG and close to 33% contain IgA. The rest secrete IgM, IgD, and IgE.

Ultrastructural Findings

The primary ultrastructural feature of the oncocytic cells of PCL is an increased amount of mitochondria. The mitochondria are prominent throughout the cytoplasm, with dense packing in the cells adjacent to the cystic lumina. The size of the mitochondria is variable with as high as three times larger sizes being observed. The cristae of the aberrant mitochondria are longer and numerous and form closely packed lamellar sheaves, rouleaux, spheric concentric rings, or they may be arranged haphazardly in villous forms. Crystalloids that appear as rectangular prisms are observed in the pyramidal cells. Tonofilaments may be observed in cells displaying squamous metaplasia. The apical surfaces of the epithelial cells exhibit microvilli besides the cilia.

Differential Diagnosis

Clinically, PCL might be mistaken for lympho-epithelial cyst, chronic lymphadenitis, caseating tuberculous lymphadenitis, AIDS related lymphadenopathy, lymphadenoma, and metastatic carcinoma.

Cellular atypia and a pseudoinfiltrative appearance of the metaplastic epithelium might mimic squamous cell or mucoepidermoid carcinoma. But, lack of true infiltrative growth into the surrounding parenchyma and identification of merging between the atypical squamous islands and the oncocytic epithelium help in diagnosis.

Papillary oncocytic cystadenoma resembles PCL, but it arises from minor salivary glands and lacks a well organized lymphoid element. Parotid lesions that might resemble PCL due to the presence of prominent lymphoid element and cystic configuration are lymphoepithelial cyst, AIDS-related lymphadenopathy, lymphadenoma, metastatic carcinoma, and tumor associated lymphoid proliferations. However, none of these lesions exhibit the characteristic bilayered epithelium of PCL.

Malignant Transformation

The epithelial or the lymphoid component of the tumor might very rarely undergo malignant transformation. The most common carcinomas in decreasing order of frequency are squamous cell carcinoma, oncocytic carcinoma, adenocarcinoma, undifferentiated carcinoma, and mucoepidermoid carcinoma. The lymphomas include Hodgkin's lymphoma and various types of non-Hodgkin's lymphoma. These lymphomas are characterized by a relatively monomorphic infiltrate with distortion of the epithelial and lymphoid architecture.

CANALICULAR ADENOMA

Canalicular adenoma is a benign salivary gland neoplasm characterized by an isomorphic architecture; made of single or bilayered columnar epithelial cells forming branching cords in a loose stroma.

Clinical Presentation

This tumor usually presents in the elderly population with an average age of 65 years, with a definite female preponderance. Canalicular adenomas represent about 4 to 6% of all salivary gland tumors in minor salivary glands, where these tumors occur exclusively. Thus, oral cavity is the most common site of canalicular adenomas, with a majority of lesions occurring in the upper lip (Figs 7.6A and B) The other common sites include buccal mucosa, parotid gland, and palate.

Canalicular adenomas present as non ulcerated painless, slow-growing, movable, and slightly compressible masses, ranging in size from 0.4 to 2 cm. Bluish coloration of the mucosa covering the tumor may be observed in few occasions. Rarely, superficial ulceration, necrosis, or multifocal nodules may be seen.

Macroscopic Features

Canalicular adenomas appear as encapsulated or non-encapsulated but circumscribed lesions that are occasionally multifocal or multinodular. The color has been reported to range from pink-tan to tan, brown, or yellow. Cut section of the tumor often reveals cystic spaces and gelatinous mucoid material.

Microscopic Features

Canalicular adenomas are well-circumscribed, with or without a capsule. The tumor is made of bilayered strands of cells that abut and separate haphazardly, giving rise to single files, double rows, beads, and pseudopapillae. These double rows of cells form a meshwork of branching and interconnecting cords and form long canals with a central lumen; hence the name 'canaliculi'. Sometimes these rows separate to form duct-like structures within the lumina.

The epithelial cells that make up these rows are isomorphic and cuboidal to columnar, with a moderate amount of amphophilic cytoplasm, which contains scattered granules that stain positive with periodic acid-Schiff stain. These granules are diastase labile, indicating they are glycogen. The basophilic nuclei are regular, ovoid, and elongated in normal sections with stippled chromatin. The nuclei appear elongated or round based on the plane of section. Variation in heights of the nuclei might sometimes impart a pseudostratified appearance. Cellular pleomorphism and mitosis are not observed.

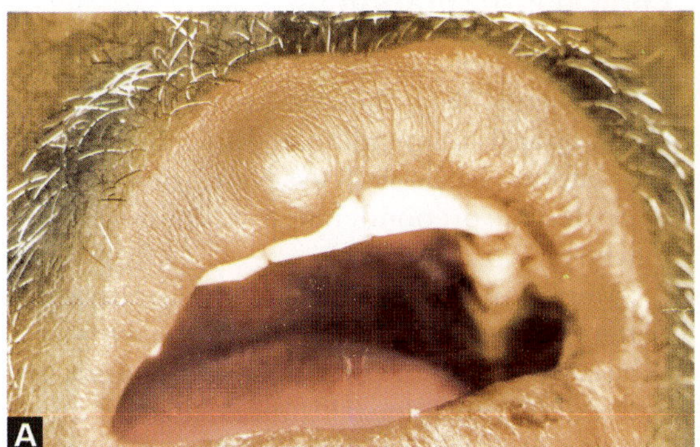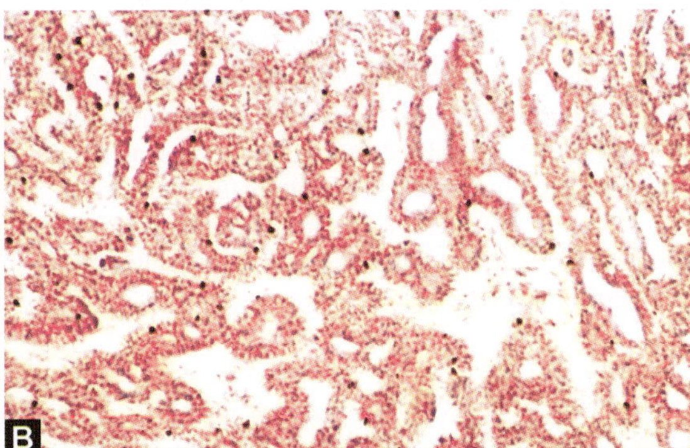

Figures 7.6A and B: Canalicular adenoma presenting as an asymptomatic mass in the upper lip. Histologically, it is made of bilayered strands of cells, giving rise to single files, double rows, beads, and pseudopapillae

In few cases, multiple cystic spaces might be observed giving the neoplasm a microcystic appearance. In such tumors, the tumor may have papillary projections into the lumina. These projections are covered by the same columnar and cuboidal cells that make up the body of the tumor. Psammoma bodies may be observed in the areas where projections are present.

Rarely, foci of basaloid cells are seen. This basaloid appearance, in most cases, results from a tangential plane of section, which produces an "online" presentation of the normal columnar cells. Solid cellular proliferations of basaloid cells may also be observed, mimicking basal cell adenomas.

The stroma is sparse, fibrillar and lacks cellularity with many capillaries and sinusoids. Fibroblasts are few and minimum to moderate collagen is present. The extremely thin nature of the stroma makes it appear as if the tumor strands are 'floating in the air'. In many areas, the stroma has an edematous, lightly basophilic appearance with few inflammatory cells. This relatively acellular stroma stains positively with mucicarmine, alcian blue, and periodic acid-Schiff, with or without diastase predigestion.

In the occasionally presenting multifocal canalicular adenomas, larger encapsulated and smaller uncapsulated foci of tumor cells are seen. These small foci should not be considered as feature of malignancy.

> **Immunohistochemical and Ultrastructural Features**
>
> Excessive luminal cell differentiation without myoepithelial cell participation has been confirmed by both immunohistochemical and ultrastructural studies. The tumor cells are positive for cytokeratin, vimentin, S-100 protein, and infrequently for EMA. They are negative for CEA, smooth muscle actin, and GFAP.

Differential Diagnosis

Most common clinical differential diagnosis include sialolith, mucous extravasation phenomenon, mucous retention cyst, and salivary gland tumor, possibly pleomorphic adenoma. Canalicular adenomas with prominent foci of basaloid cells may mimic basal cell adenomas. But the characteristic peripheral palisading of basal cell adenomas is not seen in canalicular adenomas. Further, basal cell adenomas lack the columnar cells or canaliculi seen in canalicular adenomas.

The cribriform-tubular patterns of adenoid cystic carcinoma may resemble canalicular adenoma. But adenoid cystic carcinomas lack the rows of columnar cells, have pale to clear cells with indistinct cell boundaries and irregular-shaped nuclei, have stromal pseudocysts that contain basophilic glycosaminoglycans or eosinophilic basal lamina but not capillaries, have basaloid cells with angular nuclei and clear cytoplasm, demonstrates perineural invasion, and have infiltrative destructive growth.

Other histologic similarities include ameloblastoma and basal cell carcinoma.

BASAL CELL ADENOMA

Basal cell adenoma is a benign neoplasm of salivary gland origin, composed of a uniform population of basaloid cells arranged in various histologic patterns. It has been variously referred to as tubular solid adenoma, trabecular adenoma, dermal analogue tumor, clear cell adenoma, basalioma, canalicular adenoma, and monomorphic adenoma.

Clinical Presentation

Most basal cell adenomas occur in the parotid gland (nearly 70%). The next common sites are the upper lip and submandibular gland. These tumors are common in the sixth to seventh decade of life, with a female preponderance. It is more common in whites.

Membranous basal cell adenoma, also known as *dermal analogue tumor*, is a distinctive variant of basal cell adenoma that is commonly associated with cutaneous adnexal tumors such as dermal cylindroma, trichoepithelioma, and eccrine spiradenoma. This association could signify a genetic disorder affecting the multipotential duct reserve stem cell. Membranous basal cell adenomas show a striking male preponderance and a significant multicentric development.

The tumor typically presents as a solitary, slow growing, asymptomatic, firm, and movable swelling, which might show cystic areas and compressible areas. The swelling never grows beyond three centimeters.

Macroscopic Features

The excised mass is usually a single, well-defined nodule, measuring less than three centimeter. The cut surface is gray, tan, or brown. Membranous basal cell adenoma is usually multifocal and multinodular.

Microscopic Features

The tumor is essentially made of basaloid cells characterized by round to oval basophilic nuclei, pale eosinophilic to amphophilic scanty cytoplasm and indistinct cell borders. Nuclear pleomorphism and mitoses are not seen. Two types of basaloid cells, the dark and light cells, can be made out. The small dark cells have less cytoplasm and intense basophilic nuclei. The larger light cells are uniform small pale eosinophilic cells with indistinct borders characterized by increased cytoplasm and pale basophilic nuclei. The light cells predominate with the dark cells often located in the peripheral portions of the epithelial tumor nests, cords, or islands. Few ductal structures can be seen interspersed among the basaloid cells.

The common histologic patterns seen in basal cell adenomas are the solid, tubular, trabecular, and membranous types and basal cell adenomas with myoepithelium-derived stroma. The tumors are usually dominated by one type of architecture, but a mixture of patterns can be seen in some cases. Except for the membranous type, the specific subtype does not imply any predictable biologic behavior variation.

Solid Type

The basaloid cells are arranged in the form of broad bands, smooth-contoured islands, and solid masses with palisading of the peripheral hyperchromatic columnar or cuboidal cells. The central cells of the tumor islands often appear to have a directional orientation that tends to parallel the basilar cells. They can also form scattered whorled eddies that may mature into epidermoid cells, sometimes producing keratin to give rise to the appearance of small keratin cysts, or keratin pearls. The tumor cells are separated from the surrounding loose and sometimes highly vascularized stroma by a distinct basement membrane.

Tubular Type

This histologic subtype is predominated by discrete or anastomosing tubules lined by two distinct layers of cells, with inner cuboidal ductal cells surrounded by an outer layer of basaloid cells. The ductal cells are characterized by a more eosinophilic cytoplasm and the lumen often contains PAS-positive eosinophilic secretion. Rare areas of cribriform pattern can be seen. Even though the tubular pattern is the least common of all histologic subtypes of basal cell adenoma, tubule formation can be seen alone or interspersed with basaloid areas in most basal cell adenomas, at least focally.

Trabecular Type

The tumor cells are arranged in the form of narrow or broad trabeculae of cells interconnected with one another, producing a reticular pattern. Because the trabecular type also presents with small cysts and ductal lumens occasionally, it has been suggested to consider the trabecular and tubular types as one 'tubulotrabecular' type.

Basal Cell Adenoma with Myoepithelium-Derived Stroma

This rare subtype of basal cell adenoma is characterized by spindle cell-rich stroma that separates the tumor islands and cords. The dense and fascicular arrangement of the stroma may impart a "solid" appearance to the tumor. These spindle cells are positive for S-100 protein and resemble myoepithelium ultrastructurally.

Membranous Type

The histologic appearance of this subtype is identical to that of dermal cylindroma. In low magnification, a multilobular pattern is observed, demonstrating large lobules of epithelial islands that appear to mould to the shape of the other lobules so as to fit closely together in a 'Jig-saw' puzzle appearance.

The distinctive feature of membranous basal cell adenomas is the presence of abundant, thick, eosinophilic, PAS-positive hyaline basal lamina material around the smooth-contoured tumor islands. The hyaline material also insinuates in between the individual cells, appearing as hyaline droplets. These interepithelial droplets are often associated with, or surrounded by, slightly darker and smaller epithelial cells. On some occasions, these droplets may coalesce and produce larger eosinophilic masses.

Occasional glandular spaces can also be formed in the tumour islands. Few tumor cells might show squamous metaplasia. The multinodular growth pattern of membranous basal cell adenoma results in normal salivary gland tissue often entrapped within the tumor. This should not be erroneously interpreted as a malignant lesion.

Immunohistochemistry

Basal cell adenomas show differentiation of both epithelial and myoepithelial elements. Epithelial markers (CK, CEA, EMA) as well as myoepithelial markers (calponin, actin, GFAP, S-100, vimentin) can be variably demonstrated in the luminal and basal/myoepithelial cells respectively.

Ultrastructural Findings

Several layers of basement membrane are seen to envelop the individual tumor cells. Cytoplasmic interdigitations and anchoring by membrane-bound desmosomes are present. Lumen formation by microvilli is seen at times.

Malignant Transformation

Rarely (4%) basal cell adenomas may undergo malignant transformation into basaloid cell carcinomas (basal cell adenocarcinoma, adenoid cystic carcinoma), and less commonly into non-basaloid cell carcinoma (salivary duct carcinoma, adenocarcinoma). This malignant transformation is more in the membranous subtype (as high as 28%). Invasion into the adjacent salivary gland or other structures, perineural permeation, and intravascular growth are features that signify supervening malignancy.

Differential Diagnosis

Basal cell adenomas are differentiated from pleomorphic adenomas by a distinct boundary between the tumor cells and the stroma. Further, the characteristic myxochondroid areas of pleomorphic adenomas are not seen in basal cell adenomas. The absence of plasmacytoid and spindled myoepithelial cells helps to differentiate from cellular pleomorphic adenomas and myoepitheliomas.

Adenoid cystic carcinoma is another entity to be differentiated from basal cell adenomas. Basaloid cells with irregular angled nuclei and pale to clear cytoplasm, prominent cribriform pattern, and eosinophilic basal lamina are features common in adenoid cystic carcinoma but absent in basal cell adenomas. Infiltration and perineural invasion, characteristic of adenoid cystic carcinomas, further differentiate them from basal cell adenomas. Membranous basal cell adenoma mimics adenoid cystic carcinoma because of its cellular features and hyaline production. The three features that help in differentiating membranous adenomas from adenoid cystic carcinomas are the whorled eddies of epithelial cells that are not seen in adenoid cystic carcinoma, the haphazard arrangement of the hyaline material that is seen in the membranous adenoma, and the absence of parenchymal and perineural invasion in basal cell adenoma.

Palisading of the peripheral layer of cells in basal cell adenomas mimics ameloblastomas.

But examination of radiographs for alveolar bone involvement helps in the diagnosis. Basal cell adenomas approaching the skin can mimic cutaneous basal cell carcinomas.

Basal cell adenocarcinoma is differentiated from its benign counterpart basal cell adenoma by its infiltration of parotid parenchyma and adjacent tissues such as fat, muscle, skin, bone, nerves, and vessels and its often high mitotic count.

Canalicular adenomas with prominent foci of basaloid cells may mimic basal cell adenomas. But, basal cell adenomas lack the columnar cells or canaliculi seen in canalicular adenomas. Further, the characteristic peripheral palisading of basal cell adenomas is not seen in canalicular adenomas.

ONCOCYTOMA (OXYPHILIC ADENOMA)

Oncocytes or oxyphilic cells are mature salivary gland cells seen as a component of aging. Oncocytoma is a discrete, encapsulated tumor consisting exclusively of oncocytes, with no myoepithelial or basal cell participation. It is a rare benign tumor of salivary glands, usually confined within the salivary gland tissue and is closely related to Warthin's tumor.

Pathogenesis

Various theories have been postulated to explain the pathogenesis of oncocytomas. The oncocyte has been believed to result from a 'peculiar degeneration' or to represent a metaplastic or neoplastic or hyperplastic process. The multinodular nature and bilateral occurrence of the condition has given credence to the belief that it represents a nodular hyperplasia. It has also been suggested that the salivary gland oncocyte may be an adaptive or compensatory response hyperplastic cell that occurs secondary to an undetermined somatic cell mutation rather than a purely degenerative process.

Ionizing radiation has been implicated in the causation of this condition. Nearly 20% of the patients have a history of radiation therapy to the face or upper torso or long-term occupational radiation exposure 5 to 40 years before the discovery of the tumor. Patients with previous radiation exposure are, on average, 20 years younger at tumor detection than those without a documented history of irradiation.

Clinical Features

Oncocytomas of major salivary glands commonly involve parotid gland. Few tumors are incidentally found in the salivary rests of the upper cervical lymph nodes. Among the minor salivary gland sites, the lower lip, palate, pharynx, and buccal mucosa are commonly involved.

Oncocytomas are frequently reported in the fifth and sixth decades of life with a marked female predilection. Clinically, they present as a single, often multilobulated, well-circumscribed, firm nodule of the superficial lobe of the parotid gland. They are slow growing, painless, and usually 1 to 7 cm in size. Rarely, the tumor presents bilaterally. Pain and swelling have been occasionally reported.

Macroscopic Features

On gross examination, oncocytomas are usually 3 to 4 cm in size and possess a well-defined capsule. The external surface is smooth and may be multilobular or lobulated. The cut surface is white-grey with focal areas of red-brown hemorrhage. Oncocytomas from minor salivary glands are usually solid tumors with an occasional focal cystic component.

Microscopic Features

The tumor is essentially made of tightly packed large oncocytes arranged in a solid or trabecular pattern, rounded groups, diffuse sheets, and rarely glands, with occasional microcyst formation. The cells possess granular, eosinophilic cytoplasm and distinct cell borders. The nuclei are round with dispersed chromatin and prominent nucleoli. Mitoses are rare. The supporting stroma is fine and fibrovascular and may contain lymphoid infiltrate (Figs 7.7A and B).

Rarely, oncocytomas present as large, polyhedral, clear cells with an organoid distribution. Such tumors with a predominant clear cell

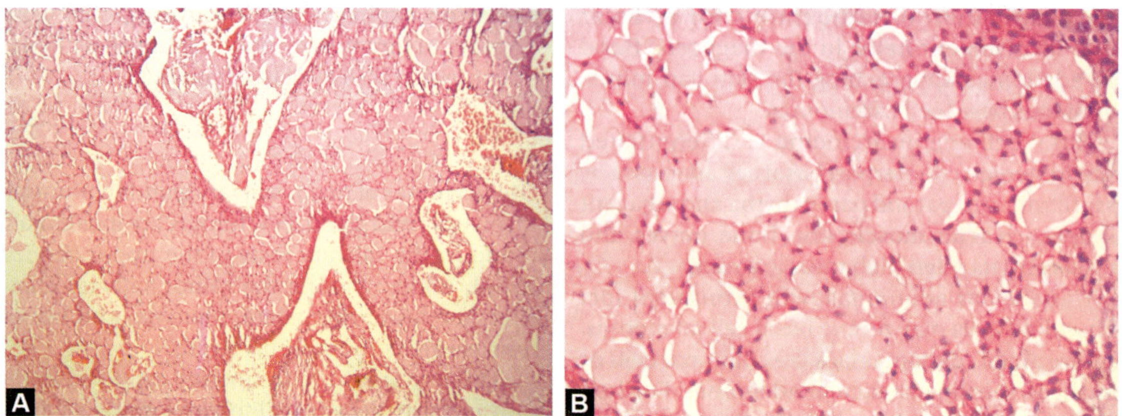

Figures 7.7A and B: Oncocytoma: Oncocytes have large eosinophilic granular cytoplasm and small dark nuclei
(*Courtesy:* Dr TR Saraswathi, Vishnu Dental College, Bhimavaram, Andhra pradesh)

component are referred to as clear-cell oncocytomas. The cytoplasmic clearing is either due to glycogen accumulation which displaces the mitochondria peripherally or might represent an artefactual change. An intimate intermixture of eosinophilic and clear-cell oncocytes can be encountered within the same tumor.

Tyrosine-rich crystals can be sometimes found in the tumor and adjacent striated ducts of some oncocytomas. These eosinophilic crystals are needle-shaped or plate-like. These crystals are seen extracellularly as well as within the oncocytic cells. These crystals are not specific to oncocytomas, but also found in Warthin's tumor and oncocytic cystadenoma. Ultrastructurally, these tyrosine-rich crystals appear as electron-dense structures with periodicity.

Compromise in the vascular supply often leads to infarction, resulting in necrotic cells presenting as ghost shadows or eosinophilic granular material. The residual viable tumor or adjacent salivary epithelium commonly undergoes squamous metaplasia with atypical (reparative) nuclei, mimicking squamous cell carcinoma. This can be overcome by extensive sampling that helps to identify focally better preserved areas.

Histochemistry

The cytoplasm of the tumor cells of oncocytoma is positive for phosphotungstic acid hematoxylin (PTAH). PAS staining before and after diastase digestion reveals a granular cytoplasm representing numerous tightly packed mitochondria. Bensley's aniline-acid fuchsin on frozen tissue stains the cytoplasmic granules of oncocytomas red. A strong Luxolfast-blue reaction and metachromatic staining with thionin and cresyl violet stains have been observed in oncocytomas.

Immunohistochemistry

Immunohistochemical staining with anti-mitochondrial antibody has been claimed to be superior in sensitivity and specificity. Oncocytes stain positively for cytokeratin and negatively for S-100 protein and muscle-specific actin.

Ultrastructure

Ultrastructurally, the mitochondria reveal elongated cristae in the tumor cells and a partial lamellae internal structure. The nuclei of the oncocytes are irregular and reveal inclusions and glycogen granules. The desmosomal cell attachments and basement membrane confirm the epithelial origin of the cells. The microvilli present on cells that border glandular lumens help identify oncocyte as a glandular cell.

Differential Diagnosis

Diffuse oncocytosis is a diffuse, oncocytic metaplastic process in the salivary gland, often associated with atrophy of the surrounding parenchyma. The lobular architecture remains intact however. Nodular oncocytic hyperplasia the parotid gland mimics multinodular oncocytoma. This condition consists of multiple nodular proliferations of closely packed oncocytes. The nodules are less circumscribed and less organized than those of oncocytoma, and a fibrous capsule is lacking. These two conditions along with oncocytoma could be described to represent a spectrum. Making great efforts to differentiate these three possibly related conditions may not be warranted given the similarities in terms of excellent prognosis and treatment.

It is difficult to differentiate oncocytoma from salivary gland tumors which show prominent oncocytic change, most notably Warthin's tumor, pleomorphic adenoma, basal cell adenoma, and mucoepidermoid carcinoma. Pleomorphic architectural patterns, myxochondroid tissue, and proliferation of non-cohesive myoepithelial type cells are typical of pleomorphic adenomas as opposed to oncocytomas. Mucous and squamous cell differentiations are features that characterize mucoepidermoid carcinoma are rare in oncocytomas. Also, the organoid architectural pattern of oncocytomas, positive PTAH staining, and the absence of intracytoplasmic sialomucin, can be useful in differentiating oncocytomas from mucoepidermoid carcinomas.

The arrangement of cells and cytoplasmic granularity may resemble acinic cell carcinoma. But the nuclei of acinic cell carcinoma are peripherally located, in contrast to the central round nuclei in oncocytoma.

Clear cell oncocytomas may be mistaken for clear cell neoplasms such as clear cell carcinoma, clear cell acinic cell adenocarcinoma, epithelial myoepithelial carcinoma, metastatic renal cell carcinoma, and the like. These tumors have characteristic histomorphologic features and are non-reactive with PTAH stain. Metastatic renal cell carcinoma does pose a diagnostic problem, considering the abundance of glycogen and mitochondria. Features such as infiltrative growth, prominent vascularity, and more extensive cellular and nuclear pleomorphism help distinguish metastatic renal cell carcinoma. Further clinical evaluation of the patient for a primary tumor in the kidney is worthy of consideration in such cases.

The pathologist has to remember that cytoplasmic granularity can also result from the presence of secretory granules, lysosomes, and endoplasmic reticulum, besides mitochondrial organelles. Thus in cases of oncocytomas where PTAH reaction is equivocal, ultrastructural observation of the cells might help in confirming the diagnosis.

DUCTAL PAPILLOMAS

Papillary configuration is not uncommon in salivary gland tumors. It might be the principal morphologic pattern as in Warthin's tumor or foci among other morphologic forms such as cystadenoma, acinic cell adenocarcinoma, polymorphous low-grade adenocarcinoma, mucoepidermoid carcinoma, and cystadenocarcinoma. Excluding Warthin's tumor, benign papillary tumors of salivary gland are rare. However, three distinct types of such papillary tumors have been recognized, namely, sialadenoma papilliferum, inverted ductal papilloma, and intraductal papilloma based on their unique histopathologic features.

There has been considerable controversy over the criteria for definition of intraductal papilloma and its differentiation from papillary cystadenomas. Based on our recent understanding, intraductal papilloma can be defined as a unicystic structure that probably represents the dilatation of a salivary gland excretory duct. In the cystic lumen, there is papillary proliferation of the lining ductal epithelium. There is no proliferation of glandular tissue outside this cystic structure.

Sialadenoma Papilliferum

Histogenesis

Various theories have been put forward to explain the histogenesis of sialadenoma papilliferum. The possible cell of origin has been variously reported as the excretory duct reserve cell, intercalated duct cells, extralobular duct cell, or salivary gland excretory duct cell. Based on the location of the tumor, it seems probable that the salivary gland excretory duct cell is the possible cell of origin.

As most of the squamous papillomas of the oral mucosa are being associated with papilloma virus infection in the recent past, there is speculation if sialadenoma papilliferum may also be of viral origin. But till date, no strong evidence points in this direction.

Clinical Features

Sialadenoma papilliferum presents uniquely as an exophytic, papillary surface lesion in contrast to nearly all benign and malignant salivary gland neoplasms, which present as subsurface nodular swellings or masses, covered by smooth, intact mucosa or skin. These exophytic tumors are commonly seen in the minor salivary glands, mostly involving the posterior hard or soft palate and characteristically presenting in the junction of the hard and soft palate. Other sites of involvement include buccal mucosa and retromolar trigone. These asymptomatic tumors usually never exceed one cm in diameter and are commonly reported in the fifth decade of life.

Macroscopic Features

The gross specimen reveals a broad based or pedunculated round to oval, well-circumscribed lesion of the surface mucosa. The surface of the tumor appears verrucous or papillary or rough and often appears reddish. Sections might reveal circumscribed nodules of tumor tissue below the level of the mucosa.

Microscopic Features

These tumors reveal both exophytic and endophytic growth patterns. The surface of the lesion is characterized by numerous papillary projections and folds extending above the level of adjacent mucosa and is covered by parakeratotic, acanthotic, and stratified squamous epithelium. These papillary projections enclose fibrovascular cores that may reveal mild to mixed infiltrate of lymphocytes, plasma cells, and neutrophils. The junction of the proliferating epithelium and the normal mucosal surface epithelium may exhibit pseudoepitheliomatous hyperplasia with wide, rounded rete ridges that push into the lamina propria. The normal mucosal epithelium may either form the stalk of pedunculated tumors or may form a lip or rolled border with more broad-based tumors.

Below the surface papillary projections, the stratified squamous epithelium merges into the ductal epithelium. The ductal epithelium encloses branched duct-like lamina that are continuous with the interpapillary clefts of the surface epithelium. On few occasions, the lining epithelium may form papillary projections into the dilated lumen of the ducts.

The base of the lesion is characterized by proliferation of small ducts. Because these structures are not surrounded by a capsule, it may appear to the untrained eye as if the ductal cells are infiltrating the lamina propria and submucosa.

The ductal epithelium that lines the ducts, cystic areas, and papillary projections is made of double layer of cells. The luminal cells are tall columnar and the basilar cells are small cuboidal. These cells resemble striated and interlobular excretory duct cells due to their prominently eosinophilic cytoplasm. The cells of the ducts at the base of the lesion appear oncocytic, owing to the deep eosinophilic cytoplasm. Mucous cells are occasionally seen.

Ultrastructural Findings

The cells at the tip of the papillary projections are consistent with typical squamous epithelium because of the demonstration of desmosomal attachments and bundles of tonofilaments in these cells. The ductal cells are characterized by numerous mitochondria, nuclei in the apical half of the cell, junctional complexes near the luminal surface, and desmosomal attachments.

Differential Diagnosis

Sialadenoma papilliferum clinically and histologicallly resembles exophytic lesions such as oral squamous cell papilloma commonly, and warty dyskeratoma and incipient verrucous carcinoma. Diagnosis of sialadenoma papilliferum is made on the presence of ductal and glandular proliferations.

Sialadenoma papilliferum and mucoepidermoid carcinoma share features such as mucous cells, squamous cells, ductal cells, cystic structures, and lack of encapsulation. However, features unique to sialadenoma papilliferum such as papillary configuration of the epithelium and the presence of squamous epithelial caps on the papillary fronds are helpful in arriving at the proper diagnosis.

The presence of pseudoepitheliomatous hyperplasia may mimic the appearance seen in necrotizing sialometaplasia. But again, branching and papillary proliferation of ducts and exophytic projections covered by ductal and squamous epithelium is unique to sialadenoma papilliferum. Further, the necrotizing lobules of salivary glands that are characteristic of necrotizing sialometaplasia are absent in sialadenoma papilliferum.

The unique exophytic growth pattern of sialadenoma papilliferum differentiates it from the other ductal papillomas.

Inverted Ductal Papilloma

Clinical Features

Inverted ductal papillomas present as asymptomatic, firm, discrete submucosal nodules, never exceeding 1.5 cm in diameter, with a predilection to involve the minor salivary glands of lower lip and buccal vestibular mucosa. Other common sites include upper lip, floor of the mouth, and soft palate. These tumors are common in the fifth decade of life.

Macroscopic Features

The gross specimen appears well-circumscribed round to oval lesion. The surface is smooth in contrast to sialadenoma papilliferum which has a papillary or verrucous surface.

Microscopic Features

Inverted ductal papilloma bears resemblance to sialadenoma papilliferum in that it occurs within the terminal portion of a minor salivary gland excretory duct. But the morphology is distinctively different. In contrast to the papillary projections of sialadenoma papilliferum, inverted ductal papilloma is characterized by a well-circumscribed tumor mass within the lamina propria, with an epidermoid appearance. The tumor cells are basaloid and squamoid, arranged in thick, bulbous proliferations, that project in papillary projections into the lumen, appearing to fill the cavity. The proliferating epithelium is also seen extending outward into the surrounding lamina propria. A well-demarcated and broad 'pushing' interface with the connective tissue stroma of the lamina propria and the submucosa is seen at the periphery. The proliferation of tumor epithelium in broad papillae into the lumen results in a constricted and branched lumen. This lumen may occasionally communicate by a constricted opening with the exterior of the mucosal surface. In such cases, the stratified squamous epithelium of the mucosal surface forms a lip at the opening and is contiguous with the tumor epithelium. Features of infiltration or invasion that suggest malignancy are never observed.

Other than the basaloid and immature epidermoid cells that make up bulk of the tumor, columnar or cuboidal, duct-like cells with eosinophilic cytoplasm are seen covering the luminal surface of the papillary proliferation.

Mucous cells may also be seen interspersed among these ductal cells.

Differential Diagnosis

Inverted ductal papillomas and inverted papillomas of nasal and paranasal sinuses share features such as papillary, and endophytic proliferation of stratified basal and epidermoid epithelium, intraepithelial microcysts, mucous cells, and columnar and cuboidal cells in areas along the luminal surface. But sinonasal papillomas frequently recur and undergo malignant transformation, features never observed in inverted ductal papillomas. Further, sinonasal papillomas are large lesions, involving extensive areas of the sinonasal mucosa in contrast to inverted ductal papillomas which are small discrete masses that appear to grow by centripetal and centrifugal expansion.

Intraductal Papilloma

Clinical Features

Intraductal papillomas present as asymptomatic, submucosal swellings that vary from 1.0 to 1.5 cm in diameter and are usually reported in the fifth decade. They are commonly found in the upper and lower lips, arising from the minor salivary glands in these areas. Other sites of occurrence include palate, buccal mucosa, parotid gland duct, and submandibular gland duct.

Macroscopic Features

The gross specimen reveals a well circumscribed cyst with a lumen partially or completely filled with friable tissue that extends from the wall of the cyst.

Microscopic Features

Intraductal papillomas arise in the duct system at a much distant site from the mucosal surface compared to the inverted ductal papillomas. They are characterized by dilated unicystic areas, lined by single or double layered cuboidal or columnar epithelium. The proliferating epithelium is characteristic of the ductal epithelium in this location. Multiple, arborising, papillary projections with thin fibrovascular cores are seen projecting into the lumen. In a cross section, the papillary projections have a complex branching structure that creates an appearance of tumor islands floating in the cyst lumen. The papillary projections are covered by the same cuboidal/columnar cells. Mucous cells may be observed as foci among the ductal cells or they may predominate. The epithelium does not proliferate into or beyond the cyst wall. Minimal to moderate inflammatory cell infiltration may be seen within the connective tissue wall.

Differential Diagnosis

Intraductal papilloma has to be differentiated form papillary cystadenoma. Cystadenoma is a benign neoplastic proliferation of salivary gland duct epithelium in the form of multiple epithelium-lined cystic structures. If the epithelium is papillary, it is referred to as papillary cystadenoma. Intraductal papillomas are unicystic structures. Further, the multiple cysts of cystadenoma appear to be proliferating in the supporting connective tissue stroma.

Intraductal papillomas are lined by columnar or cuboidal epithelium and/or mucous cells, whereas inverted ductal papillomas are characterized by epidermoid proliferating epithelium. Further, intraductal papilloma is a well-demarcated cyst, whereas inverted ductal papillomas present with epidermoid epithelium appearing to push into the surrounding stroma on a broad front.

A common salivary gland disorder such as ductal dilatation and hyperplasia of the ductal epithelium due to duct blockage may be considered in the differential diagnosis. But ductal epithelial hyperplasia hardly shows prominent papillary projections or folds. Further, in such duct blockage reactions, inflammation, fibrosis, and atrophy of the subjacent salivary gland lobules is seen.

CYSTADENOMA

Cystadenoma is a rare benign neoplastic proliferation of salivary gland duct epithelium showing unicystic or multicystic growth and focal intraluminal papillary proliferation of the lining epithelium.

Since papillary formation is almost a constant feature, cystadenoma is sometimes referred to as papillary cystadenoma. When oncocytic or mucous metaplasia is prominent, designations such as papillary oncocytic cystadenoma or papillary mucous cystadenoma can be applied.

Clinical Features

Cystadenomas most frequently involve the minor salivary glands compared to the major salivary glands. The common sites of occurrence are the lips and the buccal mucosa, unlike the other minor salivary gland tumors which are common in the palate.

Cystadenomas are commonly seen in the old age with a marked female predilection. The tumors present as well-circumscribed, slow-growing, painless, slightly compressible swellings, never exceeding one centimeter in diameter. Tumor in the oral cavity may present as smooth surfaced nodules, resembling mucoceles.

Macroscopic Features

The gross specimen reveals multiple cystic spaces or a single cyst, into which there may be nodular projections. The tumor is well circumscribed, with or without a capsule.

Microscopic Features

Cystadenomas are well-circumscribed tumors that are occasionally encapsulated. They are characterized by various-sized cystic structures that enclose proteinaceous fluid, psammoma bodies, or crystalloids. The epithelium lining the ducts may be made of cuboidal or columnar cells with uniform nuclei. Further, the lining which is usually two to three cells thick, might abruptly become focally thickened or form ramifying papillary projections with central cores of connective tissue. Extraluminal sheet-like growth is limited in cystadenomas. Mitoses are extremely rare in the epithelial cells. Rare areas of melanin deposition and occasional foci of oncocytes and mucous cells may be observed in the lining epithelium. The supporting stroma is dense and fibrous with scattered inflammatory cells.

Differential Diagnosis

Cystadenomas with oncocytic epithelium (papillary oncocytic cystadenomas) can be differentiated from Warthin's tumor by the absence of bilayered epithelium, by the presence of other types of epithelial cells admixed with the oncocytic cells and by the lack of a diffuse and dense lymphoid stroma with germinal centers.

Features such as squamous metaplasia, chronic inflammation, acinar atrophy, fibrosis, and periductal hyalinization differentiate ductal ectasia with focal epithelial proliferation from cystadenomas.

Intraductal papilloma has to be differentiated from papillary cystadenoma. Intraductal papillomas are always unicystic structures. Further, the multiple cysts of cystadenoma appear to be proliferating in the supporting connective tissue stroma.

Cystadenocarcinoma manifests frank invasion of surrounding tissues as compared to cystadenomas.

Mucoepidermoid carcinomas are differentiated from cystadenomas by the markedly thickened epithelial lining and the presence of squamous, mucous, and basaloid cells in mucoepidermoid carcinoma.

Papillary cystic patterns are very common in acinic cell adenocarcinomas. But the microcystic pattern, less uniformity of the lining epithelium, presence of large serous, acinar cells, at least focally, and cords of tumor, are features characteristic of acinic cell carcinomas and not found in cystadenomas.

Polycystic disease of the parotid gland microscopically resembles cystadenoma, but is distinguished by the more diffuse involvement of the salivary gland lobules, focal apocrine-like lining epithelial cells, and the unique presence of congophilic and eosinophilic spheroliths with concentric laminations or radial structures.

SEBACEOUS ADENOMA AND SEBACEOUS LYMPHADENOMA

Sebaceous adenomas and lymphadenomas are exceptionally rare tumors, arising almost exclusively in the parotid gland. It is of significance that the sebaceous tumors are rare in spite of the fact that sebaceous cells are relatively common in both the parotid and submandibular salivary glands.

These tumors are well-encapsulated or sharply circumscribed and vary in size from one to three centimeter. They present as asymptomatic, slow-growing masses. The average age of occurrence is approximately 60 years.

Macroscopically, the sebaceous adenomas vary in color from grayish-white to pinkish-white to yellow or yellowish-gray.

Microscopically, sebaceous adenoma is made of multiple incompletely differentiated sebaceous lobules accompanied by a fibrous stroma. Each lobule consists of groups of mature sebaceous cells surrounded by basaloid cells. Cells intermediate between these two cell types can also been observed. The sebaceous cells contain small honeycombed vacuoles of lipid that can be identified by an oil red O stain on frozen sections. Focal areas of squamous, mucous, or oncocytes arising due to metaplasia can be observed. The mature sebaceous cells may disintegrate resulting in the formation of cystic spaces within the lobule. These cystic structures lined by squamous, columnar, or cuboidal cells, with or without sebaceous cells. The well-differentiated sebaceous cells show either no or only minimal cellular atypia or pleomorphism, with practically no tendency for local invasion. The supporting stroma can be infiltrated by copious inflammatory cells, including lipogranuloma formation, probably in response to extravasated sebum.

Sebaceous lymphadenomas bear resemblance to Warthin's tumor. They are microscopically similar to sebaceous adenomas, except that lymphoid follicles and lymphocytes are seen intimately mixed with the sebaceous elements. It has been postulated that sebaceous lympha-denomas, originate from ectopic salivary gland in parotid lymph node.

It is to be noted that tumors such as pleomorphic adenoma, Warthin's tumor, and mucoepidermoid carcinoma may also show focal sebaceous differentiation.

LIPOADENOMA

Lipoadenoma is a recently reported, extremely rare tumor of the major salivary glands. This well-circumscribed, occasionally encapsulated tumor characterized by proliferated mature adipose cells, among which are interspersed sertoliform narrow tubules or acini. The tubules are lined by uniform columnar cells supported by an outer layer of basal cells. The oncocytic variant of Lipoadenoma shows an oncocytic change.

LYMPHADENOMA

Lymphadenoma is a rare benign epithelial tumor of salivary glands bearing considerable resemblance to sebaceous lymphadenomas, except for the absence of the sebaceous component. It is characterized by solid to cystic epithelial islands with bland cytomorphology, dispersed in a dense lymphoid stroma. This tumor has been often misinterpreted as metastatic carcinoma in lymph node.

BIBLIOGRAPHY

1. Agnantis NJ, Maounis N, Priovolou-Papaevangelou M, Baltatzis I. Pleomorphic adenoma of the human female breast. Pathol Res Pract 1992;188:235-40.
2. Andreadis D, Epivatianos A, Mireas G, Nomikos A, Poulopoulos A, Yiotakis J, Barbatis C. Immuno-histochemical detection of E-cadherin in certain types of salivary gland tumours. J Laryngol Otol. 2006;120(4):298-304.
3. Anjum K, Revington PJ, Irvine GH. Superficial pa-rotidectomy: Antegrade compared with modified retrograde dissections of the facial nerve. Br J Oral Maxillofac Surg. 2008;46(6):433-4.
4. Araújo VC, Demasi AP, Furuse C, Altemani A, Alves VA, Freitas LL, Araújo NS. Collagen type I may influence the expression of E-cadherin and beta-catenin in carcinoma ex-pleomorphic adenoma.

Appl Immunohistochem Mol Morphol. 2009; 17(4):312-8.

5. Auclair PL, Ellis GL. Major salivary glands. In: Silverberg SG, DeLellis RA, Frable WJ (Eds). Principles and practice of surgical pathology and cytopathology. 3rd edn. New York: Churchill Livingstone; 1997. pp. 1463-73, 1505-8.

6. Auclair PL, Ellis GL Atypical features in salivary gland mixed tumors: Their relationship to malignant transformation. Mod Pathol. 1996; 9:652–7.

7. Auclair PL, Ellis GL, Gnepp DR, Wenig BM, Janney CG. Salivary gland neoplasms: General considerations. In: Ellis GL, Auclair PL, Gnepp DR (Eds). Surgical pathology of the salivary glands. 1st edn. Philadelphia: WB Saunders Company; 1991. pp. 135-64.

8. Auclair PL, Ellis GL, Gnepp DR. Other benign epithelial neoplasms. In: Ellis GL, Auclair PL, Gnepp DR (Eds). Surgical pathology of the salivary glands. 1st edn. Philadelphia: WB Saunders Company; 1991. pp. 252-68.

9. Bablani D, Bansal S, Shetty SJ, Desai R, Kulkarni SR, Prasad P, Karjodkar FR. Pleomorphic adenoma of the cheek: A case report and review. J Oral Maxillofac Surg 2009;67(7):1539-42.

10. Badia L, Weir JN, Robinson AC. Heterotopic pleomorphic adenoma of the external nose. J Laryngol Otol 1996;110:376-8.

11. Badia L, Weir JN, Robinson AC. Heterotopic pleomorphic adenoma of the external nose. J Laryngol Otol 1996;110:376-8.

12. Barnes L, Brandwein M, Som PM. Surgical Pathology of the Head and Neck. 2nd edn. Marcel Dekker Inc: New York, 2001.

13. Barnes L, Eveson JW, Reichart P, Sidransky D. World Health Organization Classification of Tumours. Pathology and Genetics of Head and Neck Tumours. Salivary glands. Lyon, IARC Press, 2005;5.

14. Batrani M, Kaushal M, Sen AK, Yadav R, Chaturvedi NK. Pleomorphic adenoma with squamous and appendageal metaplasia mimicking mucoepidermoid carcinoma on cytology. Cytojournal 2008;6:5.

15. Batsakis JG, Luna MA, el-Naggar AK. Basaloid monomorphic adenomas. Ann Otol Rhinol Laryngol 1991;100:687-90.

16. Batsakis JG. Tumors of the head and neck: Clinical and pathological considerations, 2nd edn. Baltimore, MD: Williams and Wilkins, 1979.

17. Bradley PJ. Benign salivary gland disease. Hosp Med 2001;62:392-5.

18. Brandewein MS, Huvos AG. Oncocytic tumours of major salivary glands. A study of 68 cases with follow-up of 44 patients. Am J Surg Pathol 1991;15:514-28.

19. Brandwein M, Al-Naeif NS, Manwani D, Som P, Goldfeder L, Rothschild M, Granowetter L. Sialoblastoma: Clinicopathological/immunohistochemical study. Am J Surg Pathol 1999;23(3): 342-8.

20. Breeze J, Andi A, Williams MD, Howlett DC. The use of fine needle core biopsy under ultrasound guidance in the diagnosis of a parotid mass. Br J Oral Maxillofac Surg. 2009;47(1):78-9.

21. Bullerdiek J, Wobst G, Meyer-Bolte K, et al. Cytogenetic subtyping of 220 pleomorphic adenomas: Correlation to occurrence, histological subtype, and in vitro cellular behaviour. Cancer Genet Cytogenet 1993;65:27-31.

22. Calearo C, Pastore A. Parotid carcinoma. In: Hermarek P, Gospodarowicz M, Henson D, Hutter R, Sobin L (Eds). Prognostic factors in cancer. Berlin: Springer-Verlag; 1995. pp. 23-7.

23. Canalis RF, Mok MW, Fishman SM, Hemenway WG. Congenital basal cell adenoma of the submandibular gland. Arch Otolaryngol 1980;106:284-6.

24. Cavaliéri Gomes C, da Silveira e Oliveira C, Santos Pimenta LG, De Marco L, Santiago Gomez R. Immunolocalization of DNMT1 and DNMT3a in salivary gland neoplasms. Pathobiology. 2009; 76(3):136-40.

25. Chan JK, Tang SK, Tsang WY, Lee KC, Batsakis JG. Histologic changes induced by fine- needle aspiration. Adv Ana Pathol 1996;3:71-90.

26. Chan JK, Yip TT, Tsang WY, Poon YF, Wong CS, Ma VW. Specific association of Epstein-Barr virus with lymphoepithelial carcinoma among tumours and tumorlike lesions of the Salivary gland. Arch Pathol Lab Med 1994;118:994-7.

27. Chapnik J. The controversy of Warthin's tumor. Laryngoscope 1983;93:695-716.

28. Cheuk W, Chan JKC. Salivary gland tumours. In: Fletcher CDM (Ed). Diagnostic Histopathology of Tumours, 2/e (Vol 1), Churchill Livingstone; 2002. pp. 233-63, 290-307.

29. Daneshbod Y, Daneshbod K, Khademi B. Diagnostic difficulties in the interpretation of fine needle aspirate samples in salivary lesions: Diagnostic pitfalls revisited. Acta Cytol. 2009; 53(1):53-70.

30. Dardick I, Cavell S, Boivin M, et al. Salivary gland myoepithelioma variants. Histological, ultra-structural, and immunocytological features. Virchow's Arch [A] Pathol Anat Histopathol 1989;416:25-42.

31. Dardick I, Cavell S, Boivin M, et al. Salivary gland myoepithelioma variants. Histological, ultra-structural, and immunocytological features. Virchow's Arch [A] Pathol Anat Histopathol 1989;416:25-42.

32. Dardick I, Daley TD, van Nostrand AW. Basal cell adenoma with myoepithelial cell-derived "stroma": A new major salivary gland tumor entity. Head Neck Surg 1986;8:257-67

33. Dardick I, Thomas MJ, van Nostrand AW. Myoepithelioma-new concepts of histology and classification: a light and electron microscopic study. Ultrastruct Pathol 1989;13:187-224.

34. Darling MR, Jackson-Boeters L, Daley TD, Diamandis EP. Human kallikrein 13 expression in salivary gland tumors. Int J Biol Markers. 2006;21(2):106-10.

35. De Araujo VC, de Sousa SO, Carvalho YR, et al. Application of immunohistochemistry to the diagnosis of salivary gland tumors. Appl. Immunohistochem. Mol. Morph 2000;8:195–202.

36. De Araujo VC, de Sousa SO. Expression of different keratins in salivary gland tumours. Eur J Cancer B Oral Oncol 1996;32:14-8.

37. De Araújo VC, Furuse C, Cury PR, Altemani A, de Araújo NS. STAT3 expression in salivary gland tumours. Oral Oncol 2008;44(5):439-45.

38. Declercq J, Van Dyck F, Van Damme B, Van de Ven WJ. Upregulation of Igf and Wnt signalling associated genes in pleomorphic adenomas of the salivary glands in PLAG1 transgenic mice. Int J Oncol. 2008;32(5):1041-7.

39. DeRoche TC, Hoschar AP, Hunt JL. Immuno-histochemical evaluation of androgen receptor, HER-2/neu, and p53 in benign pleomorphic adenomas. Arch Pathol Lab Med 2008;132 (12):1907-11.

40. Di Palma S, Simpson RHW, Skalova A, Leivo I. Major and minor salivary glands. In: Pathology of the head and neck. Cardesa A, Slootweg PJ (Eds). Springer Verlag, 2006;5:132-7.

41. Doi Y, Kawamata H, Ono Y, Fujimori T, Imai Y. Expression and cellular localization of TSC-22 in normal salivary glands and salivary gland tumors: implications for tumor cell differentiation. Oncol Rep 2008;19(3):609-16.

42. Ellis GL, Auclair PL. Ductal papillomas. In: Ellis GL, Auclair PL, Gnepp DR (Eds). Surgical pathology of the salivary glands. 1st edn. Philadelphia: WB Saunders Company; 1991. pp. 238-51.

43. Ellis GL, Auclair PL, Gnepp DR. Surgical pathology of the salivary glands. 1st edn. Philadelphia: WB Saunders Company, 1991.

44. Ellis GL, Auclair Pl. Major Salivary Glands. In: Silverberg SG, DeLellis RA, Frable WJ (Eds). Principles and Practice of Surgical Pathology and Cytopathology, 3/e (Vol 2), Churchill Livingstone, 1997.

45. Ellis GL, Auclair PL. Tumours of the salivary glands. 3rd edn. Armed Forces Institute of Pathology: Washington, 1996.

46. Ellis GL. "Clear cell" oncocytoma of salivary gland. Hum Pathol 1988;19:862-7.

47. El-Naggar AK, Hurr K, Kagan J. Gillenwater A, Callender D, Luna MA, Batsakis JG. Genotypic Alterations in Benign and Malignant Salivary Gland Tumors: Histogenetic and Clinical Implications. Am J Surg Pathol 1997;21:691-7.

48. Eneroth C. Salivary gland tumours in the parotid, submandibular, and the palate region. Cancer 1971;27:1415-8.

49. Eneroth CM, Franzen S, Zajicek J. Aspiration biopsy of salivary gland tumors. A critical review of 910 biopsies. Acta Cytol 1967;11(6):470-2.

50. Eveson JW, Cawson RA. Infarcted ("infected") adenolymphomas. A clinicopathologic study of 20 cases. Clin Otolaryngol 1989;14:205-10.

51. Eveson JW, Cawson RA. Infarcted ("infected") adenolymphomas. A clinicopathologic study of 20 cases. Clin Otolaryngol 1989;14:205-10.

52. Frankenthaler RA, Luna MA, Lee SS, et al. Prognostic variables in parotid gland tumors. Arch Otolaryngol Head Neck Surg 1991;117:1251-6.

53. Fukuda M, Hiroi M, Suzuki S, Ohmori Y, Sakashita H. Loss of CYLD might be associated with development of salivary gland tumors. Oncol Rep 2008;19(6):1421-7.

54. Fukuda M, Kusama K, Sakashita H. Cimetidine inhibits salivary gland tumor cell adhesion to neural cells and induces apoptosis by blocking NCAM expression. BMC Cancer 2008;8:376.

55. Geurts JM, Schoenmakers EF, Roijer E, Astrom AK, Stenman G, van de Ven WJ. Identification of NFêB as recurrent translocation partner gene of HMGIC in pleomorphic adenomas. Oncogene 1998;16: 865-72.

56. Geurts JM, Schoenmakers EF, Roijer E, Stenman G, van de Ven WJ. Identification of NFêB as recurrent hybrid transcripts of HMGIC and FHIT in a pleomorphic adenoma of the parotid gland. Cancer Res 1998;57:13-7.

57. Gilcrease MZ, Nelson FS, Guzman-Paz M. Tyrosine-rich crystals associated with oncocytic salivary gland neoplasms. Arch Pathol Lab Med 1998; 122:644-9.

58. Gnepp DR, Brandenwein MS, Henley JD. Salivary and lacrimal glands. In: Gnepp DR (Ed). Diagnostic surgical pathology of the head and neck. WB Saunders, Philadelphia, 2001.

59. Gnepp DR. Diagnostic Surgical Pathology of the Head and Neck. WB Saunders: Philadelphia, 2001.

60. Gnepp DR. Sebaceous neoplasms of salivary gland origin: A review. Pathol Annu 1983;18:71-102.

61. Goode RK. Oncocytoma. In: Ellis GL, Auclair PL, Gnepp DR (Eds). Surgical pathology of the salivary glands. 1st edn. Philadelphia: WB Saunders Company; 1991.pp.225-37.

62. Grisius MM, Fox PC. Salivary gland diseases. In: Greenberg MS, Glick M (Eds). Burket's Oral Medicine Diagnosis and Treatment. BC Decker Inc, Ontario, 2003.

63. Gürbüz Y, Yildiz K, Aydin O, Almaç A. Immuno-phenotypical profiles of salivary gland tumours: A new evidence for their histogenetic origin. Pathologica 2006;98(2):147-52.

64. Guo Y, Yang MC, Weissler JC, Yang YS. Modulation of PLAGL2 transactivation activity by Ubc9 co-activation not SUMOylation. Biochem Biophys Res Commun 2008;374(3):570-5.

65. Handa U, Dhingra N, Chopra R, Mohan H. Pleomorphic adenoma: Cytologic variations and potential diagnostic pitfalls. Diagn Cytopathol. 2009;37(1):11-5.

66. Hickman RE, Cawson RA, Duffy SW. The prognosis of specific type of salivary gland tumors. Cancer 1992;54:1620-54.

67. Hirokawa M, Shimizu M, Manabe T, Ito J, Ogawa S. Oncocytic lipoadenoma of the submandibular gland. Hum Pathol 1998;29:410-2.

68. Hoch BL, Wu M, Lewis M, Gan L, Burstein DE. An immunohistochemical study of XIAP expression in pleomorphic adenoma and carcinoma ex-pleomorphic adenoma. J Oral Pathol Med 2008;37(10):634-8.

69. Horiuchi C, Tsukuda M, Taguchi T, Ishiguro Y, Okudera K, Inoue T. Correlation between FDG-PET findings and GLUT1 expression in salivary gland pleomorphic adenomas. Ann Nucl Med 2008;22(8):693-8.

70. Hseuh C, Gonzalez-Crussi F. Sialoblastoma: A case report and review of the literature on congenital epithelial tumours of salivary gland origin. Pediatr Pathol 1992;12:205-14.

71. Huvos AG, Paulino AFG. Salivary glands. In: Sternberg SS, Antonioli DA, Carter D, Mills SE, Oberman HA (Eds). Diagnostic surgical pathology. 3rd edn. Philadelphia: Lippincott Williams and Wilkins; 1999. pp. 857-80.

72. Jansisyanont P, Blanchaert Jr RH, Ord RA. Intraoral minor salivary gland neoplasm: A single institution experience of 80 cases. Int J Oral Maxillofac Surg 2002;31:257–61.

73. Kas K, Voz ML, Roijer E, et al. Promoter swapping between the genes for a novel zinc finger protein and beta-catenin in pleomorphic adenomas with t(3;8)(p21;q12) translocations. Nat Genet 1997;15:170-4.

74. Kilpatrick SE, Hitchcock MG, Kraus MD, Calonje E, Feltcher CDM. Mixed tumors and myoepi-theliomas of soft tissue: A clinicopathologic study of 19 cases with a unifying concept. Am J Surgical Pathol 1997;21:13-22.

75. Klijanienho J, Vielh P. Salivary gland tumours: Monographs in clinical cytology. Karger: Basel, 2000;15.

76. Kondo T. A case of lipomatous pleomorphic adenoma in the parotid gland. Diagn Pathol. 2009;4(1):16.

77. Kotwell C. Smoking as an etiologic factor in the development of Warthin's tumour of the parotid gland. Am J Surg 1992;164:646-7.

78. Kratochvil FJ. Canalicular adenoma and basal cell adenoma. In: Ellis GL, Auclair PL, Gnepp DR (Eds). Surgical pathology of the salivary glands. 1st edn. Philadelphia: WB Saunders Company; 1991. pp. 203-24.

79. Lam KH, Wei WI, Ho HC, Ho CM. Whole organ sectioning of mixed parotid tumors. Am J Surg 1990;160:377-81.

80. Lee KC, Chan JK, Chong YW. Ossifying pleomorphic adenoma of the maxillary antrum. J Laryngol Otol 1992;106:50-2.

81. Lewis JE, Olsen KD, Sebo TJ. Carcinoma ex-pleomorphic adenoma: Pathologic analysis of 73 cases. Hum Pathol 2001;32(6):596-604

82. Li Y, Li LJ, Huang J, Han B, Pan J. Central malignant salivary gland tumors of the jaw: retrospective clinical analysis of 22 cases. J Oral Maxillofac Surg. 2008;66(11):2247-53.

83. Little JW. The histogenesis of papillary cystadenoma lymphomatosum. Oral Surg Oral Med Oral Pathol 1966;22:72-81.

84. Lopes MA, Kowalski LP, da Cunha Santos G, Paes de Almeida O. A clinicopathologic study of 196 intraoral minor salivary gland tumours. J Oral Pathol Med 1999;28:264-7.

85. Mantravadi J, Roth L, Kafrawy A. Vascular neoplasms of the parotid gland. Parotid vascular tumors. Oral Surg Oral Med Oral Pathol 1993;75:70-5.

86. Manucha V, Ioffe OB. Metastasizing pleomorphic adenoma of the salivary gland. Arch Pathol Lab Med. 2008;132(9):1445-7.

87. Mardi K, Sharma J. Oncocytic pleomorphic adenoma of the parotid gland. Indian J Pathol Microbiol 2007;50(4):840-1.

88. Maruyama S, Cheng J, Yamazaki M, Liu A, Saku T. Keratinocyte growth factor colocalized with perlecan at the site of capsular invasion and vascular involvement in salivary pleomorphic adenomas. J Oral Pathol Med 2009;38(4):377-85.

89. McDaniel RK. Benign mesenchymal neoplasms. In: Ellis GL, Auclair PL, Gnepp DR (Eds). Surgical pathology of the salivary glands. 1st edn. Philadelphia: WB Saunders Company; 1991. pp. 489-513.

90. Meer S, Altini M. CK7+/CK20- immunoexpression profile is typical of salivary gland neoplasia. Histopathology. 2007;51(1):26-32.

91. Monk JJ, Church J. Warthin's tumour. A high incidence and no sex predominance in central Pennsylvania. Arch Otolaryngol Head Neck Surg 1992;118:477-8.

92. Mostafapour SP, Folz B, Barlow D, Manning S. Sialoblastoma of the submandibular gland: Report of a case and review of the literature. Int J Pediatr Otorhinolaryngol 2000;53(2):157-61.

93. Muramatsu K, Kusafuka K, Watanabe H, Mochizuki T, Nakajima T. Ultrastructural immunolocalization of a cartilage-specific proteoglycan, aggrecan, in salivary pleomorphic adenomas. Med Mol Morphol 2009;42(1):47-54.

94. Nagarkar NM, Bansal S, Dass A, Singhal SK, Mohan H. Salivary gland tumours-Our experience. Indian J Otolaryngol Head Neck Surg 2004;56:31-4.

95. Navarro Rde L, Martins MT, de Araujo VC. Maspin expression in normal and neoplastic salivary gland. J Oral Pathol Med 2004;33:435-40.

96. Neville BW, Damm DD, Allen CM, Bouquot JE. Oral and Maxillofacial Pathology, 2nd edn, WB Saunders Co., 2002.

97. Nordkvist A, Roijer E, Bang G, Gustafsson H, Behrendt M, Ryd W, Thoresen S, Donath K, Stenman G. Expression and mutation patterns of p53 in benign and malignant salivary gland tumours. Int J Oncol 2000;16(3):477-83.

98. Ogata T, Hongfang Y, Kayano T, Hirai K. No significant role of Epstein-Barr virus in the tumorigenesis of Warthin's tumour. J Med Dent Sci 1997;44:45-52.

99. Palmer TJ, Gleeson MJ, Eveson JW, Cawson RA. Oncocytic adenomas and oncocytic hyperplasia of salivary glands: A clinicopathologic study of 26 cases. Histopathology 1990;16:487-93.

100. Pantelis A, Wenghoefer M, Haas S, Merkelbach-Bruse S, Pantelis D, Jepsen S, Bootz F, Winter J. Down regulation and nuclear localization of human beta-defensin-1 in pleomorphic adenomas of salivary glands. Oral Oncol 2009;45(6):526-30.

101. Persson F, Andrén Y, Winnes M, Wedell B, Nordkvist A, Gudnadottir G, Dahlenfors R, Sjögren H, Mark J, Stenman G. High-resolution genomic profiling of adenomas and carcinomas of the salivary glands reveals amplification, rearrangement, and fusion of HMGA2. Genes Chromosomes Cancer 2009;48(1):69-82.

102. Perzin KH. A systematic approach to the diagnosis of salivary gland tumours. In: Fenoglio CM, Wolff M (Eds). Progress in surgical pathology. New York: Masson; 1982;4:137-80.

103. Pinkston JA, Cole P. Cigarette smoking and Warthin's tumor. Am J Epidemiol 1996;144:183-7.

104. Pinkston JA, Cole P. Incidence rates of salivary gland tumours: Results from a population-based study. Otolaryngol Head Neck Surg 1999;120(6):834-40.

105. Ponniah I, SureshKumar P, Karunakaran K, Shankar KA, Kumaran MG, Preeti LN. Hemangioma in minor salivary glands: Real or illusion. Diagnostic Pathology 2006;1:21.

106. Prabhu S, Kaveri H, Rekha K. Benign and malignant salivary gland tumors: Comparison of immunohistochemical expression of e-cadherin. Oral Oncol. 2009;45(7):594-9.

107. Prasad AR, Savera AT, Regezi JA, Gown AM, Zarbo RJ. Immunohistochemcal demonstration of myoepithelial cell participation in salivary gland basal cell and canalicular adenomas. Mod Pathol 1999;12:130A (abstract).

108. Pusztaszeri M, Braunschweig R, Mihaescu A. Pleomorphic adenoma with predominant plasma-cytoid myoepithelial cells: A diagnostic pitfall in aspiration cytology. Case report and review of the literature. Diagn Cytopathol 2009;37(1):56-60.

109. Queimado L, Obeso D, Hatfield MD, Yang Y, Thompson DM, Reis AM. Dysregulation of Wnt pathway components in human salivary gland tumors. Arch Otolaryngol Head Neck Surg 2008;134(1):94-101.

110. Qureshi A, Barakzai A, Sahar NU, Gulzar R, Ahmad Z, Hassan SH. Spectrum of malignancy in mixed tumors of salivary gland: A morphological and immunohistochemical review of 23 cases. Indian J Pathol Microbiol 2009;52(2):150-4.

111. Rajendran R, Sivapathasundharam B. Diseases of salivary gland. In: Shafer's textbook of oral pathology, 5th edn. Elsevier, 2005.

112. Sadetzki S, Oberman B, Mandelzweig L, Chetrit A, Ben-Tal T, Jarus-Hakak A, Duvdevani S, Cardis E, Wolf M. Smoking and risk of parotid gland tumors: A nationwide case-control study. Cancer 2008;112(9):1974-82.

113. Sakamoto K, Ono T, Nakamura Y, Harada H, Nakashima T. Expression of cluster of differentiation 9 glycoprotein in benign and malignant parotid gland tumours. J Laryngol Otol. 2009;123(31):58-63.

114. Saku T, Hayashi Y, Takahara O, et al. Salivary gland tumours among atomic bomb survivors, 1950-1987. Cancer 1997;79:1465-75.

115. Savera AT, Gown AM, Zarbo RJ. Immuno-localization of three novel smooth muscle-specific proteins in salivary gland pleomorphic adenoma: Assessment of morphogenetic role of myoe-pithelium. Mod Pathol 1997;10:1093-100.

116. Schwarz S, Ettl T, Kleinsasser N, Hartmann A, Reichert TE, Driemel O. Loss of Maspin expression is a negative prognostic factor in common salivary gland tumors. Oral Oncol 2008;44(6):563-70.

117. Seifert G, Brocheriou C, Cardesa A, Eveson JW. WHO International Histological classification of tumors. Tentative histological classification of salivary gland tumors. Pathol Res Pract 1990;186: 555-81.

118. Seifert G, Bull HG, Donath K. Histologic subclassification of the cystadenolymphoma of the parotid gland. Analysis of 275 cases. Virchow's Arch [A] 1980;388:13-38.

119. Seifert G, Miehlke A, Haubrich J, Chillar R. Disease of the salivary glands. Stuttgart: George Thieme; 1986.

120. Seifert G, Sobin LH. Histological typing of salivary gland tumors. World Health Organization international histological classification of tumors. 2nd edn. New York: Springer-Verlag; 1991.

121. Seifert G, Sobin LH. The World Health Organi-zation's Histological classification of salivary gland tumors. A commentary on the Cancer 2nd edn. 1992;70:379-85.

122. Seifert G. Tumor- like lesions of salivary glands. The new WHO classification. Pathol Res Pract 1992;188:836-46.

123. Shigeishi H, Yoneda S, Taki M, Nobumori T, Ohta K, Higashikawa K, Yasui W, Kamata N. Correlation of human Bub1 expression with tumor-proliferating activity in salivary gland tumors. Oncol Rep 2006;15(4):933-8.

124. Shintaku M, Honda T. Identification of oncocytic lesions of salivary glands by anti-mitochondrial immunohistochemistry. Histopathology 1997;31: 408-11.

125. Siddiqi SH, Solomon MP, Haller JO. Sialoblastoma and hepatoblastoma in a neonate. Pediatr Radiol 2000;30(5):349-51.

126. Simpson RH, Jones H. Beasley P. Benign myoepithelioma of the salivary glands. A true entity? Histopathology 1995;27:1-9.

127. Skalova A, Leivo I, Michal M, Saksela E. Analysis of collagen isotypes in crystalloid structures of salivary gland tumours. Hum Pathol 1992;23:748-54.

128. Skalova A, Michal M, Ryska A, Simpson RHW, Kinkor Z, Walter J, Leivo I. Oncocytic myoepi-thelioma and pleomorphic adenoma of the salivary glands. Virchows arch 1999;1434:537-46.

129. Skalova A, Simpson RH, Lehtonen H, Leivo I. Assessment of proliferative activity using the MIB1 antibody helps to distinguish polymorphous low adenocarcinoma from adenoid cystic carcinoma of salivary glands. Pathol Res Pract 1997;193:695-703.

130. Smith BC, Ellis GL, Meis-Kindblom JM, Williams SB. Ectomesenchymal chondromyxoid tumour of the anterior tongue. Nineteen cases of a new clinicopathologic entity. Am J Surg Pathol 1995;19:519-30.

131. Speight PM, Barrett AW. Salivary gland tumours. Oral Dis 2002;8(5):229-40.

132. Spiro RH. Salivary neoplasms: Overview of a 35-year experience with 2,802 patients. Head Neck Surg 1986;8:177-84.

133. Subhashraj K. Salivary gland tumors: A single institution experience in India. Br J Oral Maxillofac Surg 2008;46:635-8.

134. Sweeney EC, Mc Dermott M. Pleomorphic adenoma of the bronchus. J Clin Pathol 1996;49: 87-89.

135. Takahashi H, Fujita S, Okabe H, Tsuda N, Tezuka F. Immunohistochemical characterization of basal cell adenomas of the salivary gland. Pathol Res Pract 1991;187:145-56.

136. Taxy JB. Necrotizing squamous / mucinous metaplasia in oncocytic salivary gland tumours. A potential diagnostic problem. Am j Clin Pathol 1992;97:40-5.

137. Thompson AS, Bryant HC. Histogenesis of papillary cystadenoma lymphomatosum (Warthin's tumor) of the parotid salivary gland. Am J Pathol 1950; 26:807-49.

138. Thompson LD, Wenig BM, Ellis GL. Oncocytomas of the submandibular gland. A series of 22 cases and a review of the literature. Cancer 1996; 78:2281-7.

139. Tobón-Arroyave SI, Flórez-Moreno GA, Jaramillo-Cárdenas JF, Arango-Uribe JD, Isaza-Guzmán DM, Rendón-Henao J. Expression of hMLH1 and hMSH2 proteins in pleomorphic adenoma of minor salivary glands: Relationship with clinical and histologic findings. Oral Surg Oral Med Oral Pathol Oral Radiol Endod. 2009;108(2):227-36.

140. Toida M, Shimokawa K, Makita1 H, et al. Intraoral minor salivary gland tumors: A clinicopathological study of 82 cases. Int J Oral Maxillofac Surg 2005;34:528–32.

141. Tyagi N, Abdi U, Tyagi SP, Maheshwari V, Gogi R, Pleomorphic adenoma of skin (chondroid syringoma) involving the eye lid. J Postgrad Med 1996;42:125-6.

142. Vargas H, Sudilovsky D, Kaplan MJ, Regezi J, Weidner N. Mixed tumor, polymorphous low grade adenocarcinoma, and adenoid cystic carcinoma of the salivary gland: Pathogenic implications and differential diagnosis by Ki67 {MIB1}, BCL2, and S100 immunohistochemistry. Appl Immuno-histochem 1997;5:8-16.

143. Vargas PA, Cheng Y, Barrett AW, Craig GT, Speight PM. Expression of Mcm-2, Ki-67 and geminin in benign and malignant salivary gland tumours. J Oral Pathol Med 2008;37:309-18.

144. Vargas PA, Speight PM, Bingle CD, Barrett AW, Bingle L. Expression of PLUNC family members in benign and malignant salivary gland tumours. Oral Dis. 2008;14(7):613-9.

145. Vargas PA, Torres-Rendon A, Speight PM. DNA ploidy analysis in salivary gland tumours by image cytometry. J Oral Pathol Med. 2007;36(6):371-6.

146. Vawter G, Tefft M. Congenital tumours of the parotid gland. Arch Pathol 1966;82:242-5.

147. Waldron CA. Mixed tumor (Pleomorphic adenoma) and myoepithelioma. In: Ellis GL, Auclair PL, Gnepp DR (Eds). Surgical pathology of the salivary glands. 1st edn. Philadelphia: WB Saunders Company; 1991. pp. 165-86.

148. Wang D, Li Y, He H, Liu L, Wo L, He Z. Intraoral minor salivary gland tumors in a Chinese population: A retrospective study on 737 cases. Oral Surg Oral Med Oral Pathol Oral Radiol Endod 2007;104:94-100.

149. Warnock GR. Papillary cystadenoma lympho-matosum (Warthin's tumour). In: Ellis GL, Auclair PL, Gnepp DR (Eds). Surgical pathology of the salivary glands. 1st edn. Philadelphia: WB Saunders Company; 1991. pp. 187-201.

150. Yim YM, Yoon JW, Seo JW, Kwon H, Jung SN. Pleomorphic adenoma in the auricle. J Craniofac Surg. 2009;20(3):951-2.

151. Yoo GH, Eisele DW, Askin FB, Driben JS, Johns ME. Warthin's tumour: A 40-year experience at The Johns Hopkins Hospital. Laryngoscope 1994;104:799-803.

152. Yu GY, Ussmuller J, Donath K. Histogenesis and development of membranous basal cell adenoma. Oral Surg Oral Med Oral Pathol Oral Radiol Endod 1998;86:446-51.

153. Zhang X, Cairns M, Rose B, O'Brien C, Shannon K, Clark J, Gamble J, Tran N. Alterations in miRNA processing and expression in pleomorphic adenomas of the salivary gland. Int J Cancer. 2009;124(12):2855-63.

8

Malignant Tumors of the Salivary Glands

Kanthimathi Sekhar, B Sivapathasundharam

Malignant salivary gland tumors are a morphologically and clinically diverse group of neoplasms accounting for >0.5% of all malignancies and approximately three to five percent of all head and neck cancers. The annual incidence of malignant salivary gland tumors has been recorded to range from 0.4 to 13.5 cases per 100,000 people and several large studies have shown that malignant tumors comprise between 35 and 40% of all salivary gland tumors.

CLINICAL FEATURES

Although it is generally stated that most salivary gland neoplasms are more common in females, males have been reported to have a higher proportion of malignant tumors especially with respect to parotid and submandibular tumors. But these differences are not so evident in case of minor glands. In older children, malignant neoplasms are common (60%) especially the epithelial tumors. However, these tumors are usually low grade and mortality and morbidity are low.

Malignant tumors may arise from major as well as minor salivary glands. In the parotid gland the proportion of benign tumors were found to be more than malignant tumors. Conversely, the proportion of malignant tumors reported to occur in the submandibular, sublingual and all minor gland sites (except for the lip) were more than that of benign tumors. In the tongue, the most common area for malignant salivary tumor is the base of the tongue regardless of the histologic type.

About one-third of major salivary gland tumors are malignant whereas nearly one-half of those occurring in the minor glands are malignant; the sites with the highest proportion of malignant tumors being the retromolar area, and floor of the mouth followed by the tongue and sublingual gland. It appears to be that the smaller the gland, the higher the proportion of malignant tumors.

Among the specific histologic types of malignant salivary gland tumors, according to the Armed Forces Institute of Pathology (AFIP) case files, the most common is mucoepidermoid carcinoma followed by adenocarcinoma Not Otherwise Specified (NOS), acinic cell carcinoma, polymorphous low grade adenocarcinoma, adenoid cystic carcinoma and carcinoma ex pleomorphic adenoma. Other series have reported adenoid cystic carcinoma to be the second most common malignant salivary gland tumor.

Most of the malignant salivary gland tumors are clinically indistinguishable from benign tumors except when they show rapid increase in size, pain, fixation to adjacent structures, ulceration, or cervical lymph node involvement. Neurological signs, such as numbness or weakness caused by nerve involvement typically indicate malignancy. Facial nerve paralysis is a more consistent sign of malignancy (rarely occurs in Warthin's tumor) and is especially seen in high grade tumors such as squamous cell carcinoma and undifferentiated carcinoma.

BEHAVIOR OF MALIGNANT SALIVARY GLAND TUMORS

The behavior of malignant salivary gland tumors is largely influenced by tumor size, histological grade and clinical stage. Exceptions are undifferentiated carcinomas and poorly differentiated mucoepidermoid carcinomas, where the prognosis is poor regardless of the size, extension, fixation or consistency of the tumor. Some studies have shown that Ki-67 index, S-phase fraction, DNA ploidy and expression of p53 protein to be of prognostic significance.

Grading

Malignant salivary gland tumors can be broadly categorized into low, intermediate and high grade according to their behavior (Table 8.1). The low grade tumors are locally invasive with a tendency to recur, especially with incomplete excision, but distant metastasis and mortality are rare. The five-year survival rate is in the range of 80 to 95%. The intermediate grade tumours have five year survival rates ranging from 50 to 75%. The high grade tumors grow rapidly and are often bulky at presentation. Spread to regional lymph nodes and distant sites often occur early and the 5-year survival rate ranges from 5 to 45%.

Staging

The staging criteria for carcinoma of the major salivary glands were proposed by the American Joint Committee on Cancer in 2002 (Table 8.2). The staging system uses four variables, namely size, local extension, palpability of the tumor, suspected metastasis to regional lymph nodes and presence or absence of distant metastasis. Regional lymph nodes are those within or immediately adjacent to the salivary glands and the deep cervical lymph nodes. Infiltration to other nodes is considered as distant metastases. Local extensions in smaller tumors are considered less ominous than those of larger tumors and so the presence or absence of local extension was designated by a suffix within each T group. Hence T1 and T2 lesions with local extension are considered Stage II rather than Stage III.

MORPHOLOGY

Histologically, salivary gland tumors represent the most heterogeneous group of tumors of any tissue in the body posing a diagnostic challenge. Hence, it becomes imperative the basic cytoarchitectural features of each tumor type so that a diagnosis can be made logically through analysis of the cellular components, cell arrangements and extracellular components.

Malignant tumors of the salivary glands may be broadly categorized into malignant mixed tumors, carcinomas, adenocarcinomas and others which include the mesenchymal tumors, lymphomas and metastatic tumors.

Table 8.1: Grading of malignant salivary gland neoplasms

Low grade	Intermediate grade	High grade
• Acinic cell carcinoma	• Mucinous adenocarcinoma	• Mucoepidermoid carcinoma, high grade
• Mucoepidermoid carcinoma low to intermediate grade	• Adenoid cystic carcinoma	• Adenocarcinoma NOS-high grade
• Polymorphous low grade adenocarcinoma	• Sebaceous adenocarcinoma	• Squamous cell carcinoma
• Basal cell adenocarcinoma	• Malignant myoepithelioma	• Salivary duct carcinoma
• Hyalinizing clear cell carcinoma	• Lymphoepithelioma like carcinoma	• Malignant mixed tumor, high grade
• Epithelial-myoepithelial carcinoma		• Oncocytic carcinoma
• Malignant mixed tumors, low grade		• Large cell undifferentiated carcinoma
• Cystadenocarcinoma		• Small cell carcinoma
• Adenocarcinoma NOS-low grade		• Dedifferentiated acinic cell or adenoid cystic carcinoma
• Clear cell carcinoma		

Table 8.2: Staging system for major salivary gland tumors

Primary tumor (T)

TX	Primary tumor cannot be assessed
T0	No evidence of primary tumor
T1	Tumor 2 cm or less in greatest dimension without extraparenchymal extension*
T2	Tumor more than 2 cm but not more than 4 cm in greatest dimension without extraparenchymal extension*
T3	Tumor more than 4 cm and/or tumor with extraparenchymal extension*
T4a	Tumor invades skin, mandible, ear canal, or facial nerve
T4b	Tumor invades base of skull, pterygoid plates, or encases carotid artery

Note: *Extraparenchymal extension is clinical or macroscopic evidence of invasion of soft tissues or nerve, except those listed under T4a and 4b. Microscopic evidence alone does not constitute extraparenchymal extension for classification pur poses.

Regional lymph nodes (N)

NX	Regional lymph nodes cannot be assessed
N0	No regional lymph node metastasis
N1	Metastasis in a single ipsilateral lymph node, 3 cm or less in greatest dimension
N2	Metastasis as specified in N2a, 2b, 2c below
N2a	Metastasis in a single ipsilateral lymph node, more than 3 cm but not more than 6 cm in greatest dimension
N2b	Metastasis in multiple ipsilateral lymph nodes, none more than 6 cm in greatest dimension
N2c	Metastasis in bilateral or contralateral lymph nodes, none more than 6 cm in greatest dimension
N3	Metastasis in a lymph node more than 6 cm in greatest dimension

Note: Midline nodes are considered ipsilateral nodes.

Distant metastasis (M)

MX – Distant metastasis cannot be assessed
M0 – No distant metastasis
M1 – Distant metastasis

Stage grouping

Stage I	T1	N0	M0
Stage II	T2	N0	M0
Stage III	T3	N0	M0
	T1, T2, T3	N1	M0
Stage IV A	T1, T2, T3	N2	M0
	T4a	N0, N1, N2	M0
Stage IV B	T4b	Any N	M0
	Any T	N3	M0
Stage IV C	Any T	Any N	M1

ACINIC CELL ADENOCARCINOMA

Acinic cell adenocarcinoma is a malignant epithelial neoplasm in which at least some of the tumor cells demonstrate serous acinar differentiation. Although tumors with cells resembling acinar cells were described as early as 1892, the term acinic cell adenocarcinoma was first used by Foote and Frazell, and Godwin et al in the 1950s. It is the third most common epithelial malignancy of the salivary gland and the incidence is about 17% among primary malignant salivary gland tumors or 6% of all salivary gland neoplasms.

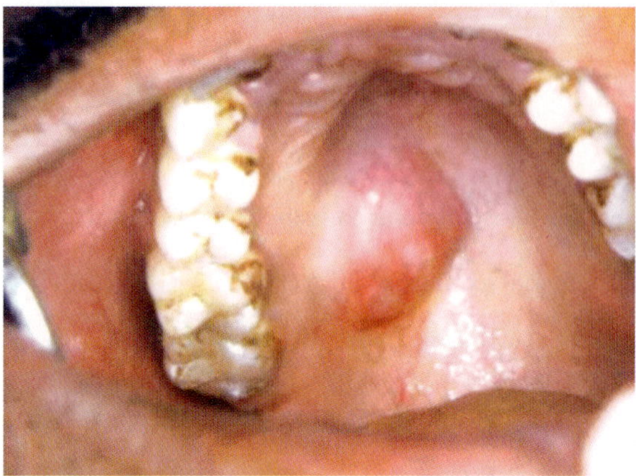

Figure 8.1: Acinic cell adenocarcinoma presenting as a painless mass on the palate *(Courtesy: Dr S Karthinga Kannan, Sree Mookambika Institute of Dental Sciences, Kanyakumari District*

Clinical Features

The mean age of presentation was about 44 years with a slight female predominance. The tumors typically present as a slowly growing mass with or without pain. Facial muscle weakness is seen in about 5 to 10% of tumors. It is the most common malignant tumor that may present bilaterally (3%). These tumors have a recurrence rate of 35% and a metastatic rate of 16%. Acinic cell carcinomas arising in minor salivary glands are less aggressive than those that arise in major salivary glands. The most frequent sites of occurrence are the parotid gland (84%) and submandibular gland (4%), followed by the buccal mucosa, upper lip, and palate (Fig. 8.1).

Macroscopic Features

Acinic cell carcinoma is often circumscribed with an incomplete capsule, but can be multinodular or infiltrative. Most tumors are about one to three centimeters in size. The cut surface is grayish white to reddish gray and may be firm to soft in consistency. There may be solid or cystic areas.

Microscopic Features

Acinic cell carcinoma is cellular with little fibrous stroma and variable number of lymphoid aggregates.

One half of the tumors have a fine vascularized fibrous connective tissue stroma while others have areas of collagenization. Prominent vascularity, areas of hemorrhage, and psammoma-type calcifications may be found. The tumor is composed of cells arranged in varying patterns which include solid, microcystic, papillary-cystic, and follicular. These may contain acinar, intercalated ductal, vacuolated, clear, and nonspecific glandular cells. Any or all of these morphologic patterns and cell types may be seen (Figs 8.2A to F).

The acinar cells are polygonal and have abundant, pale, basophilic cytoplasm with purplish cytoplasmic granules, and eccentrically placed, basophilic to vesicular nuclei. The zymogen-type secretory granules are PAS positive, diastase resistant and mucicarmine positive. These cells are the predominant cell type in 40% of tumors.

The intercalated duct-like cells are smaller with a greater nuclear/cytoplasmic ratio than the acinar cells. They are cuboidal and have eosinophilic to amphophilic cytoplasm and central, basophilic to vesicular nuclei surrounding luminal spaces. They are the predominant cell type in one-third of the tumors.

Vacuolated cells have cytoplasmic vacuoles and nuclear features similar to those of the intercalated duct-like cells. They are found in less than 10% of acinic cell adenocarcinomas. Clear cells are seen in about 6% of acinic cell adenocarcinomas. They have nonstaining cytoplasm that does not contain glycogen and probably represent dilatation of endoplasmic reticulum or tissue processing artifacts.

The nonspecific glandular cells are rounded to polygonal with amphophilic to eosinophilic cytoplasm and round, basophilic to vesicular nuclei. They do not have cytoplasmic granules and are PAS negative. Nuclear pleomorphism and mitoses are more in these cells than in the other cell types.

Solid Pattern

This is seen in one-third of acinic cell adnocarcinomas. The tumor is composed mainly of acinar cells arranged in sheets, nodules, or aggregates (Fig. 8.2A).

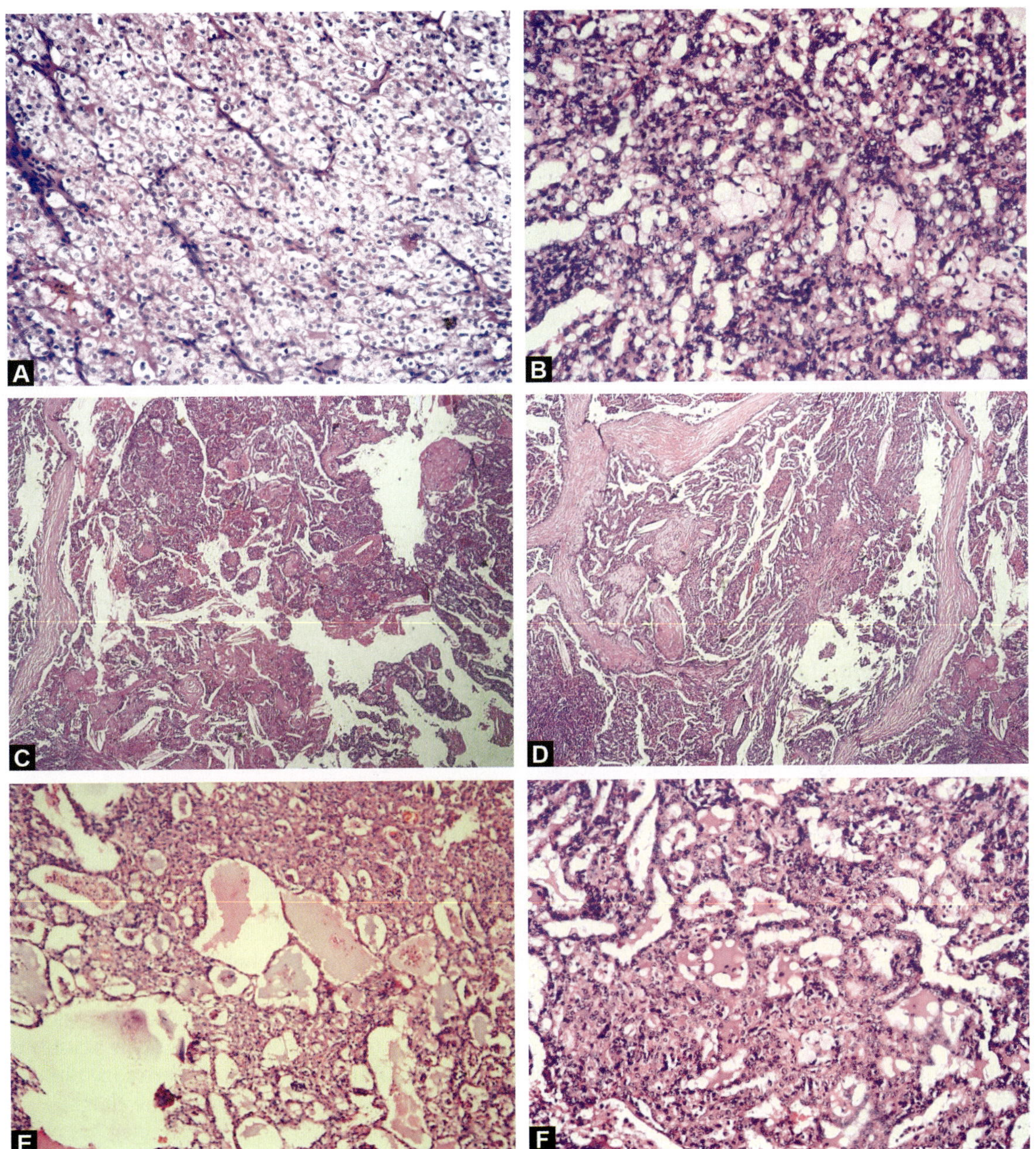

Figures 8.2A to F: Acinic cell adenocarcinoma: (A) Solid growth of polygonal tumor cells separated by delicate blood vessels; (B) Clumps of acinar cells seen in an area showing the characteristic microcystic pattern of growth; (C and D) Acinic cell adenocarcinoma showing papillary cystic growth pattern; (E and F) Tumor cells arranged in a follicular pattern resembling thyroid follicles

Microcystic Pattern

This pattern is more frequent than the solid pattern. Many small spaces varying in size from few microns to a millimeter within sheets or nodules of tumor cells are seen giving rise to a lacy appearance. The microcystic spaces differ from microglandular spaces in that the surrounding cells lack orientation around the spaces. The spaces may be empty or contain amorphous eosinophilic or pale basophilic, PAS positive material (Fig. 8.2B).

Papillary-cystic Pattern

In this pattern, there are large cystic lumens lined by simple or cuboidal epithelium and filled with papillary epithelial growths. The papillae are covered by hobnail cells, intercalated duct-like cells, vacuolated cells, nonspecific glandular cells and nondescript cells with eosinophilic to amphophilic cytoplasm, central nuclei, and indistinct cell borders. Some of the epithelial cells bulge into the lumen producing a "tombstone row" luminal surface. Intraluminal mucinous material may be present (Figs 8.2C and D).

Follicular Pattern

The tumor is composed of multiple, large, round, cystic spaces lined by intercalated duct-like cells and nonspecific glandular cells. These spaces are filled with eosinophilic material giving a thyroid-like appearance. This colloid like material is PAS positive. This pattern is prominent in only about 5% of the tumors (Figs 8.2E and F).

Dedifferentiated Acinic Cell Carcinoma

Dedifferentiation of acinic cell carcinoma to a high grade adenocarcinoma, poorly differentiated carcinoma or undifferentiated carcinoma can occur rarely. It is a bulky and is associated with rapid tumor growth, significant pain and facial palsy. The prognosis is poor.

Immunohistochemistry

Immunohistochemically most tumor cells show positivity for low molecular weight cytokeratin especially CK 18 where there is a membranous staining, CEA and amylase. Other markers found reactive are transferrin lactoferrin, alpha 1 antitrypsin, alpha 1 chymotrypsin, IgA and LeuM1 antigen. CK 7 staining is negative which helps in differentiating from adenocarcinoma where it is strongly positive. Vasoactive intestinal polypeptide is reported to be specifically reactive in acinic cell adenocarcinoma. There is no immunohistochemical evidence of myoepithelial differentiation. Ultra-structural studies reveal zymogen granules in the form of multiple, round, electron dense cytoplasmic granules in the acinar cells. Ductal cells often border lumen and have apical junctional complexes and microvilli.

Cytogenetics

In one study, it has been reported that 84.0% of acinic cell adenocarcinomas had chromosomal alterations. In general, chromosomal regions at chromosomes 4p, 5q, 6p, and 17p were more frequently altered than those on chromosomes 1p and 1q, 4q, 5p, and 6q. Certain markers at 4p15-16, 6p25-qter, and 17p11 regions showed the highest incidence of LOH, suggesting the presence of tumor suppressor genes associated with the oncogenesis of these tumors.

Differential Diagnosis

Cystadenocarcinoma has to be differentiated from papillary cystic acinic cell adenocarcinoma. The presence of numerous vacuolated areas and/or areas of microcyst formation favor acinic cell adenocarcinoma while the presence of intensely stained mucous cells is against the diagnosis of this condition.

The presence of clear cells should alert to the possibility of clear cell tumors like mucoepidermoid carcinoma, epithelial-myoepithelial carcinoma, clear cell variant of oncocytoma and metastatic renal cell carcinoma. Mucoepidermoid carcinomas have many mucicarminophilic cells, not seen in acinic cell adenocarcinoma while epithelial-myoepithelial carcinomas have a typical biphasic pattern and glycogen in the cells. Unlike the clear cell variant of oncocytoma, the clear cells of acinic cell adenocarcinoma do not contain glycogen and are unreactive with the PTAH stain. The clear cells of metastatic renal cell carcinoma are diastase sensitive PAS positive and the vascular pattern of this is typical.

Metastatic thyroid carcinoma is differentiated from the follicular pattern of acinic cell adeno-carcinoma by positive staining for thyroglobulin in the cells of the former. In all cases recognition of acinar differentiated cells with the help of special stains or electron microscopy is a key to diagnosis.

Prognosis

The most important prognostic factors for acinic cell carcinoma are clinical stage and status of the resection margin. Other poor prognostic factors include pain, fixation of the tumor, frequent mitoses, high proliferative index (Ki67 greater than five percent), focal necrosis, perineural invasion, gross invasion, desmoplasia, atypia, and depletion of lymphocytes in the stroma. These have been associated with more frequent recurrences and metastases. In an AFIP study it was seen that 12% of patients had recurrences while 8% had metastasis. In acinic cell carcinoma, a pre-dominantly solid architecture is believed to be a predictor of recurrence.

MUCOEPIDERMOID CARCINOMA

Mucoepidermoid carcinoma is a malignant epithelial tumor composed of varying proportions of mucus secreting cells, epidermoid cells and intermediate cells forming cysts and solid islands. This was, at first, termed mucoepidermoid by Stewart, Foote and Becker in 1945 and the tumors were divided into benign and malignant forms. Subsequently it was found that those tumors classified as benign, yielded metastases. Hence all mucoepidermoid tumors were considered carcinomas.

This is the most common malignant salivary gland tumor and has the second highest frequency of occurrence among all salivary gland tumors. It represents 22 and 41% of malignant tumors occurring in the major and minor glands respectively. Mucoepidermoid carcinoma is the principal histologic type of radiation related salivary gland carcinoma, as seen in the survivors of the atomic bombing of Hiroshima and Nagasaki and children treated with radiotherapy for cranial leukemia and tinea capitis.

Clinical Features

The mean age of presentation of mucoepidermoid carcinoma is about 43 years. However, the average age of patients with these tumors in the lower lip is about a decade more than that mentioned above. In the hard palate, about 44% of patients are found to be under the age of 20 years and 63% are younger than 40 years. Females are affected more than males. With regard to the anatomic location, in the submandibular gland, females are affected at a younger age than males. The converse is true in the case of lesions of the hard palate, where males are affected at a younger age. Mucoepidermoid carcinomas are the most common malignant tumors to arise in children and adolescents under 20 years of age.

In the major salivary glands, they present as solitary painless masses which are well circumscribed and movable. Rarely tenderness, pain, drainage from the ipsilateral ear, dysphagia, trismus, fixation to the overlying skin, or facial paralysis may be present, the latter often occurring in high grade tumors.

Minor salivary gland tumors may be detected as incidental findings during a dental examination. Those of the palate present as fluctuant, blue, smooth surfaced swellings and may be mistaken for a mucocele. Some have a magenta color resembling a hemangioma.

A small mucosal opening may be present simulating draining dental abscesses (Fig. 8.3). Dysphagia, pain, paresthesia, numbness of teeth, ulceration or hemorrhage may be present. In both major and minor salivary glands, high-grade

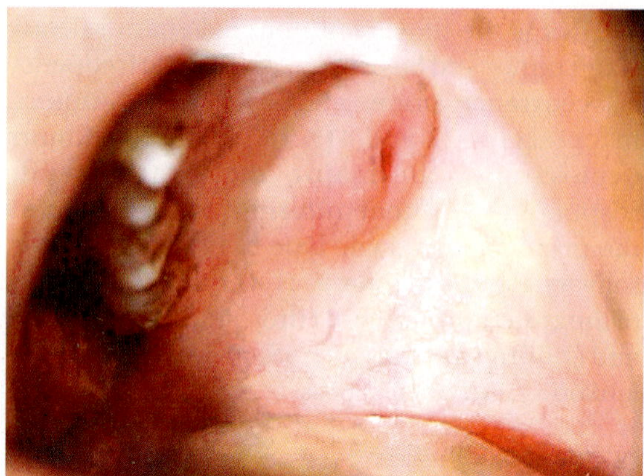

Figure 8.3: Mucoepidermoid carcinoma of the palate mimicking dental abscess

tumors are more likely to be symptomatic. Central mucoepidermoid carcinoma typically presents as an asymptomatic radiolucent lesion.

Most of these tumors occur in the parotid gland (45%) followed by the palate (21%), buccal mucosa, upper and lower lips and retromolar region. Central mucoepidermoid carcinoma arises in the jaws with mandibular to maxillary predilection of approximately 3:1.

Macroscopic Features

Mucoepidermoid carcinoma usually presents as an ill-defined mass which may be partially encapsulated with a firm to hard consistency. The size of the parotid tumors is between 1 and 4 cm but may be much larger. The cut surface is gray, tan-yellow or pink, lobulated and may have cysts containing mucus or blood stained fluid. Focal areas of hemorrhage are sometimes seen.

Microscopic Features

The tumor is composed of haphazardly dispersed mucin filled cysts and irregular tumor nests of mucus, epidermoid, intermediate, columnar and clear cells in variable combinations. It is the relative proportion of these cells that helps to determine the grade.

Mucous Cells

Mucous cells are large, columnar, goblet shaped or polygonal with copious mucin giving a frosted glass appearance to the cytoplasm. They may form closely packed nests, line cysts or lie scattered amidst the squamous cell islands. These mucous cells should be differentiated from large edematous squamoid cells with pale eosinophilic granular cytoplasm. Sebaceous cells may rarely be seen in mucoepidermoid carcinomas. The epithelial mucin produced by the mucous cells stain positively for mucicarmine and shows diastase resistant PAS positivity. Tumors with predominantly mucous cells are seen more in the minor salivary glands (Figs 8.4A to D).

Epidermoid or Squamoid Cells

These cells occur in nests or line cystic spaces. They may have a stratified appearance and intercellular bridges are inconspicuous. Keratin pearls are not common. These epidermoid zones may be sharply demarcated from the intermediate cells or they may blend imperceptibly with other cell types.

Intermediate Cells

They are the putative precursors of mucous and epidermoid cells. They are so called because they are intermediate in size and appearance between basal cells and epidermoid cells and range from small basal cells to medium sized cells. They are polygonal in shape with a wide rim of cytoplasm or ample cytoplasm. These cells may form nests and sheets merging into the other cell types and in some areas have a syncytial arrangement. Intermediate cells may have cytoplasmic mucin and diastase labile PAS positive granules which have been identified ultrastructurally to be glycogen.

Clear Cells

Clear cells are large and polygonal cells having sharply defined cytoplasmic borders. They resemble squamous cells in spite of their clear cytoplasm. Only traces of cytoplasmic mucin are seen.

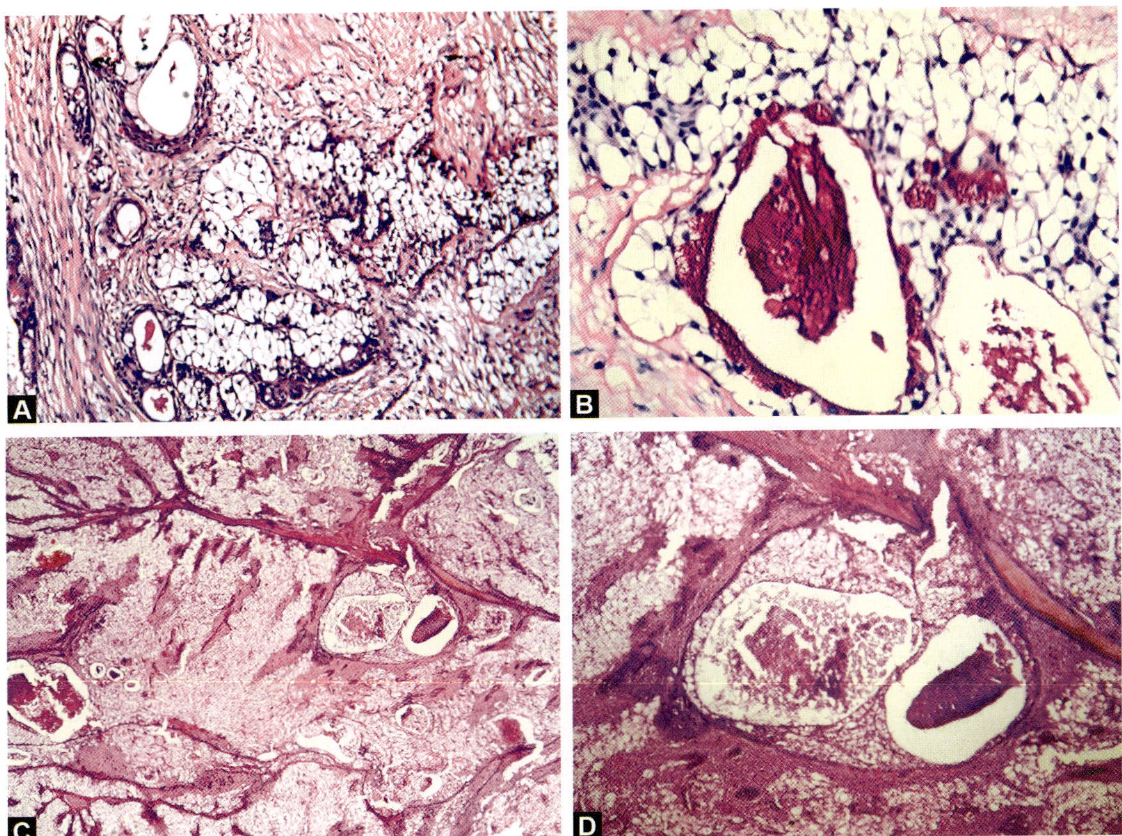

Figures 8.4A to D: Mucoepidermoid carcinoma, low grade. Islands consisting of cystic space that are lined by mucous cells and epidermoid cells: (A) The same in higher magnification; (B) The cystic spaces contain PAS positive material; (C) The same in higher magnification; (D) *Courtesy:* Dr I Ponniah, Tamil Nadu Government Dental College and Hospital, Chennai

The stroma is typically sclerotic and abundant with chronic inflammatory cells and occasional extravasated pools of mucin.

Grading of Mucoepidermoid Carcinomas

Mucoepidermoid carcinomas are divided into low, intermediate, and high grade types on the basis of morphologic and cytologic features. For grading, it is imperative to have an adequate quantity of properly fixed and stained tissue. Rarely, there may be differences in the degree of differentiation in different areas of a tumor. In such cases, if 20% or more exhibit a higher grade it is better to give a higher grade even if the predominant pattern is of a lower grade. The two grading systems used are AFIP grading system and three tier grading system (Table 8.3). The AFIP grading system is applicable to intraoral and parotid tumors.

Armed Forces Institute of Pathology Grading

Grading parameters with point values include:

- Intracystic component (+2)
- Neural invasion present (+2)
- Necrosis present (+3)
- Mitosis ($\geq$ 4 per 10 high power field) (+3)
- Anaplasia present (+4)

Table 8.3: Three tier grading system for mucoepidermoid carcinoma

Histologic parameters for grading	Low grade	Intermediate grade	High grade
Cysts	Many macro and micro cysts	Some cysts	Few cysts
Mucinous cells	Many	Some	Few
Mitoses	Few	Few or some	Many
Cytology	Bland	Some atypia	Significant cellular pleomorphism

Total point scores are 0 to 4 for low grade, 5 to 6 for intermediate grade and 7 to 14 for high grade. This grading system correlated well with prognosis for tumors of the parotid gland.

Low Grade Mucoepidermoid Carcinoma

A large proportion of the tumor is made of mucin filled cysts, abundant mucous cells and irregular mature epithelial cell islands. The lining of the cysts varies from one to three cells in thickness. The lining of the cysts and epithelial islands either consist of only mucous cells or a mixture of mucous, intermediate, and epidermoid cells. Large sheet like proliferations and neural invasion are not usually seen. Nuclei are bland and mitotic figures are rare. The mucous cysts may rupture and the mucus escaping into the stroma elicits an inflammatory cell response. This may allow the tumor to spread more easily and make complete surgical excision difficult. Later there is fibrosis and lymphoid infiltration seen in the stroma.

Intermediate Grade Mucoepidermoid Carcinoma

The distinction between the low and intermediate grades is based primarily on the relative proportion of cystic and solid cellular areas. Cystic spaces comprise less than 20% of the entire tumor and there is a predominance of intermediate cells with scattered mucus cells and foci of epidermoid cells. Positivity for mucin is readily demonstrable in many of the cells. Nuclear atypia and mitotic figures are rare, but nucleoli are seen more often than in low grades.

High Grade Mucoepidermoid Carcinoma

In this type, there are more solid areas of squamoid and intermediate cells and less cystic areas exhibiting cytologic atypia. Cellular pleomorphism, nuclear hyperchromasia, prominent nucleoli, numerous mitotic figures, areas of coagulative necrosis and individual cell keratinization may be present. There are two patterns seen in high grade mucoepidermoid carcinomas. One resembles a moderately differentiated squamous cell carcinoma. Glandular, small cystic structures and the presence of sparse mucous cells must be identified to differentiate mucoepidermoid carcinoma from a squamous cell carcinoma. Stains for mucin may be helpful.

The second pattern shows a mixture of the different cell types usually seen in mucoepidermoid carcinoma with intermediate cell being predominant. Most of these cells display anaplastic features. Perineural and intravascular invasion may be present. There is less fibrosis and chronic inflammatory cell infiltrate in the stroma when compared to infiltrate low grade tumors.

Histological Variants of Mucoepidermoid Carcinoma

Clear cells, with glycogen in the cytoplasm may be abundant. The others are a spindle cell variant, oncocytic variant and sclerotic variant. The sclerosing variant of mucoepidermoid carcinoma is characterized by an intense central sclerosis that occupies the entirety of an otherwise typical tumor along with an inflammatory infiltrate of plasma cells, eosinophils, and/or lymphocytes at its peripheral regions. The sclerosis associated with these tumors can obscure their typical morphologic features and cause difficulties in diagnosis. Tumor infarction and extravasation of mucin causing a reactive fibrosis are the two mechanisms that have been proposed as underlying this morphologic variant. A new subtype that has been proposed is mucoepidermoid carcinoma with stromal fibrosis and eosinophilic infiltration, which has low malignant potential.

Central Mucoepidermoid Carcinoma

These tumors arise centrally in the mandible or maxilla and represent about 4.3% of mucoepidermoid carcinomas from all sites. They are unique in that arise in sites that do not normally contain salivary gland tissue and present clinically as radiolucent lesions. They believed to arise either from ectopic rests of salivary gland tissue or from neoplastic transformation of the epithelial lining of odontogenic cysts. Central mucoepidermoid carcinomas occur more frequently in the molar area and have been found to be associated with impacted third molars. They are either asymptomatic or produce a painless swelling. Rarely there may be pain, paresthesia or dysphagia. Most of them are low grade lesions with one study showing a 30% recurrence rate and two-year and five-year survival rates of 100%.

Immunohistochemistry

The tumor cells of mucoepidermoid carcinoma are positive for cytokeratin and variably stain for EMA, CEA, actin and S-100 protein. Immunostaining for mucin is also used in the characterization of salivary gland mucoepidermoid carcinomas. Normal salivary glands frequently express MUC1 and MUC4, mainly in ductal cells; while MUC5B and MUC7 stain the mucous and serous acini respectively of submandibular and minor salivary glands; and MUC5AC and MUC2 were poorly detected in excretory ducts. Mucin expression in mucoepidermoid carcinomas differs from that in normal salivary glands. Most mucoepidermoid carcinomas express MUC1 and MUC4. Both these membrane-bound mucins stain membranes and cytoplasm of all cell types (epidermoid, intermediate, mucous, clear and columnar). MUC5AC is reported to be expressed in more than 50% of high grade tumors. In addition, high expression of MUC1 has been found to be related to higher histologic grades, high recurrence and metastasis rates and a shorter disease-free interval. On the other hand, high expression of MUC4 has been reported to be related to low grade tumors, lower recurrence rates and a longer disease-free interval indicating a better prognosis.

Cytogenetics

Cytogenetically, several mucoepidermoid carcinomas are reported to pose t(11;19)(q14-21;p12-13) translocation. This translocation creates a new fusion product, MECT1-MAML2, which disrupts a Notch signaling pathway. (Notch signaling plays a key role in the normal development of many tissues and cell types through effects on cellular differentiation, survival and/or proliferation). These tumors also show loss of chromosomal arms 2q, 5p, 12p and 16q in more than 50% of cases.

Differential Diagnosis

Cystadenomas have large cystic structures predominantly lined by cuboidal cells whereas in mucoepidermoid carcinomas the cysts are of varying sizes and lined by different cell types. However, it has to be borne in mind that mucoepidermoid carcinomas may develop from the epithelial lining of cystadenomas and extensive sampling of the tumor should be done to differentiate these two lesions.

Mucoepidermoid carcinomas having solid sheets of intermediate cells may resemble pleomorphic adenomas. But ducts with central lumina, chondroid and myxoid areas which are characteristic of pleomorphic adenoma are not seen in mucoepidermoid carcinomas.

The adenocarcinomatous component of adenosquamous carcinoma may resemble mucoepidermoid carcinoma, however in the former, the surface epithelium is dysplastic and the intermediate cells characteristic of mucoepidermoid carcinoma are absent.

Polymorphous low grade adenocarcinoma may have cellular proliferations and pools of mucoid substance. However, these tumors have concentrically arranged cords of cells and foci of perineural invasion which are rare in mucoepidermoid carcinoma. Epidermoid cells are not seen in polymorphous low grade adenocarcinoma.

Primary or metastatic squamous cell carcinomas have a greater degree of individual cell keratinization and keratin pearl formation than high grade mucoepidermoid carcinomas. The presence of intracytoplasmic mucin has to be demonstrated to differentiate mucoepidermoid carcinomas from these tumors.

Cellular adenocarcinomas NOS and cystadenocarcinomas may resemble intermediate grade mucoepidermoid carcinomas but do not have the mixed cell population seen in latter. Mucoepidermoid carcinomas with numerous clear cells will show focal clusters of epidermoid, mucous or intermediate cells permitting the differentiation from clear cell carcinomas.

Prognosis

The behavior of mucoepidermoid carcinoma strongly correlates with the clinical stage and histologic grade. Mucoepidermoid carcinoma in general are reported with recurrence rates of about 25%. Low grade and high grade tumors are reported with recurrence rates of 10% and 74% respectively. Recurrences are more common if the margins of resection are positive.

The prognosis is good for low and intermediate grade tumors with the five-year survival rate being about 92% for low grade and 70 to 83% for intermediate grade tumors. On the other hand, high grade tumors, submandibular tumors and tumors in the base of the tongue have a poorer outlook, as do those with evidence of bony invasion. The five-year survival rate is about 22 to 42% for high grade tumors.

High proliferative index (mitotic count greater than two or 10 HPF or Ki67 index greater than ten percent), vascular invasion, advanced stage of disease and aneuploidy are also associated with poor prognosis. Studies using p27, a universal cyclin-dependent kinase inhibitor, has shown that low expression of the same is indicative of a worse prognosis especially when combined with large size in mucoepidermoid carcinoma of the intraoral minor salivary gland.

Metastasis to regional lymph nodes are more frequent with submandibular tumors and distant metastases are seen more in parotid and submandibular tumors rather than the lesions of minor glands. Distant metastases have been reported to occur more commonly to the lung, skeleton and brain; however no site may be spared.

ADENOID CYSTIC CARCINOMA

Adenoid cystic carcinoma is an invasive neoplasm composed of basaloid cells with a predominant myoepithelial/basal cell differentiation accompanied by interspersed ductal structures. Although the tumor was originally described by Theodor Billroth it was called cylindroma; the term adenoid cystic carcinoma was first proposed by Foote and Frazell in 1953. According to the AFIP, it is the fifth most common malignant epithelial tumor of the salivary gland; however other series report adenoid cystic carcinoma to be the second most common malignancy. It constitutes 7.5% of all epithelial malignancies and 4% of all benign and malignant epithelial salivary gland tumors.

Clinical Features

Adenoid cystic carcinoma usually occurs between the fourth and sixth decades of life. It presents as a slow growing swelling with larger tumors showing fixation to the skin or deeper tissues. Pain and tenderness are usually seen during the growth of the tumor. The occurrence of facial nerve palsy is an ominous feature (Figs 8.5A to C). Palatal tumors often ulcerate

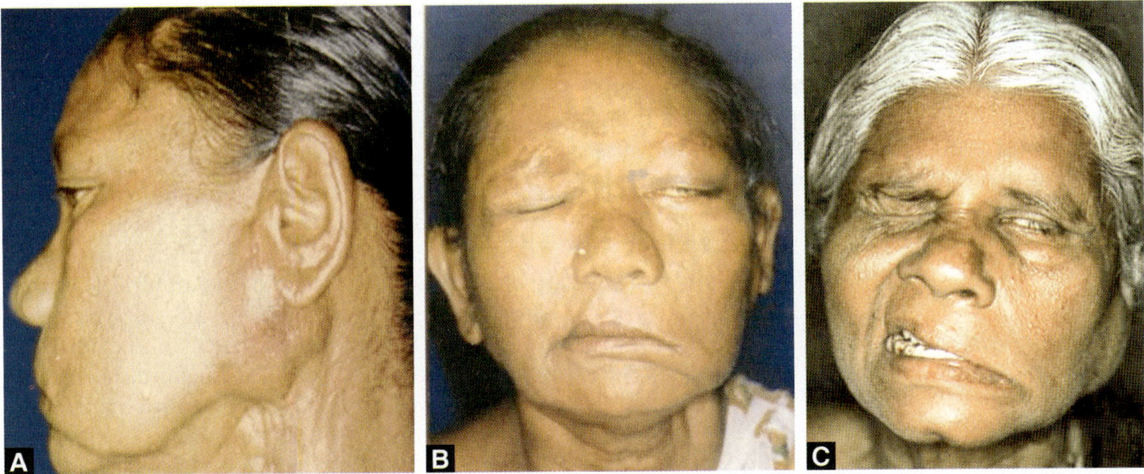

Figures 8.5A to C: Adenoid cystic carcinoma of the parotid presenting as irregular mass over the angle of the mandible along with facial nerve paralysis *(Courtesy:* Dr S Karthiga Kannan, Sree Mookambika Institute of Dental Sciences, Kanyakumari District

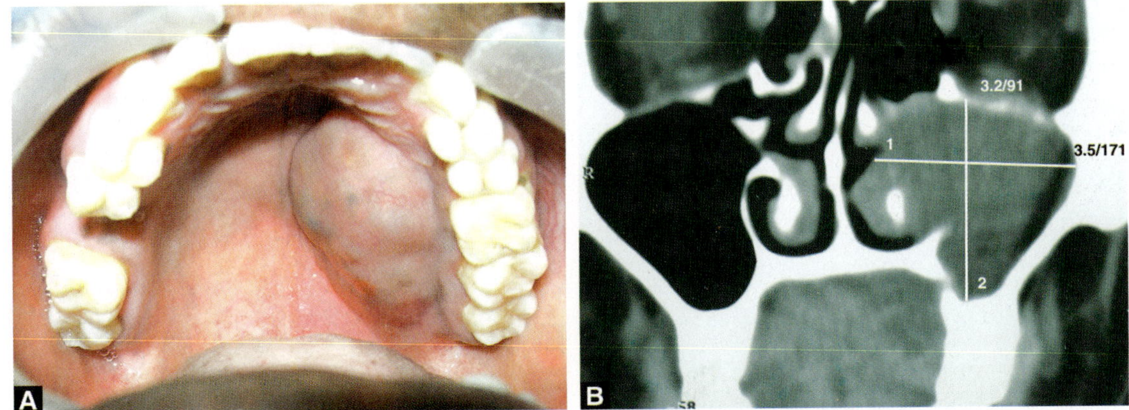

Figures 8.6A and B: (A) Adenoid cystic carcinoma of the palate presenting as a smooth submucosal mass; (B) that has invaded into the maxillary sinus

and bone invasion may occur through infiltration of the marrow spaces (Figs 8.6A and B). Neural invasion is characteristic. The parotid gland, submandibular gland, and palate are more commonly involved. Sublingual glands are rarely affected. Other sites in which they have been reported are the tongue (they constitute the third most common malignancy of the tongue), buccal mucosa, and lips.

Macroscopic Features

Adenoid cystic carcinomas are usually firm, white or grayish-white and lack encapsulation. However, small tumors may appear well circumscribed, although the circumscription is deceptive as the tumor tissue often infiltrates beyond the tumor margin.

Microscopic Features

Adenoid cystic carcinoma is characterized by basaloid cells arranged in variable combinations of cribriform, tubular, or solid patterns but there is no melting of the basaloid cells into the stroma as seen in pleomorphic adenoma. The stroma is fibrous with variable amounts of myxohyaline material which may compress the tumor islands to form a lace-like pattern (Figs 8.7A to H).

Cribriform Pattern

This pattern is the most characteristic feature of adenoid cystic carcinoma. They are almost always found in all cases of this tumor. The tumor is made of small, uniform basaloid cells having round or angulated dark nuclei and scanty cytoplasm arranged in discrete to coalescent islands punctuated by round rigid spaces, giving rise to a "Swiss cheese" appearance (Fig. 8.7A). Some cells may have pale to clear cytoplasm. Nuclear pleomorphism is mild and mitotic figures are few. These cribriform spaces often constitute stromal invaginations (pseudocysts) and contain eosinophilic hyaline material (PAS positive, diastase resistant) and/or lightly basophilic myxoid, ground substance (alcian blue positive). This material represents glycosaminoglycans and duplicated basal lamina. Within the cribriform spaces, occasional, small, true glandular lumina lined by low cuboidal spaces with eosinophilic cytoplasm and a thin eosinophilic cuticle along the luminal border. The lumen may contain PAS positive, diastase resistant, eosinophilic secretion (Figs 8.7C to G).

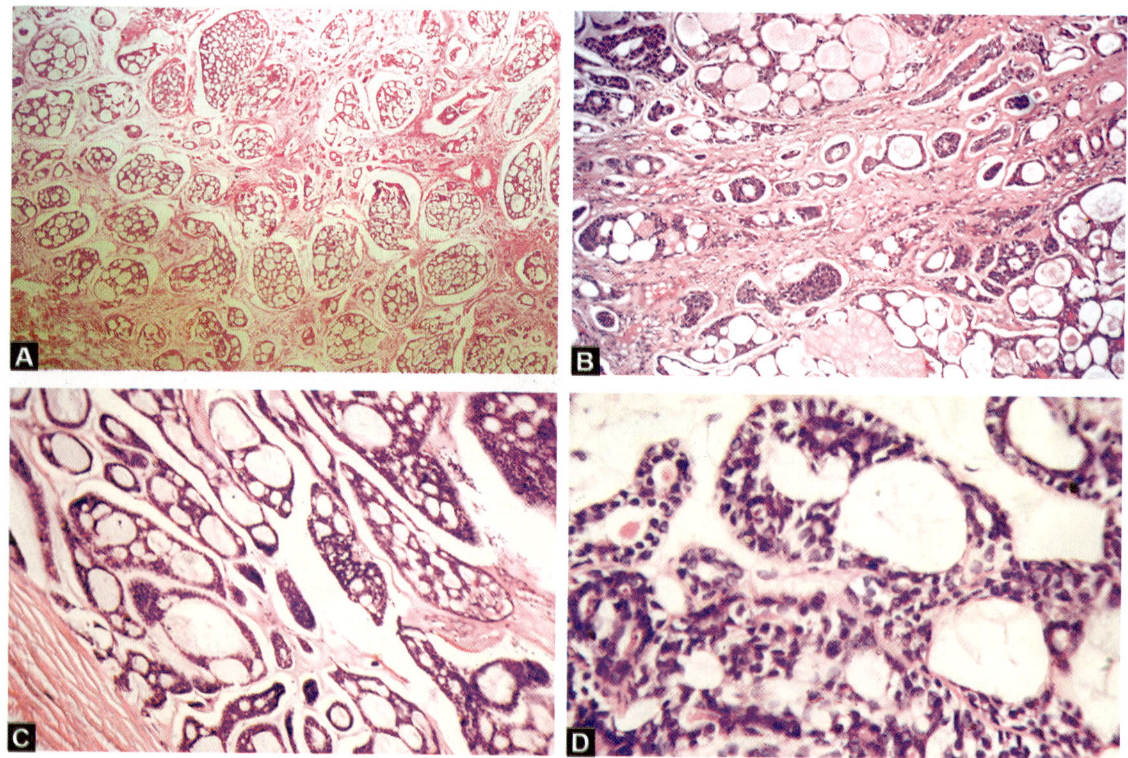

Figs 8.7 A to D

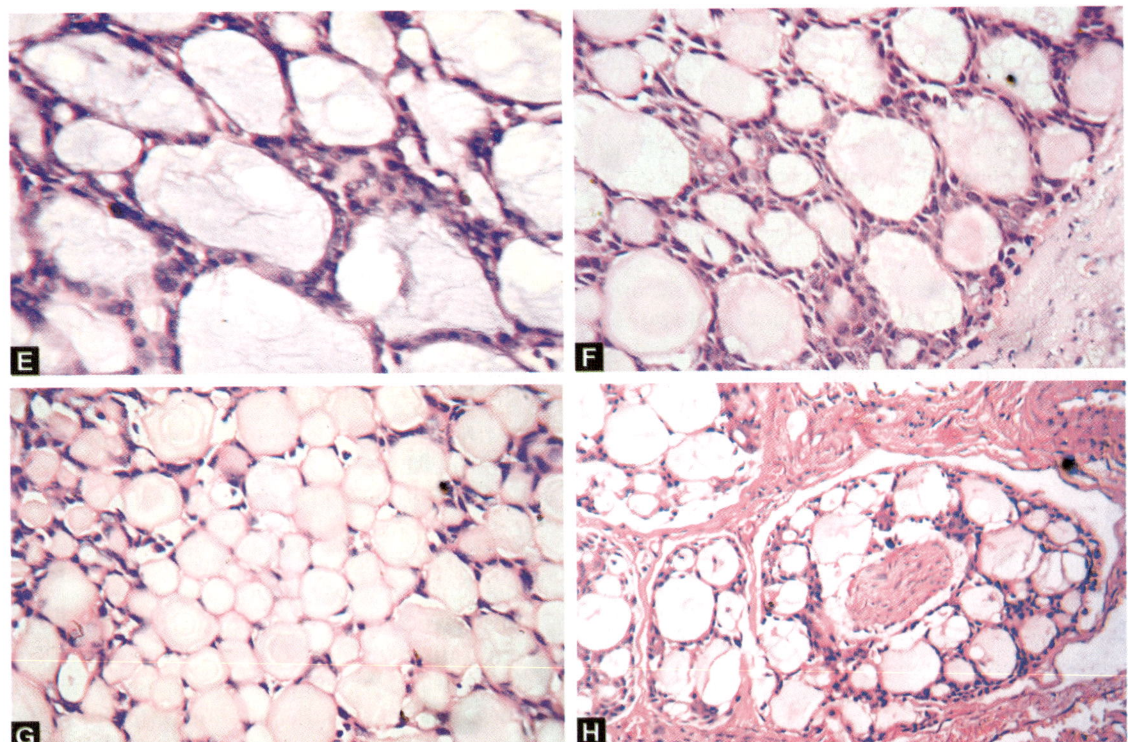

Figures 8.7A to H: Adenoid cystic carcinoma: (A) Variable sized cribriform spaces formed by small, deeply basophilic cells in cribriform pattern; (B) A single tumor exhibits areas of cribriform and tubular (center) paterns; (C) The cribriform spaces may contain a faintly basophilic material; (D) eosinophilic material; (E, F and G) or eosinophilic hyalinized material; (H)Adenoid cystic carcinoma characteristically exhibits perineural invasion. *(Courtesy:* Dr I Ponniah, Tamil Nadu Government Dental College and Hospital, Chennai

Tubular Pattern

This is the second most common microscopic pattern and consists of elongated tubules lined by a single layer of ductal epithelial cells and a single or multiple layers of basaloid cells. Glandular lumens are easily seen and they may be dilated and empty or contain faintly eosinophilic, PAS positive diastase resistant substance. Some tubules are coiled upon themselves giving rise to a necklace-like appearance. The surrounding stroma is abundant and hyalinized. Both the cribriform and tubular patterns may coexist along with transitions between the two (Fig. 8.7B).

Solid Pattern

This is composed of sheets and islands of closely packed basaloid cells with small interspersed pseudocysts. Nuclear palisading is absent and the basaloid cells exhibit more nuclear pleomorphism and increased mitotic figures unlike the other patterns. Coagulative necrosis may occur in the center of the islands.

In most adenoid cystic carcinomas, all the above three patterns may be observed and the tumors are classified according to the histologic pattern that predominates. A characteristic feature of adenoid cystic carcinomas is the propensity to invade perineural spaces and peripheral nerves (Fig. 8.7H).

Dedifferentiated Adenoid Cystic Carcinoma

Dedifferentiation is defined as transformation of adenoid cystic carcinoma into another high grade neoplasm and is associated with an aggressive clinical course and rapidly fatal outcome. The dedifferentiated component is composed of poorly differentiated adenocarcinoma or sarcomatoid carcinoma and there may be a loss or acquisition of immunohistochemical markers.

Immunohistochemically, the basaloid cells are positive for low molecular weight cytokeratin, vimentin, S-100 protein, actin, and calponin. The ductal epithelial cells show positivity for low molecular weight cytokeratin, CEA and EMA. The stromal hyaline material stains for Type IV collagen and laminin. Estrogen, progesterone and progesterone receptor have also been demonstrated.

Variants

A sclerosing variant of adenoid cystic carcinoma has been described recently in which the tumors were composed predominantly of varying-sized large sclerotic and hypocellular nodules containing myoepithelial cells and pseudovascular spaces, with numerous small globules or spherules surrounded by myoepithelial cells similar to those of collagenous or mucinous spherulosis. Electron microscopy has revealed that both the large nodules and small globules or spherules were composed of excessive amounts of basement membrane and thick-banded collagen fibers.

Immunohistochemistry and Cytogenetics

Allelic loss of chromosomal arm 19q has been reported in adenoid cystic carcinoma. In addition, mutations in 14-3-36, CTNNB1 (b-catenin gene), AXIN1 (axis inhibition protein 1) and APC (adenomatosis polyposis coli tumor suppressor) genes have been found. Increased expression of PCNA with higher expression in submandibular derived malignancies has been noted. It has been postulated that cumulative mutations in the p53 and retinoblastoma genes are associated with transformation from cribriform and tubular areas to solid areas. Overexpression of Cyclin D1, p53 mutations, HER-2/neu, overexpression or loss of pRb expression is considered to be associated with transformation to dedifferentiated adenoid

cystic carcinoma. Decreased expression of E cadherin is also seen in high grade tumors. Brain derived neurotropic factor (BDNF), a growth factor involved in neurogenesis has been found to be uniformly expressed by adenoid cystic carcinomas and is presumed to play a causative role in the predilection of these tumors for perineural invasion. Expression of c-kit, a transmembrane receptor tyrosine kinase, has recently been reported to be expressed in adenoid cystic carcinoma but not in polymorphous low grade adenocarcinoma.

Differential Diagnosis

The differential diagnosis of adenoid cystic carcinoma includes polymorphous low grade adenocarcinoma (PLGA), epithelial-myoepithelial carcinoma, pleomorphic adenoma, basal cell adenocarcinoma, and basaloid squamous carcinoma. Under low power, PLGA often has a swirled appearance and the nuclei of the tumor cells are round rather than angulated. The pseudocystic, cribriform and tubular patterns are less prominent than in adenoid cystic carcinoma. In epithelial-myoepithelial carcinoma, the periductal cells have rounded nuclei and large clear cells are present predominantly. Myxochondroid areas, plasmacytoid and spindled myoepithelial cells seen in pleomorphic adenomas are not evident in adenoid cystic carcinoma. Basaloid squamous carcinoma has a squamous component that distinguishes it from the solid type of adenoid cystic carcinoma.

Prognosis

Adenoid cystic carcinomas are slow growing tumors with a protracted course and an ultimately poor outcome. These tumors typically show frequent recurrences and late distant metastasis. Metastasis to the lung, bone, and soft tissue occurs more commonly than lymph node metastasis. The prognosis depends on the histologic grade of the tumor, which is determined by the proportion of the various growth patterns. The tubular and cribriform patterns represent lower grade growths and the cumulative 5- and 15-year survival rates are about 92% and 39% respectively. The solid pattern is associated with a poorer prognosis and five year and 15-year survival rates of 14% and 5% respectively. Other factors associated with a poor prognosis include advanced clinical stage, location in a minor salivary gland, and tumor size above four centimeter, bone invasion, involved excision margins, non-diploid DNA content, high S-phase fraction, and high Ki-67 index.

POLYMORPHOUS LOW GRADE ADENOCARCINOMA

(Terminal duct carcinoma, lobular carcinoma, low grade papillary adenocarcinoma)

Polymorphous low grade adenocarcinoma (PLGA) is an infiltrative malignant epithelial tumor characterized by diverse architectural patterns but unified by the presence of bland looking tumor cells. The term was used by Evans and Batsakis in 1984. In the AFIP series they form the fourth most common malignant salivary gland tumors. They represent about 11 percent of all minor salivary gland tumors and 26% of those that were malignant. The importance of recognizing this lies in the fact that it may mimic many benign and malignant salivary gland tumors and for many years was probably misdiagnosed as tumors such as adenoid cystic carcinoma and mixed tumors. The term polymorphous refers to the variety of growth patterns that may be identified within the same lesion and among different lesions (Figs 8.8A to F).

Clinical Features

The peak age of presentation is the fifth and sixth decades but children can also be affected. The female to male ratio is about 2:1. The tumor presents as an asymptomatic mass with or without mucosal ulceration. It is locally invasive with infrequent recurrences (12–25%) or lymph node metastasis (9–29%). PLGA occurs almost exclusively in the minor salivary gland sites, the commonest site being the hard and soft palate (60–70%) followed by the buccal mucosa (16%), upper lip (12%), retromolar area, and base of tongue.

Microscopic Features

Polymorphous low grade adenocarcinoma presents as an unencapsulated, circumscribed mass with a light tan to gray glistening cut surface. The tumor is composed of tumor cells arranged in solid sheets, trabeculae, ductular, tubular, glandular, papillary or papillary-cystic, and cribriform patterns. These cells have uniform round, oval or fusiform nuclei with finely stippled chromatin and inconspicuous nucleoli and a moderate amount of eosinophilic cytoplasm. Cell borders are indistinct. Mucinous cells or clear cells are occasionally seen. Myoepithelial cells are a minor component.

Small tubular structures with central lumens lined by a single layer of cuboidal cells are seen close to the periphery of the tumor infiltrating the surrounding tissue. There may also be concentric, streamlined or swirling columns and trabeculae of cells arranged around the tubules giving a target-like appearance—targetoid lesion, which is a relatively diagnostic pattern of growth in polymorphous low grade adenocarcinoma. In the papillary or papillary cystic patterns, dilated cysts with small intraluminal papillary projections lined by a single layer of cells are seen. Complex tubuloglandular or tubulopapillary structures may be present. Perivascular and perineural infiltration is seen in many tumors. Variability of growth pattern is the most consistent architectural feature of this tumor.

The stroma is often hyalinized, collagenous or mucinous. Intratubular calcifications resembling psammoma bodies, squamous metaplasia and pseudoepitheliomatous hyperplasia of the overlying epithelium may be seen. Mitosis and necrosis are rare.

Two cases of dedifferentiated polymorphous low grade adenocarcinoma have been reported. These had solid and cystic areas and had high nuclear grade and tumor necrosis.

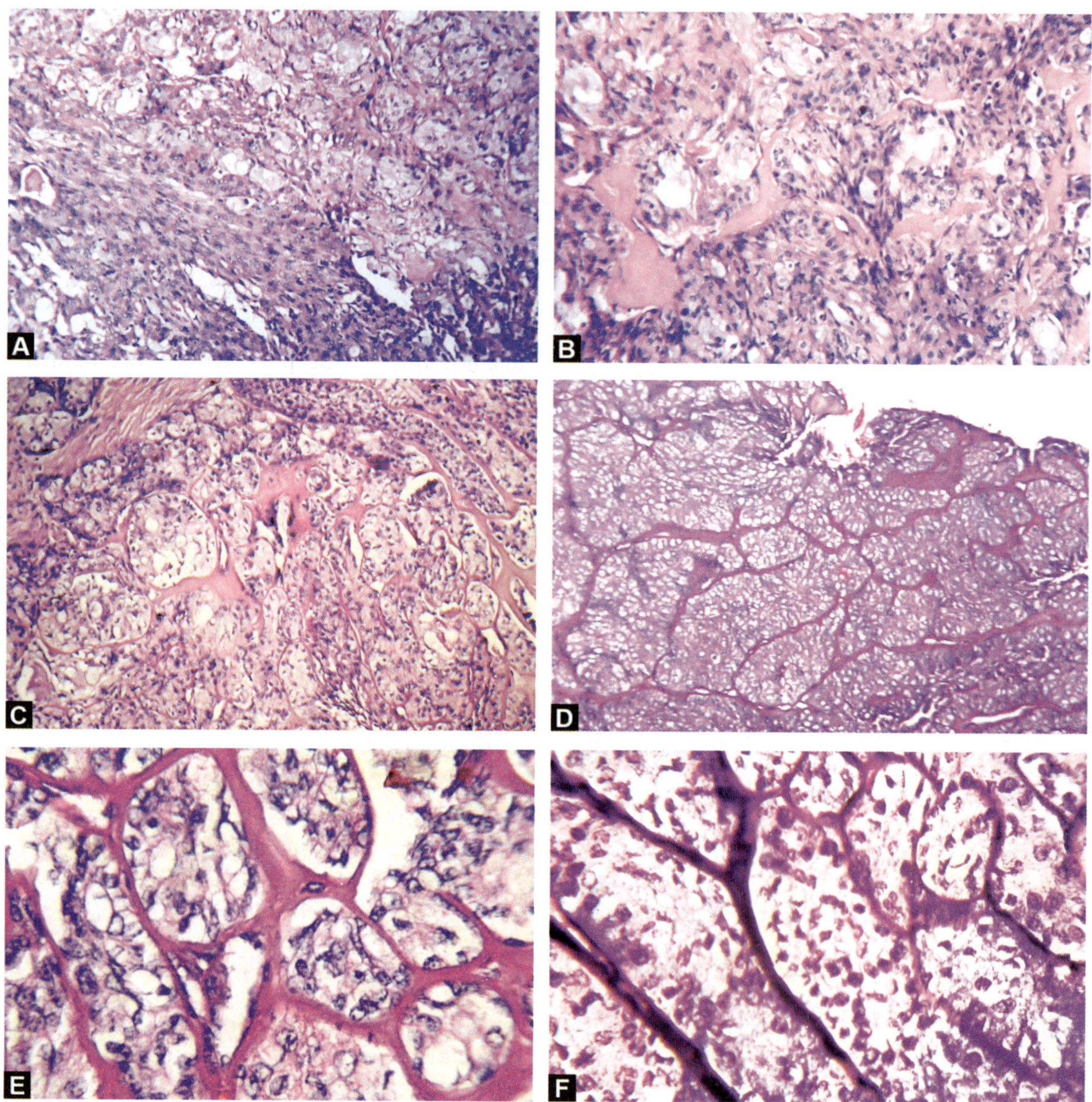

Figures 8.8A to F: Polymorphous low grade adenocarcinoma *(Courtesy:* Dr I Ponniah, Tamil Nadu Government Dental College and Hospital, Chennai)

Immunohistochemistry

The tumor cells in PLGA are immunoreactive for both low and high molecular weight cytokeratin, EMA and S-100 protein, vimentin and variably reactive for CEA and muscle specific actin. GFAP is usually negative. Overexpression of bcl-2 protein and a low proliferative index (mean Ki-67 index about 1.56–7%) are usually seen.

Differential Diagnosis

Polymorphous low grade adenocarcinoma should be distinguished from pleomorphic adenomas and adenoid cystic carcinomas. Benign mixed tumors do not show infiltration into surrounding tissues or nerves and blood vessels like PLGA; hence the need to include the tumor interface with surrounding tissue in the biopsy specimen. Further, the tubular or ductular structures in PLGA are often isolated from the solid areas unlike pleomorphic adenomas. Positive staining for GFAP in a mesenchymal-like cell population adjacent to epithelial nests is seen only in pleomorphic adenoma.

The nuclei of the tumor cells in PLGA are slightly larger and more round and uniform than the angular hyperchromatic nuclei of adenoid cystic carcinoma and the cytoplasm of the cells in PLGA stain eosinophilic whereas those of adenoid cystic carcinoma are clear. PLGA shows only focal areas of cribriform growth and does not show the large spaces containing hematoxyphilic glycosaminoglycans. In contrast to PLGA, EMA staining is confined to the glandular lumina in adenoid cystic carcinoma. S-100 protein staining is patchy and the proliferative index is much higher in adenoid cystic carcinoma.

Prognosis

Polymorphous low grade adenocarcinoma is an indolent neoplasm. Recurrence may occur and has been reported to be about 17%. The regional metastasis occurs to the cervical lymph nodes and the rate is about 6 to 10%. Although PLGAs were considered to be indolent tumors recently three cases of PLGA with microscopically confirmed distant metastases have been reported, one with metastasis to the lung, another to the orbit and skin and the third with multiple pleural and pulmonary parenchymal metastases and metastases in the para-esophageal lymph nodes.

EPITHELIAL-MYOEPITHELIAL CARCINOMA

(Adenomyoepithelioma)
Epithelial-myocpithclial carcinoma is a biphasic low grade malignant neoplasm composed of ductal and myoepithelial cells in which large, clear, myoepithelial cells predominate. Donath et al introduced the term epithelial-myoepithelial carcinoma of intercalated duct origin in 1972. This is a rare tumor and constitutes less than one percent of all salivary gland neoplasms.

Clinical Features

The peak incidence is in the seventh and eighth decades with a female predominance (60%). Localized swelling may be the only symptom but occasionally patients present with facial weakness or pain. Local recurrences occur in about 30% of cases. Facial paralysis may occur and patients with maxillary involvement may present with nasal obstruction and facial deformity. Some studies have suggested that patients with these tumors are at risk of a second malignancy in the salivary gland itself or other sites like the breast or thyroid. The association of epithelial myoepithelial carcinoma with another primary salivary gland neoplasm has also been reported. It is predominantly a tumor of the parotid gland (75%), the remainder develop equally in the submandibular and intraoral minor salivary glands, mainly the palate and tongue.

Macroscopic Features

The tumor is typically single, well circumscribed, lobulated and may even be partially encapsulated. The size may vary from two to eight centimeters. The cut surface is multinodular with irregular cystic spaces.

Microscopic Features

Histologically, the tumor is made up of multiple nodules of tumor cells separated by a dense fibrous stroma. Within the tumor nodules, the stroma can be scanty and loose, myxoid, hyalinized or fibrous. The islands show a distinct bicellular differentiation and the architecture consists of small duct-like structures lined by an inner layer of cuboidal, intercalated duct-like cells with eosinophilic or amphophilic cytoplasm, round central or basal nuclei, and an outer layer of large, columnar to ovoid, clear myoepithelial cells with eccentrically placed vesicular nuclei, enveloped by a well-defined basement membrane. Rarely there can be squamous differentiation in the duct-like cells. The clear cells contain glycogen and that can be demonstrated with PAS staining. The ductal lumen may have material that stains positive with mucicarmine and alcian blue but there is no intracytoplasmic mucin.

In some tumors there may be more complex glandular structures, papillary cystic structures, trabeculae, nests, and large sheets of clear cells delineated by a thick basement membrane. Rarely fascicles of spindle shaped myoepithelial cells may be present. Cytologic atypia is minimal with low mitotic count. Tumors with greater nuclear atypia, solid growth patterns and frequent mitoses belong to a higher grade.

Immunohistochemistry

Immunohistochemical studies of epithelial-myoepithelial carcinomas show the ductal cells to be strongly positive for cytokeratin and variably positive for S-100 protein. The clear cells are variably immunoreactive for S-100 protein, calponin and actin. The proliferation index (Ki-67) is low; <1% for ductal cells and <3% for myoepithelial clear cells.

Differential Diagnosis

Neoplasms that should be differentiated from this are pleomorphic adenoma, acinic cell adenocarcinoma, adenoid cystic carcinoma, mucoepidermoid carcinoma, sebaceous carcinoma and metastatic renal cell carcinoma. Epithelial-myoepithelial carcinoma does not exhibit the varying growth patterns and chondromyxoid areas that are characteristic of pleomorphic adenoma. The clear cells of acinic cell adenocarcinoma are negative for PAS stain and these clear cells are believed to occur due to a processing artifact.

Adenoid cystic carcinoma is differentiated from epithelial-myoepithelial carcinoma by the paucity of large clear cells and the presence of

cyst-like structures containing basement membrane-like intercellular substance. Although mucoepidermoid carcinomas may have areas of clear cells like epithelial-myoepithelial carcinomas, the former also have mucous and epidermoid cells not seen in the latter. Further, myoepithelial cells are not seen in mucoepidermoid carcinoma. The clear cells of sebaceous carcinoma stain positive for lipid and not glycogen. Metastatic tumors having clear cells are differentiated from epithelial-myoepithelial carcinoma by a careful clinical history and special stains.

Prognosis

Generally it is a low grade tumor but local recurrences may occur. It has been reported that nuclear atypia in more than 20% of the tumor cells indicates a poorer prognosis. Metastasis may occur to the periparotid and cervical lymph nodes. However, distant metastasis (lung, kidney, and brain) is uncommon (9%).

CLEAR CELL ADENOCARCINOMA

(Glycogen rich carcinoma, clear cell carcinoma, glycogen rich monomorphic clear cell carcinoma)
Clear cell adenocarcinoma is a very rare malignant epithelial neoplasm composed of a monomorphous population of cells that have optically clear cytoplasm with standard hematoxylin and eosin stains and lack features of other specific neoplasms. They comprise less than one percent of epithelial salivary gland neoplasms reviewed at the AFIP. It was Batsakis and Regezi who first stated that majority of nonmucinous epithelial clear cell neoplasms were malignant and since then the classification of this group of tumors has undergone significant modifications over the last decade.

Clinical Features

The peak incidence of this tumor is in the fifth to seventh decades and occurs mainly in females. Most of them present as painless slow growing masses while the others may ulcerate or show fixation to underlying tissues. Only rarely do they metastasize to the cervical lymph nodes.

Clear cell adenocarcinoma occurs mainly in the minor salivary glands of the oral cavity (57%) especially in the palate, buccal mucosa, tongue, floor of the mouth, lip, and retromolar and tonsillar areas. Cases have also been reported in the parotid and submandibular glands.

Macroscopic Features

The tumor is usually about 3 cm in size and is poorly circumscribed but not encapsulated with a grayish-white to grayish-tan cut surface. It may infiltrate the mucosal surface, bone and nerves.

Microscopic Features

Clear cell adenocarcinoma is composed of cords, nests, sheets, or streaming columns of large monomorphic clear cells separated by a stroma that may comprise interconnecting fibrous septae, thick cellular collagenous bands, short feathery strands or dense, eosinophilic, hyaline ground substance. Microcysts may occur but ductular structures are usually absent. The cells are polygonal to round with discrete cell membranes and the abundant clear cytoplasm are due to the accumulation of glycogen (PAS positive-diastase sensitive, mucicarmine negative). The nuclei are centrally or eccentrically located with fine, granular chromatin, inconspicuous nucleoli and exhibiting mild to moderate atypia. Foci of polygonal cells with eosinophilic cytoplasm may be found. Mitotic figures are rare.

Immunohistochemistry

Clear cell adenocarcinomas exhibit focal or diffuse immunoreactivity for high molecular weight cytokeratin and both positive and negative immunostaining for S-100 protein, GFAP, actin and vimentin have been reported. Ultrastructural studies show features of only duct differentiation and no myoepithelial differentiation.

Differential Diagnosis

Clear cell adenocarcinoma is a diagnosis of exclusion of other specific tumor types having clear cells. In mucoepidermoid carcinoma, mucicarmine and Alcian blue positive mucocytes and epidermoid cells are seen.

In acinic cell adenocarcinomas, the clear cells have PAS positive-diastase resistant, intracytoplasmic granules with microcystic, papillary-cystic and follicular patterns.

Unlike clear cell adenocarcinoma, epithelial-myoepithelial carcinoma has a biphasic cell population wherein lumina lined by small cuboidal, eosinophilic, lumen-lining cells are surrounded by clear cells. Oncocytomas with clear cells are not infiltrative and are reactive with PTAH and have excessive mitochondria in the cytoplasm. Sebaceous adenomas and adenocarcinomas have lipids rather than glycogen in the cytoplasm. Metastatic renal cell carcinoma has prominent cytologic atypia and dilated vascular channels with hemorrhage and hemosiderin. Moreover, lipid may be demonstrated in the cytoplasm of the clear cells of metastatic clear cell carcinoma by using frozen sections.

Those tumors arising from near the maxillary or mandibular alveolar ridges have to be differentiated from clear cell odontogenic carcinoma. Radiographic evidence of a centralized destructive osseous lesion indicates odontogenic rather than salivary gland origin.

Prognosis

Clear cell adenocarcinoma is a low grade malignant neoplasm and may recur and metastasize.

BASAL CELL ADENOCARCINOMA

Basal cell adenocarcinoma is an epithelial neoplasm that is cytologically and immunohistochemically similar to basal cell adenoma but is infiltrative and has a potential for metastasis. It comprises about 1.6% of all salivary gland neoplasms and 2.9% of malignant salivary gland neoplasms in the AFIP case files. Most of them arise *de novo* but a small percentage is believed to have developed in basal cell adenomas especially the membranous subtype.

Clinical Features

The average age of presentation of basal cell adenocarcinoma is about 60 years with no sex predilection. Most patients present with swelling of the affected gland and a sudden increase in size may occur in some patients. The tumors are infiltrative and locally destructive. Ninety percent of these tumors occur in the parotid gland usually in the superficial lobe and are rare in the minor salivary glands.

Microscopic Features

Basal cell adenocarcinomas also show the same solid, membranous, trabecular and tubular patterns seen in their benign counterpart. Among these the solid pattern is the most common followed by the membranous, trabecular and tubular types. It may be difficult to distinguish basal cell adenocarcinoma from basal cell adenoma on the basis of cytomorphologic features alone and hence the growth of the tumor in relation to the surrounding tissues is used to distinguish adenoma from carcinoma.

Under low power, basal cell adenocarcinomas resemble eccrine cylindromas of the skin. Under higher magnification, two types of epithelial cells may be seen, one which is small, round with scanty cytoplasm and a dark basophilic nucleus and the other which is large polygonal to elongated with eosinophilic/amphophilic cytoplasm and a large pale basophilic nucleus (Figs 8.9A and B).

The dark cells are located peripheral to the large pale cells and may have a palisading pattern. The pale cells may form swirls or eddies with a squamoid appearance with occasional keratinization. Small tubules or lumina may be seen in many of the epithelial islands. Eosinophilic, PAS positive material may be seen around the islands. Cytologic atypia varies from minimal to moderate and mitotic figures vary from zero to nine or ten per HPF. The amount of intervening fibrous stroma varies from inconspicuous to extensive and it frequently contains lymphocytic and plasmacytic infiltrates. Infiltrative growth along with perineural and vascular invasion are seen.

Immunohistochemistry

Immunohistochemically basal cell adeno-carcinomas exhibit reactivity for smooth muscle actin and vimentin. Tumors are positive for cytokeratin and often focally reactive for S-100 protein, EMA and CEA.

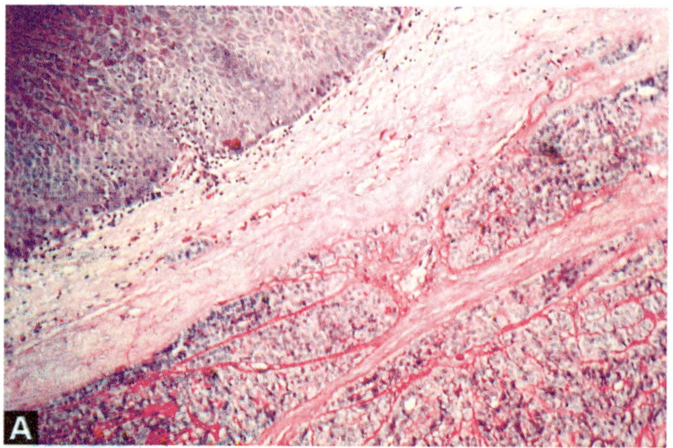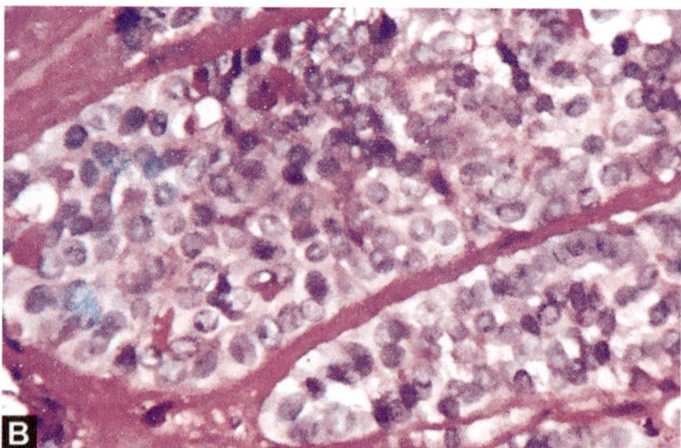

Figures 8.9A and B: Basal cell adenocarcinoma: (A) Islands of basaloid cells that surrounded by PAS positive material; (B) The peripheral cells of the islands are columnar and exhibit palisaded arrangement *(Courtesy:* Dr I Ponniah, Tamil Nadu Government Dental College and Hospital, Chennai)

Differential Diagnosis

The tumors to be ruled out are basal cell adenoma, adenoid cystic carcinoma, polymorphous low grade adenocarcinoma and basaloid squamous cell carcinoma. Neither ultrastructural characteristics nor immunohistochemistry findings appear to distinguish basal cell adenocarcinoma from basal cell adenoma; however basal cell adenoma does not show infiltration of surrounding tissue and lacks significant cytologic atypia and mitosis. Most basal cell adenocarcinomas are positive for p53 and EGFR while bcl2 expression is seen in basal cell adenomas.

Basal cell adenocarcinomas and polymorphous low grade adenocarcinoma show bland cytologic features, infiltrative growth and low grade malignant behavior. However basal cell adenocarcinomas do not have the myriad morphologic patterns and swirling formations seen in the latter.

Basal cell adenocarcinoma does not show the cribriform pattern, pseudocysts and hyperchromatic cells with angular nuclei and pale cytoplasm seen in adenoid cystic carcinoma. Basaloid squamous cell carcinoma has a malignant squamous component and is unreactive for smooth muscle actin.

Prognosis

Basal cell adenocarcinomas are generally low grade carcinomas that are locally destructive with infrequent occurrence of regional lymph node or distant metastases to the lung. The tumors arising in the minor salivary glands appear to have a higher local recurrence rate (71%), metastatic rate (21%) and mortality (29%) compared to those arising in the major glands.

SEBACEOUS ADENOCARCINOMA

Sebaceous adenocarcinoma is a rare malignant epithelial tumor composed of islands and sheets of cells with morphologically atypical nuclei, infiltrative growth pattern and focal sebaceous differentiation. Only a few cases have been reported in literature.

Clinical Features

There is a biphasic age distribution with cases occurring in the third and in the seventh and eight decades of life. These tumors occur equally in males and females. Patients present with a painless, asymptomatic, slow growing swelling or with pain and a few have facial paralysis. Occasionally there may be fixation to the skin over the tumor. Almost all the cases reported have occurred in the parotid gland.

Macroscopic Features

The tumor size ranges from 0.6 to 8.5 cm and the color varies from yellow, tan-white, grayish-white and white to pale pink. It is usually well circumscribed with partial encapsulation and pushing or focal infiltrative margins.

Microscopic Features

Islands, sheets and cords of basaloid, squamous and sebaceous cells are seen along with duct-like or cystic spaces. Sebaceous cells are seen among the islands of cytomorphologically atypical basaloid and squamous cells. Cellular pleomorphism, nuclear atypia, frequent mitoses, tumor necrosis and perineural invasion (20%) may be seen. Vascular invasion is unusual.

Prognosis

Sebaceous adenocarcinomas are considered to be intermediate grade malignancies. Recurrences occur in about 33% of cases. Out of 20 cases reported, 6 have died as a result of the tumor within 5 years of diagnosis.

SEBACEOUS LYMPHADENOCARCINOMA

Sebaceous lymphadenocarcinoma is a very rare malignant tumor which represents carcinomatous transformation of a sebaceous lymphadenoma. It is the rarest tumor of the salivary glands and till date about three cases have been reported in literature. One was a sebaceous lymphadenoma with transition to a sebaceous lympadenocarcinoma.

Clinical Features

All the three cases reported have occurred in patients in the seventh decade. Two of them were males and one was a female. The masses were asymptomatic. All the tumors reported arose in the parotid gland or in a periparotid lymph node.

Macroscopic Features

The tumors vary from yellow, tan to gray and show focal encapsulation, and areas of local invasion.

Microscopic Features

The tumor contains areas of typical sebaceous lymphadenoma juxtaposed with a malignant component which may be a sebaceous carcinoma, undifferentiated carcinoma, adenoid cystic carcinoma or epithelial myoepithelial carcinoma. The malignant component lacks the lymphoid stroma. Perineural invasion, collections of histiocytes, and a foreign body giant cell reaction have all been reported.

Prognosis

These tumors behave more aggressively than their orbital counterparts with a five year survival rate of about 62.2%.

CYSTADENOCARCINOMA

(Malignant papillary cystadenoma, mucus producing adenopapillary carcinoma, low grade papillary adenocarcinoma of the palate, papillary adenocarcinoma)

Cystadenocarcinoma is a rare malignant epithelial neoplasm characterized histologically by prominent cystic and frequent papillary growth, but lacking the features that are seen in the cystic variants of other more common salivary gland neoplasms. It is the malignant counterpart of cystadenoma. The term cystadenocarcinoma was first applied to these tumors in 1978 by the AFIP.

Clinical Features

The average age of the patients has been reported to be about 59 years with both men and women being affected equally. The patient usually presents with a painless, slow-growing, asymptomatic mass. Pain and facial nerve weakness may be seen in the parotid gland but fixation to overlying structures is usually not seen. Most of the tumors arise in the major salivary glands (65%) and primarily in the parotid. The minor gland sites include the lips, buccal mucosa, palate, tongue, retromolar area, and floor of the mouth.

Macroscopic Features

The tumor ranges in size from 0.4 to 6 cm. The cut surface may show single or multiple cysts containing clear or brown fluid.

Microscopic Features

Cystadenocarcinomas are composed of numerous irregular cystic spaces and duct like structures separated by connective tissue. Intraluminal papillary processes (seen in 75% of cases) and foci of solid growth and extraluminal extension may be seen. The cysts are lined by small cuboidal, large cuboidal or columnar cells showing mild to moderate cellular atypia and prominent nucleoli. Mucus, clear, oncocytic and rarely epidermoid cells can be present focally.

The stroma shows fibrosis with foci of sclerosis and hyalinization. Desmoplastic change may be seen. Invasion of surrounding tissue and perineural invasion (9%) may be present. Cystadeno-carcinomas may show small focal areas with features of acinic cell adenocarcinoma, epithelial-myoepithelial carcinoma or mucoepidermoid carcinoma.

Differential Diagnosis

The differential diagnosis includes cystadenomas, polymorphous low grade adenocarcinoma and papillary-cystic acinic cell carcinoma. Differentiation of cystadenocarcinoma from cystadenomas depends largely on identifying infiltration of the salivary gland parenchyma or surrounding stroma. Polymorphous low grade adenocarcinoma usually arises in the minor salivary glands and has whirling fascicles of cells encircling the islands. Acinic cell carcinomas show a microcystic growth pattern and large round cells with deeply basophilic, granular cytoplasm with diastase-resistant PAS positive material both of which are not seen in cystadenocarcinomas.

Prognosis

Cystadenocarcinoma is a low grade tumor with a good prognosis. In a series of cases studied, 7.7% had recurrence and 10% had metastases to the regional lymph nodes. Tumors arising in the minor glands and those composed predominantly of pseudostratified tall columnar cells may be associated with a higher rate of metastasis.

MUCINOUS ADENOCARCINOMA

Mucinous adenocarcinoma is a rare malignant neoplasm characterized by large amounts of extracellular epithelial mucin amidst which are seen the tumor cells. It represents the salivary gland counterpart of mucinous or colloid carcinoma of other sites such as the breast and skin. Only a few cases have been reported so far.

Clinical Features

All cases reported have occurred in adults with no gender predilection. The tumor may be associated with dull pain and tenderness. Few cases reported have occurred in the submandibular gland.

Macroscopic Features

The gross specimens were mucoid and slimy and were circumscribed.

Microscopic Features

This tumor is characterized by clusters of tumor cells floating in pools of extracellular mucin. The tumor cells may also be arranged in ducts, papillae, cysts, and cribriform structures. The cells are moderately large, cuboidal or polygonal with eosinophilic to amphophilic cytoplasm and vesicular nuclei. Few mitotic figures and minimal pleomorphism can be seen. The mucoid substance stains with mucicarmine, PAS and Alcian blue at a pH of 2.0. Many of the cells are mucicarminophilic.

Differential Diagnosis

The main differential diagnosis would be mucus producing cystadenocarcinoma. In mucinous adenocarcinoma the epithelial cells are surrounded by mucoid substance and epithelium lined cysts are minimal while in mucus producing cystadenocarcinomas, the epithelial cells surround the mucoid substance and there are many epithelium lined cystic structures.

It is difficult to differentiate between mucinous carcinomas of eccrine origin and mucinous adenocarcinomas.

Prognosis

Mucinous adenocarcinoma is a low grade tumor. Patients with similar tumors in the skin and breast have a better prognosis than those with other types of carcinomas.

ONCOCYTIC CARCINOMA

Oncocytic carcinoma is a rare oncocytic tumor that demonstrates malignant histologic features and/ or behavior. This tumor represents about less than one percent of all salivary gland tumors and 11% of all oncocytic salivary gland neoplasms. It was first reported by Langhans in 1907 and was previously termed malignant oncocytoma and malignant oxyphilic granular cell tumor.

Clinical Features

The average age of patients with this tumor is about 63 years. It has a male predilection and appears to occur at an earlier age. It may arise from a pre-existing oncocytoma or *de novo*. Parotid gland is the common site of occurrence but may involve other major and minor salivary glands also.

Macroscopic Features

Oncocytic carcinoma is an unencapsulated, single or multinodular tumor.

Microscopic Features

The tumor is composed of trabeculae, sheets, nests or clusters of large round or polyhedral cells with abundant, granular, eosinophilic cytoplasm and moderately pleomorphic medium sized or large central nuclei with large, irregular nucleoli. The tumor cells infiltrate the salivary gland parenchyma, adjacent connective tissue and also show perineural and vascular invasion. Frequent atypical mitoses and coagulative tumor necrosis are seen. PTAH stain effectively demonstrates numerous mitochondria in the oncocytes which stain as deep blue cytoplasmic granules. Immunohistochemical staining with anti-mitochondrial antibody is also useful.

Differential Diagnosis

The infiltrative growth pattern and presence of coagulative tumor necrosis distinguishes oncocytic carcinoma from an incompletely excised or recurrent benign oncocytoma. However, a history of prior local excision should be sought in these cases.

Special stains and electron microscopic examination for the presence of mitochondria in oncocytic carcinoma help to differentiate this from other adenocarcinomas. Salivary duct carcinomas, which have large cells with granular cytoplasm, do not stain with PTAH and do not show mitochondrial hyperplasia under the electron microscope. Acinic cell adenocarcinomas have more prominent zymogen granularity and PAS positivity than oncocytic carcinomas while mucoepidermoid carcinomas have intracytoplasmic mucin which is not seen in oncocytic carcinomas. Pleomorphic adenoma with oncocytic features will have evidence of myoepithelial, chondromyxoid and osseous features.

Prognosis

Oncocytic carcinoma is high grade neoplasm and it has been reported that tumors less than 2 cm have a better prognosis. Frequent recurrences are common (56%) and are believed to be an indicator of metastatic potential. The occurrence of regional lymph node metastasis carries a grave prognosis and distant metastases (80%) occur to the lungs, kidney, liver, thyroid, mediastinum, and bone. The mortality rate at 15 years is about 40%.

SALIVARY DUCT CARCINOMA

(Salivary duct adenocarcinoma)

Salivary duct carcinoma is a rare highly aggressive malignant neoplasm composed of structures that resemble expanded salivary gland ducts and is considered as counterpart of invasive ductal carcinoma of the mammary gland. This entity was first described by Kleinsasser et al who first used the term salivary duct carcinoma in 1968. Salivary duct carcinomas comprise about 0.5 to 3.9% of all salivary gland carcinomas.

Clinical Features

The tumor most frequently occurs in the sixth and seventh decades of life with a male predilection. Patients commonly present with a rapidly enlarging parotid with facial palsy (42%), pain (23%), and cervical lymphadenopathy (35%). About 80% of the salivary duct carcinomas arise in the parotid gland with the remaining occurring in the submandibular gland and very rarely in the minor glands. Salivary duct carcinomas may arise *de novo* or comprise the malignant component of a carcinoma ex-pleomorphic adenoma.

Macroscopic Features

The tumors vary in size from 1 cm to greater than 6 cm. They are usually poorly demarcated, yellowish gray to grayish white in color and solid with foci of necrosis.

Microscopic Features

The tumor is composed of variably sized, circular nodules resembling ductal carcinoma of the breast. These nodules are either cystic or solid with central comedonecrosis in the cystic nodules (Figs 8.10A to C). Both intraductal and infiltrative components are seen. The intraductal cells are arranged in band-like, papillary, and cribriform patterns while the infiltrative component consists of cords, nests,

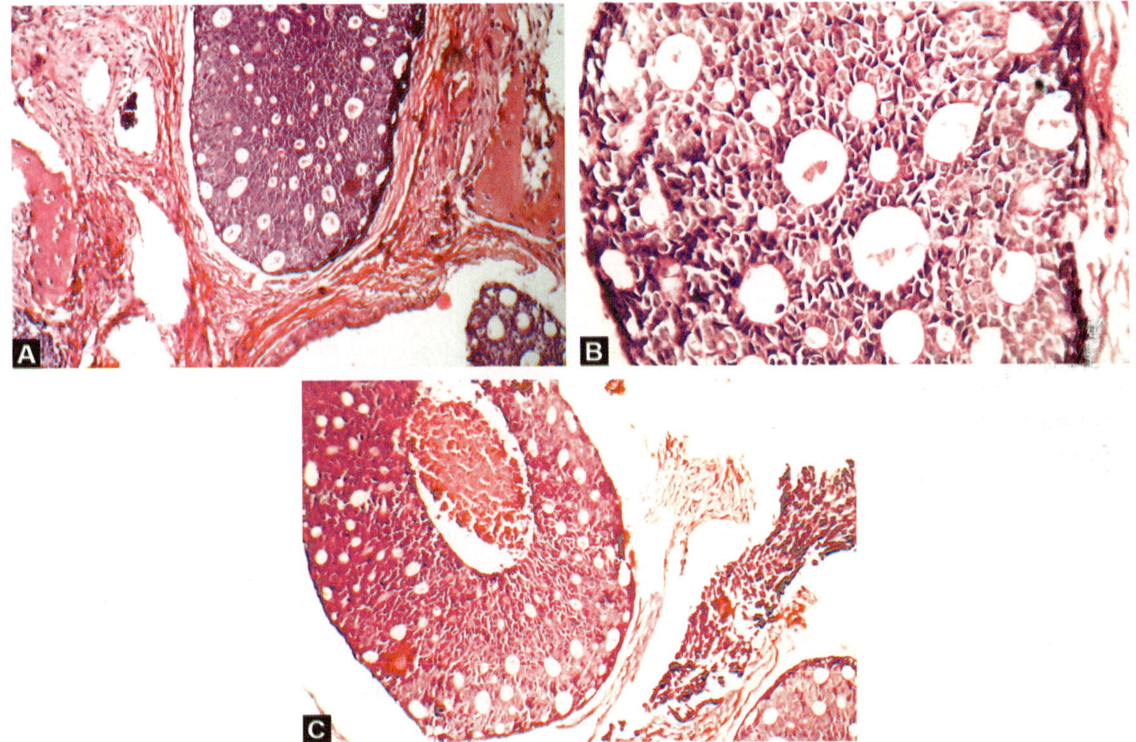

Figures 8.10A to C: Salivary duct carcinoma. Islands with cribriform pattern (A) with central comedonecrosis (C) is a characteristic features of salivary duct carcinoma. But comedonecrosis is not a requisite. The tumor cells are cuboidal (B) and polygonal ductal cells. *(Courtesy:* Dr I Ponniah, Tamil Nadu Government Dental College, Chennai)

small glands, and single cells. In both components the tumor cells are polygonal or cuboidal with moderately abundant eosinophilic cytoplasm with large pleomorphic, vesicular nuclei and prominent nucleoli and may have an apocrine appearance. Cytologic pleomorphism and mitotic activity vary from slight to marked and the stroma is densely fibrous or desmoplastic with focal areas of hyalinization. Perineural (75%) and vascular invasion (66%) with infiltration of adjacent structures are common.

Variants

The variants that have been recently described are, salivary duct carcinoma with invasive micropapillary component, mucin rich variant and sarcomatoid salivary duct carcinoma.

Immunohistochemistry

The tumor cells in salivary duct carcinomas show diffuse strong staining for cytokeratin, EMA and CEA. Reactivity for S-100 protein is variable. Most cases express GCDFP-15 (BRST-2) and c-erbB-2. Rarely there may be positivity for progesterone receptor, androgen receptor or prostate specific antigen. Ki-67 index is high: the mean being about 21.3 percent. A high expression of peroxisome proliferator-activated receptor gamma (PPAR gamma) has been reported in a recent study. 79 percent of the tumors are non diploid and the mean S phase fraction is 11%. Inactivation of the p16 gene probably plays a role in the development or progression of this tumor type.

Differential Diagnosis

The major differential diagnoses are metastatic breast carcinoma, acinic cell adenocarcinoma, high grade mucoepidermoid carcinoma, oncocytic carcinoma, cystadenocarcinoma and polymorphous low grade adenocarcinoma.

A thorough clinical history and physical examination should be done to rule out metastatic breast disease. Negative staining for estrogen receptor with diffuse intense staining for CEA favors a diagnosis of salivary duct carcinoma.

In addition to a papillary cystic pattern of growth, acini cell adenocarcinomas also have microcystic, solid and follicular patterns. Salivary duct carcinomas have only one cell type whereas a number of cell types namely, acinar, intercalated duct, vacuolated, clear and non- specific glandular cells are seen in acinic cell adenocarcinomas. Hyalinized fibrous stroma and an intraductal component are not seen in acinic cell adenocarcinoma.

The mixture of cell types seen in mucoepidermoid carcinoma is not seen in salivary duct carcinoma. High grade mucoepidermoid carcinomas lack cribriform and papillary growth patterns. Both oncocytic carcinoma and cystadenocarcinoma lack the comedonecrosis and intraductal pattern seen in this tumor. Polymorphous low grade adenocarcinoma occurs almost exclusively in the minor salivary glands whereas salivary duct carcinoma is seen principally in the major glands. The cytologic pleomorphism, increased mitotic figures, and comedonecrosis are not seen in PLGA.

Prognosis

Salivary duct carcinoma is one of the most aggressive salivary gland carcinomas. Tumor size of less than 3 cm and an intraductal component of more the 90% are believed to be associated with a more favorable prognosis. Recurrence rates are high with local recurrences occurring in about 35 to 66% of patients. Lymph node metastases occur in 66% of cases and distant metastases to the lung, bone and brain occur in 50 to 70% of cases. A few cases of metastasis to the skin and one rare case of metastasis to the bowel have been reported.

INTRADUCTAL CARCINOMA

Intraductal carcinoma of the salivary gland is an *in situ* form of salivary duct carcinoma that is very rare and has the potential to develop into an invasive salivary duct carcinoma. The term intraductal carcinoma was first introduced by Chen in 1983 and till date, about 16 such cases have been reported, many under the term low grade salivary duct carcinoma. The existence of this entity is considered controversial by some authors while others believe that by using strict criteria for diagnosis, intraductal carcinoma is a distinctive entity which may represent the preinvasive phase of some invasive salivary duct carcinomas but by itself is nonmetastasizing and having an excellent prognosis.

Clinical Features

Intraductal carcinoma of the salivary gland occurs in adults with a mean age of 60 years. There is a slight female predominance. Patients usually present with a mass. The tumor predominantly affects the parotid gland, although the minor glands can also be involved.

Microscopic Features

The tumor consists of multiple smooth contoured dilated ducts with tumor cells arranged in a cribriform, pseudocribriform, solid comedo, micropapillary or Roman bridge pattern similar to that of atypical hyperplasia or intraductal carcinoma of the breast with the cells ranging from bland looking to highly pleomorphic and in some areas apocrine. The defining feature, however, is the preservation of pre-existing myoepithelial cells around these epithelial units. The stroma is sclerotic and may have foci of hemorrhage, chronic inflammation, and calcification.

Differential Diagnosis

This tumor should be differentiated from salivary duct carcinoma which is a highly lethal neoplasm. This is facilitated by strictly using the following diagnostic criteria:

1. Resembling mammary intraductal carcinoma with islands of epithelial proliferation exhibiting a cribriform, micropapillary, solid, comedo or clinging pattern.
2. Cytologic grade which may be low, intermediate or high.
3. Exclusion of an invasive component by:
   - Thorough sampling, and
   - Immunohistochemical staining (such as actin or p63 antibody) to demonstrate myoepithelial or basal cells around all epithelial islands.

Prognosis

Following surgical excision, the recurrence rate is about 20%.

ADENOCARCINOMA NOT OTHERWISE SPECIFIED

Adenocarcinoma not otherwise specified (ANOS) refers to a group of primary carcinomas of the salivary glands that exhibit ductal and glandular differentiation but lack sufficient histologic features of the currently recognized categories of salivary gland carcinoma to allow for a more specific diagnosis. There is a wide variation in the reporting of the incidence of these neoplasms. According to an AFIP review, it is the second most common malignant salivary gland neoplasm, accounting for about 9% of all salivary gland tumors and 17% of all carcinomas.

Clinical Features

Average age of occurrence is about 58 years of age with a male predilection for high grade tumors. Patients usually present with an asymptomatic mass or fast growing painful mass associated with ulceration and fixation to the underlying structures. Facial nerve palsy is common. Pain occurs more frequently in the submandibular tumors and ulceration in case of involvement of the minor gland. Recurrence and distant metastasis to the lung occur more commonly in the case of high grade tumors. Most of the tumors occur in the parotid gland (90%) followed by the submandibular gland. The most common minor gland sites are the palate, buccal mucosa, and the lips.

Macroscopic Features

Grossly the tumors are poorly circumscribed with irregular, infiltrative borders. The cut surface is tan and solid with areas of hemorrhage or necrosis.

Microscopic Features

Adenocarcinoma NOS is characterized by glandular or ductal structures with variable organization and variable amounts of intervening connective tissue. Apart from this, cystic and papillary formations have been shown to be occasionally present. There is typically a complete lack of epidermoid differentiation. The glandular structures are composed of cuboidal cells with other areas showing polygonal epithelial cells forming solid nests or tumor islands. The tumor cells may also be columnar, polygonal or oval. Mucinous, clear, and oncocytic cells are also not uncommon. There is also a report of tumors with plasmacytoid and melanoma-like phenotypes and true sebaceous differentiation and areas resembling salivary duct carcinomas. The AFIP has reported that ANOS could exhibit foci of adenoid cystic carcinoma, acinic cell carcinoma, and epithelial-myoepithelial carcinoma. Infiltration of the normal parenchyma and perineural and perivascular invasion is also common.

Grading of ANOS

On the basis of histologic features the tumor has been graded into low grade, intermediate grade and high grade categories as follows:

It has been also recommended that high-grade tumors be distinguished from low grade tumors by the presence of one or more of the following

Table 8.4: Grading of adenocarcinoma not otherwise specified (ANOS)		
Low grade	*Intermediate grade*	*High grade*
• Well formed ductal and tubular structures • Few mitoses • Minimal variation in size, shape and staining of nuclei • Coagulative necrosis is uncommon	• Moderate nuclear morphologic variability • Frequent mitoses	• Large cells with pleomorphic, hyperchromatic nuclei • Frequent mitoses, often atypical • Coagulative necrosis is common

features: nuclear atypia, high mitotic rate, atypical mitotic figures, necrosis, perineural invasion, bony invasion, angiolymphatic invasion, and an aggressive pattern of invasion. An aggressive pattern of invasion is seen as infiltration at the tumor interface composed of small islands or strands, or 1 mm or more of normal tissue intervening tumor islands (Table 8.4).

Variants

Other types that have been reported are adenocarcinoma of tubular type which has prominent duct formation, signet-ring cell (mucin-producing) and the sclerosing type which has prominent fibrous desmoplasia.

Differential Diagnosis

Since lack of recognizable patterns seen in other salivary gland tumors is the single unifying feature in the diagnosis of this neoplasm, the diagnosis of adenocarcinoma NOS is one of exclusions. The bland cytologic features of low grade adenocarcinoma NOS, may cause misinterpretation as pleomorphic adenoma. However, unequivocal demonstration of infiltration of surrounding tissues helps in the differentiation.

The presence of clear cells in adenocarcinoma NOS, may warrant a differential diagnosis of clear cell adenocarcinoma or epithelial-myoepithelial carcinoma but adenocarcinoma NOS lacks the biphasic pattern of epithelial-myoepithelial carcinoma and the prominent presence of clear cells in clear cell adenocarcinoma. Polymorphous low grade adenocarcinoma differs from adenocarcinoma NOS in having a characteristic concentric, whirling of cells and variable growth patterns and cell types with focal myxoid areas. Adenocarcinomas NOS are distinguished from hybrid carcinomas in that the latter term is reserved for tumors showing two or more disparate architectural patterns that are both prominent and none are focal.

Prognosis

The prognosis is dependent on the grade, stage, and site of the tumor. The 15-year survival rates for low, intermediate, and high grade tumors are 54%, 31% and 3% respectively. The 10 year cure rate is about 75% for stage I tumors, irrespective of grade. Further, tumours involving the oral cavity have a more favorable outcome than those of the parotid and submandibular gland. Distant metastases have been reported to occur in 37% of patients.

MYOEPITHELIAL CARCINOMA

(Malignant Myoepithelioma)
Myoepithelial carcinoma is a rare, malignant salivary gland neoplasm in which the tumor cells almost exclusively manifest myoepithelial differentiation. Cytologic abnormalities and infiltrative growth distinguish them from myoepithelioma. They constitute about 0.2% of all epithelial neoplasms of the salivary glands.

Clinical Features

The peak age at presentation is the sixth decade and occurs equally in both males and females. It can arise *de novo* or from a pre-existing pleomorphic adenoma or myoepithelioma. Most patients present with a painless mass. Recurrence rates range from 8 to 59%. The most common site of distant metastases is the lung followed by the liver and vertebra. The parotid gland is primarily involved (66%), while the minor glands and submandibular gland are involved in about 25 and 10% of cases. The palate is the most common intraoral site.

Macroscopic Features

The tumor ranges from 2 to 20 cm in size. It is usually unencapsulated and may show areas of necrosis and cystic degeneration.

Microscopic Features

The cellular morphology is similar to that of benign myoepithelioma and includes the spindle cell, plasmacytoid, clear and epitheloid types. The cell types are often intermixed but the spindle cell type is the most common. Solid, fascicular, trabecular and lace-like growth patterns are common with variable amounts of myxoid, collagenous, or hyaline stroma. There may also be sheets of tumor cells with a cellular periphery and a necrotic or myxoid central zone. Nuclear atypia ranges from mild to marked and mitotic figures may range from 3 to 51/10 HPF. Necrosis, perineural, and vascular invasion are frequent and some may have areas of chondroid, squamous, or sebaceous metaplasia.

The clear cell variety has tight nests, hyalinized cords and trabeculae with vacuolated signet ring cell-like and lipoblast-like morphologies. This is usually seen mixed with other histological forms of myoepithelial carcinoma. They tend to have a more aggressive behavior with a 50% recurrence rate and a 40% metastatic rate to the lung and scalp.

Immunohistochemistry

The tumor cells show immunoreactivity for cytokeratin (90%), CK14 (100%), actin (70-80%), calponin (100%), S-100 protein (100%), GFAP (50%), EMA (100%), and are negative for CEA and HMB-45.

Differential Diagnosis

The spindle cell type has to be differentiated from sarcomas and metastatic amelanotic melanomas. Immunohistochemistry is useful in distinguishing between these two conditions. The absence of ductal, acinar or squamous cell differentiates this from carcinosarcoma and other salivary gland carcinomas.

Prognosis

Myoepithelial carcinoma is an intermediate to high grade carcinoma and has a potential for aggressive behavior. Tumors with marked cellular pleomorphism, perineural invasion, mitotic count > 7/10 HPF, Ki67 index > 50%, and p53 protein over expression are associated with worse prognosis. Mortality rates vary from 29 to 50%.

MALIGNANT MIXED TUMORS

The classification of malignant mixed tumors includes three distinct clinicopathologic entities: carcinoma ex-pleomorphic adenoma, carcinosarcoma, and metastasizing pleomorphic adenoma. Among these most common one is carcinoma ex-pleomorphic adenoma.

CARCINOMA EX-PLEOMORPHIC ADENOMA

(Carcinoma ex-mixed tumor)
This term refers to malignant transformation of a pre-existing pleomorphic adenoma which is untreated or a tumor with multiple local recurrences. Diagnosis of this tumor requires at least one focus of benign mixed tumor or a previously operated benign mixed tumor had been excised from the site in which the recurrent tumor is carcinomatous.

It accounts for about 4.6% of all malignant salivary gland tumors and is the sixth most common malignant salivary gland tumor. The risk of malignant transformation ranges from 1.9 to 23.3% and is about 1.6% for tumors less than 5 years duration and 9.5% for those present for more than 15 years.

Clinical Presentation

The mean age of presentation is 56 to 69 years, i.e. about 13 years more than that of pleomorphic adenoma. Malignant transformation is usually indicated by sudden rapid growth of the tumor. Pain has been reported to occur in a small percentage of patients and appears more common in submandibular tumors. Other features that may also be seen are fixation to surrounding tissues, ulceration, facial nerve palsy and regional node and distant metastases. Only the malignant component is seen in the metastatic deposit.

Among the major salivary glands it occurs most often in the parotid (81%), followed by the submandibular gland (16.5%), and sublingual gland (0.4%). In minor glands palate is the most common site (63%) followed by the upper lip (10.5%), tongue, cheek, and oropharyngeal regions (7% each).

Macroscopic Features

The tumor is usually more than twice the size of its benign counterpart, ranging in size from 1.5 to 25 cm and usually presents as a poorly circumscribed, infiltrative, hard mass and has white or tan-gray color.

Microscopic Features

Microscopically, malignant cells are present adjacent to a typical appearing pleomorphic adenoma. These cells have high nuclear-cytoplasmic ratio, nuclear pleomorphism, prominent nucleoli, coagulative tumor necrosis and show an infiltrative growth pattern. Among these characteristics, destructive infiltrative growth is the most reliable histologic criterion for the diagnosis of carcinoma ex-pleomorphic adenoma. The malignant portion of the tumor can take the form of any epithelial malignancy except acinic cell carcinoma. Most commonly this will be in the form of an undifferentiated carcinoma (30%) or poorly differentiated adenocarcinoma (25%); occasionally polymorphous low grade adenocarcinoma, salivary duct carcinoma, squamous cell carcinoma, mucoepidermoid carcinoma, malignant myoepithelioma, adenoid cystic carcinoma, clear cell carcinoma, and papillary carcinoma.

When a salivary gland carcinoma is not easily classifiable into recognized entities, the diagnosis of carcinoma ex-pleomorphic adenoma should be considered. At times, carcinoma ex- pleomorphic adenoma may have only very small areas of residual benign mixed tumor necessitating a thorough examination of the entire specimen for a proper histological classification. When the carcinoma is still within the confines of the capsule, it is known as carcinoma-*in situ* ex pleomorphic adenoma.

Immunohistochemistry

A study on about 73 cases of carcinoma ex- pleomorphic adenoma has shown an immunohistochemical profile that included positive staining reactions in the malignant component for AE1/AE3 in 97% of cases, CK7 in 94%, Epithelial Membrane Antigen (EMA) in 86%, Carcino Embryonic Antigen (CEA) in 75%, vimentin in 52%, and S-100 protein in 29%.

Cytogenetics

Mutations of p53, Rb and chromosome 5q have been implicated in the malignant transformation of mixed tumors. Overexpression or activation of c-erb B-2 and H-ras have been reported. Recently the overexpression of mdm2 and HMGIC has also been shown to lead malignant change in pleomorphic adenoma and comparative genomic hybridization using microarrays has found overexpression due to gene amplification of the genes MGC2177, PLAG1, PSMC6P and LYN on bands 8q11.2~q13 in these tumors.

Differential Diagnosis

Carcinoma arising in other types of salivary gland adenomas and carcinosarcoma are considered as important lesions in differential diagnosis. Carcinoma arising in other adenomas is differentiated by the nature of the benign elements present. Moreover, these tumors lack the chondromatous and myxoid areas seen in pleomorphic adenomas. Stromal atypia with areas of osteosarcoma, chondrosarcoma or undifferentiated sarcoma, which are characteristic of carcinosarcoma, are not seen carcinoma ex-pleomorphic adenoma. In other words, there is no evidence of stromal malignancy.

Prognosis

Carcinoma-*in situ* ex-pleomorphic adenoma has an excellent prognosis with no metastatic potential. In case of invasive tumors the outcome depends on the extent of extracapsular invasion and the histologic grade of the tumor. In addition to histologic grading, Ki67 is a useful prognostic marker in the evaluation of malignant mixed tumor. The 5 year survival rates for those with different malignant components are: undifferentiated carcinoma 55%, myoepithelial carcinoma 50%, ductal carcinoma 62%, and polymorphous low grade adenocarcinoma 96%.

CARCINOSARCOMA

(True malignant mixed tumor)

Carcinosarcoma is a very rare tumor that comprises frankly malignant epithelial and mesenchymal elements. It accounts for less than 0.1% of salivary gland neoplasms. Some develop *de novo* while others arise in association with benign mixed tumors.

Clinical Features

The mean age of presentation is about 57 years with no sex predilection. The mode of presentation may be swelling, pain, nerve palsy, or ulceration. The patient may have distant metastases on presentation. Parotid is the most frequent site of occurrence (65%), followed by the submandibular gland (22%). These tumors have also been reported to occur in the palate and tongue.

Macroscopic Features

The neoplasms are grossly infiltrative with poorly defined margins and occasionally show partial or total encapsulation. The size may range from about 2 to 13 cm. Cut surface is usually grayish in color with yellowish areas, rare areas of cystic change, hemorrhage or calcification.

Microscopic Features

The tumor is biphasic and has both carcinomatous and sarcomatous elements with the latter being dominant. Though the sarcomatous component may be a chondrosarcoma (commonest), osteosarcoma or rhabdomyosarcoma, fibrosarcoma, myxosarcoma, malignant fibrous histiocytoma, and liposarcoma have also been identified. The most frequent carcinomatous element is a high grade ductal adenocarcinoma, but squamous cell carcinoma and undifferentiated carcinoma have also been identified. The most common carcinomatous elements are high grade ductal adenocarcinoma or undifferentiated carcinoma. Prominent stromal hyalinization, diffuse areas of calcification and prominent areas of necrosis have been reported. Metastatic deposits and recurrent tumors manifest both sarcomatous and carcinomatous elements.

Ultrastructural studies have described both chondrocytic and epithelial differentiation with myoepithelial features in chondrocytic areas suggesting that the sarcomatous component is derived from modulation of myoepithelial cells.

Immunohistochemistry has shown reactivity for cytokeratin, epithelial membrane antigen and S-100 protein in the carcinomatous cells and vimentin and S-100 protein in the sarcomatous elements. Reactivity for GFAP has been reported in carcinosarcoma from the upper lip.

According to one study, loss of heterozygosity (LOH) analysis at 12 genomic locations detected complete deletion of one allele at 17p13.1, 17q21.3, and 18q21.3 indicating allelic loss in both components of the tumor favoring a monoclonal origin of the tumor from a common stem cell.

Differential Diagnosis

This includes benign mixed tumor, carcinoma ex-pleomorphic adenoma, primary sarcomas, especially synovial sarcoma and spindle cell carcinoma of the oral mucosa in the region of minor salivary glands. Presence of marked cytologic atypia, cellular and nuclear pleomorphism, hyperchromatism and mitotic figures and invasive growth differentiate carcinosarcoma from benign mixed tumors. Carcinoma ex-pleomorphic adenoma has only carcinomatous elements and no sarcomatous elements. Synovial sarcomas have uniform stromal cells arranged in tight bundles along with simple gland like structures that differentiate them from carcinosarcomas. In addition, the stromal and epithelial elements of carcinosarcoma are more pleomorphic than those of synovial sarcoma. Primary sarcomas will not show carcinomatous elements. Hence a diagnosis of primary sarcoma of the salivary gland requires careful sampling of the tumor to demonstrate the absence of foci of carcinoma. Staining for cytokeratin will be useful in this situation. Spindle cell carcinoma will show areas of epidermoid carcinoma of the mucosal epithelium and continuity with the basilar cells of the surface epithelium and the overlying is often dysplastic in spindle cell carcinoma and normal in carcinosarcoma.

Prognosis

Carcinosarcoma is an aggressive, high-grade neoplasm with a mean survival of about 29.3 months. Lung is the most common site of metastases followed by the hilar and cervical lymph nodes. Distant metastasis may be rarely found in soft tissue sites, bone, liver, and the central nervous system.

METASTASIZING PLEOMORPHIC ADENOMA

Metastasizing pleomorphic adenoma is a very rare histologically benign salivary gland neoplasm that inexplicably metastasizes. The metastases contain both epithelial and stromal components found in typical pleomorphic adenoma. The diagnosis is usually established retrospectively after metastasis. These tumors were earlier referred to as benign metastasizing mixed tumors, but since they may be lethal, the term benign is no longer in use.

Clinical Features

There is no sex predilection and the mean age of diagnosis is about 29.9 years. Patients usually present with painless masses similar to the benign mixed tumors and symptoms related to the site of metastases. The metastasis develops some time after excision of the pleomorphic adenoma of the salivary gland and may even be about 20 years. Radiotherapy and vascular infiltration, natural or iatrogenic have been suggested as factors contributing to metastasis, but no definite etiologic factors have been found. The most common primary site is the parotid gland (80%) followed by the submandibular gland (12%).

Macroscopic Features

The primary neoplasm is typically a single well-defined mass, the size of which ranges from 0.5 to 15 cm.

Microscopic Features

The histologic features of the primary tumor and the metastasis are those of benign mixed tumors with mesenchymal-like myxoid and myxochondroid tissue intermixed with epithelial areas. Characteistics of malignancy are not seen. Several primary tumors have had a primarily mucoid appearance. Both epithelial and stromal-like components and rarely myoepithelial cells are seen in the metastases.

Differential Diagnosis

Skeletal and extraskeletal chondrosarcomas, chondroid chordoma and chondroid hamartoma of the lung may be diagnostic considerations. The presence of a ductal epithelial component distinguishes metastatic mixed tumor from chondrosarcoma. Chondromas occur almost exclusively in the spheno-occipital region whereas metastasizing mixed tumors involve the spine distal to the thoracic vertebrae. Areas of ductal differentiation are seen only in mixed tumors while physaliferous cells are seen only in chordomas. Chondroid hamartomas are more common than mixed tumors metastasize to the lung and in the former the cartilage nests are usually surrounded by cellular fibrous tissue. Chondroid hamartomas also show merging of the epithelial elements with adjacent alveoli or bronchioles. However, an accurate and complete medical history is most helpful in establishing the diagnosis.

Prognosis

Almost 22% of patients die of metastasis at about 2 to 8 years after diagnosis of the metastases. The course is more aggressive in immunocompromised hosts. The common sites of metastases are the bone (50%) (middle to lower spine, iliac region, rib, skull, mandible, femur and humerus), lungs (30%) and lymph nodes (30%); oral cavity, pharynx, skin, retroperitoneum, kidney, central nervous system, scalp, abdominal wall and liver metastases have also been rarely reported. Recurrences in the primary site precede or coincide with metastases in 90% of cases.

PRIMARY SQUAMOUS CELL CARCINOMA

Primary salivary gland squamous cell carcinoma is composed of malignant squamous cells and is a rare malignant epithelial neoplasm of the major salivary glands. The diagnosis requires the exclusion of primary squamous cell carcinoma in other head and neck sites as most squamous cell carcinomas of the major salivary glands represent a metastatic lesion. This diagnosis is not made in the minor salivary glands as it is not possible to distinguish from the more common mucosal squamous cell carcinoma. The reported frequency is about 0.9 to 4.7% of all major salivary gland tumors and 4.4% of all the malignant epithelial salivary gland tumors.

Clinical Features

The average age of occurrence of this tumor is about 64 years. Males are affected more frequently than females. Previous exposure to ionizing radiation appears to increase the risk of developing this tumor, the median time between exposure and tumor occurrence being about 15.5 years. About 50% of patients are asymptomatic. They may present as a firm, rapidly enlarging mass, fixed to the surrounding tissues. Pain or facial nerve palsy may occur. Cervical lymph node metastases are common.

The tumor occurs more frequently in the parotid gland (90%), followed by submandibular and sublingual glands. In the case of submandibular lymph nodes great care has to be taken to ensure that the primary site is the submandibular gland and not an extension of metastatic disease from adjacent lymph nodes.

Macroscopic Features

These tumors are large (> 3 cm) and poorly encapsulated and it may be difficult to grossly distinguish the tumor from the salivary parenchyma.

Microscopic Features

The microscopic features are similar to those of squamous cell carcinoma of other sites. Majority of the tumors are well or moderately differentiated keratinizing squamous cell carcinomas with prominent intracellular keratin and keratin pearl formation. The tumor may be separated into multiple nodules by desmoplastic fibrous connective tissue which may at times be so extensive as to replace entire salivary gland lobules. Islands of squamous cell carcinoma may have marked infiltrates of lymphocytes in close apposition. Special stains show no intracytoplasmic mucin.

Differential Diagnosis

Ductal squamous metaplasia may resemble salivary gland squamous cell carcinoma and is distinguished by the presence of lumina with lack of marked cytologic atypia and infiltrative growth pattern. Mucoepidermoid carcinoma has a variety of cell types and cytoplasmic mucin may be demonstrated at least focally. Moreover basaloid intermediate cells may dominate many areas of the tumor in mucoepidermoid carcinoma.

In squamous cell carcinoma, the neoplastic epithelium shows obvious squamous differentiation in contrast to lymphoepithelial carcinoma. Differentiating metastatic squamous carcinoma from primary squamous cell carcinoma may pose a diagnostic challenge. If the tumor is located only within an intraparotid lymph node with no parenchymal involvement, it is unlikely to be a metastatic squamous cell carcinoma. A careful clinical examination of the most probable sites for the primary, namely the skin of the head and neck region or nasopharynx, will help in clinching the diagnosis.

Prognosis

This tumor is aggressive and tends to invade and spread rapidly. Primary squamous cell carcinoma has been reported with 5 and 10 years survival rates of 24 and 18% respectively. Ulceration, fixation, advanced patient age, advanced tumor stage and facial nerve palsy are unfavorable prognostic factors. Various studies have reported the metastasis to cervical nodes to be high, ranging from 21 to 45%.

ADENOSQUAMOUS CARCINOMA

Oral adenosquamous carcinoma is a rare neoplasm in which there is co-existence of squamous cell carcinoma arising from dysplastic surface mucosa and adenocarcinoma originating from the ductal epithelium of the excretory duct of a minor salivary gland. Whether the tumor arises simultaneously from both the mucosal and ductal epithelium or begins in the salivary duct and spreads to the surface is not clearly known.

Clinical Features

The tumor occurs in the sixth to seventh decade and there is a male predilection. The tumor produces swelling, erythema, mucosal ulceration, pain and induration. About 80% of patients show regional lymphadenopathy at the time of presentation.

The posterior tongue, tonsillar pillars and floor of the mouth are the sites commonly involved. Other sites include the buccal mucosa, retromolar region and lower lip. These tumors are often unencapsulated, infiltrative, and destructive.

Microscopic Features

Microscopically, the squamous cell component ranges from severe dysplasia and carcinoma *in situ* to invasive squamous cell carcinoma of the surface epithelium and superficial portion of the excretory duct. Infiltrative, poorly to moderately well differentiated squamous cell carcinoma is usually present in the lamina propria and submucosa. The better differentiated tumors exhibit intercellular bridges, individual cell keratinization and keratin pearls. The deeper portion of the tumor exhibits the adenocarcinomatous component apparently arising from the excretory or interlobular salivary gland ducts and is composed of ductal and tubular structures lined by one to several layers of pleomorphic cuboidal or basaloid cells in a desmoplastic stroma with a lymphocytic infiltrate. Intraluminal and intracellular mucin may be present in some tumors. Perineural and vascular invasion are often seen.

Immunohistochemistry

The squamous or epidermoid component of adenosquamous carcinoma is reactive for high molecular weight cytokeratin while the adenocarcinoma portions are reactive for high and low molecular weight cytokeratins and CEA.

Differential Diagnosis

The most important lesions to be considered in the differential diagnosis of adenosquamous carcinoma are mucoepidermoid carcinoma and adenoid (acantholytic) squamous carcinoma of the oral mucosa. Unlike adenosquamous carcinoma, well-defined and separate areas of adenocarcinoma and squamous cell carcinoma and carcinomatous changes in the surface mucosal epithelium are not seen in mucoepidermoid carcinoma. In addition, individual cell keratinization and keratin pearl formation are infrequent in mucoepidermoid carcinoma. Aggregates of mucous cells and cyst lined by rows of mucous cells seen in mucoepidermoid carcinoma are not present in adenosquamous carcinoma.

Adenoid squamous cell carcinoma is a histologic variant of squamous cell carcinoma of the mucosal squamous epithelium that exhibits acantholysis of cells. It occurs more commonly in the vermilion border of the lower lip and does not have mucin or the true glandular spaces seen in the adenocarcinomatous component of adenosquamous carcinoma.

Prognosis

This is a highly aggressive neoplasm with a poor prognosis. Survival rates for patients with squamous cell carcinoma of the posterior tongue, floor of the mouth, and tonsillar pillars are poorer that for patients with squamous cell carcinoma of similar grades in other sites.

UNDIFFERENTIATED CARCINOMAS

Undifferentiated carcinomas of the salivary glands are a group of uncommon malignant epithelial neoplasms that lack the specific light microscopic morphologic features of other types of salivary gland carcinomas. The incidence of these epithelial tumors has been estimated to be about 0.4% (AFIP files) of all salivary gland tumors and about 6.5% of all malignant tumors Undifferentiated carcinomas can be further subclassified into small cell undifferentiated carcinoma, large cell undifferentiated, carcinoma and lymphoepithelial carcinoma.

Small Cell Undifferentiated Carcinoma

Small cell undifferentiated carcinoma is a rare primary malignant tumor composed of undifferentiated small cells (<30 μm in diameter) by light microscopy but showing neuroendocrine differentiation on ultrastructural and immunohistochemical analysis. It represents about 1.8 percent of all major salivary gland malignancies. Biologically there appear to be three types of salivary gland small cell carcinomas namely Merkel cell carcinoma type, pulmonary type, and ductal type.

Clinical Presentation

The mean age of presentation is about 56 years and occurs more commonly in men. Most patients present with an asymptomatic rapidly growing mass with or without cervical lymphadenopathy. Facial nerve palsy is seen in 60% of patients. Pain is occasionally present. Local recurrence and distant metastasis occurs in more than 50% of patients 2 to 26 months after diagnosis. Small cell undifferentiated carcinoma occurs more frequently in the parotid gland and less commonly in the submandibular and sublingual glands.

Macroscopic Features

The tumor may be up to 8 cm in size and presents as a widely infiltrative mass with a firm to hard consistency and with varying colors like gray, gray-white, pink-gray, yellow-white, tan and yellow.

Microscopic Features

Histologically the tumor cells are slightly larger than lymphocytes with the nucleus showing finely stippled chromatin and inconspicuous nucleoli arranged in a diffuse or cord like pattern. Mitoses are frequent and vascular invasion is seen only occasionally.

In the Merkel cell type, the nuclei tend to be round and non-molded with pale and washed out chromatin. In the pulmonary type, the tumors cells are short and spindle with molding and pseudo-rosette formation. In the ductal type small cell carcinoma, focal glandular lumen formation is seen and foci of squamous differentiation with keratinization. Necrosis as well as vascular and perineural invasion are common.

Immunohistochemistry

All small cell carcinomas exhibit immuno-histochemical evidence of neuroendocrine differentiation. The Merkel cell type and pulmonary type are positive for synaptophysin/chromogranin while the ductal type is negative for them. The Merkel cell type is also positive for CK20 while the pulmonary and the ductal type are negative. Paranuclear staining with anticytokeratin and immunoreactivity with anti-Leu-7 and neuron-specific enolase is also seen in these tumors. Ultrastructurally, the Merkel cell and pulmonary type show neurosecretory granules.

Differential Diagnosis

The differential diagnoses include non-Hodgkin's lymphoma, poorly differentiated adenocarcinoma, solid-type adenoid cystic carcinoma, and metastatic cutaneous Merkel cell carcinoma. Lymphoma cells show positive staining for leukocyte common antigen while a positive mucin stain favors a diagnosis of adenocarcinoma. The tumor cells of adenoid cystic carcinoma are positive for S-100 protein, actin, and calponin. Metastatic small cell carcinoma or Merkel cell carcinoma are differentiated by a careful clinical history, examination and detailed work-up.

Prognosis

Salivary gland small cell carcinomas are aggressive tumors. However, the prognosis for patients with small cell carcinoma of the salivary gland is better than that for those with small cell carcinomas of the lung or larynx. Tumor size is considered the most important prognostic factor with tumors of 4 cm or less in size having a better prognosis. The five year survival for tumors in the major salivary glands is about 46%.

Large Cell Undifferentiated Carcinoma

Large cell undifferentiated carcinoma is defined as any tumor of salivary gland origin that exhibits a predominant poorly differentiated large cell component that occurs in island and sheets with minor foci within the adenoid or squamous differentiation. By definition, the tumor cells are 2 to 3 times bigger than the size of the cells of small cell carcinoma. This neoplasm accounts for approximately 1% of all epithelial salivary gland neoplasms.

Clinical Features

The peak incidence of this tumor is in the seventh and eighth decades with no gender predilection or association with EBV infection. The patients usually present with a rapidly growing firm mass with infiltration of and fixation to adjacent tissues and cervical lymphadenopathy. Large cell undifferentiated carcinomas occur mainly in the parotid and submandibular gland. Cases have been reported to occur in the accessory salivary glands including the palate, floor of the oral cavity, pharynx and tongue.

Macroscopic Features

The tumors range in size from 2 to 10 cm in diameter and lack encapsulation. They usually present as grayish white, infiltrative, and solid masses.

Microscopic Features

Large cell undifferentiated carcinomas consist of sheets, nests, cords, and irregular islands of large, pleomorphic cells. Cell borders are well defined with copious amphophilic to eosinophilic cytoplasm, which is sometimes vacuolated and large, has vesicular nuclei with one or two prominent nucleoli. Multinucleated tumor giant cells may be evident and mitosis, tumor necrosis, and lymphatic and vascular invasion are commonly seen. The stroma is desmoplastic and may have a variable number of scattered lymphocytes, plasma cells and osteoclastic giant cells.

Differential Diagnosis

Large cell undifferentiated carcinoma should be distinguished from metastatic poorly differentiated squamous cell carcinoma, adenocarcinoma NOS, large cell and anaplastic lymphoma and malignant melanoma. Careful sampling of the entire lesion should also be done to look for a pre-existing component of pleomorphic adenoma, acinic cell carcinoma or adenoid cystic carcinoma to exclude the possibility that it may be a transformed or dedifferentiated neoplasm.

Poorly differentiated squamous cell carcinoma is ruled out by identifying another primary tumor site. Focal ductal, organoid, papillary, or cystic architectural features distinguish adenocarcinoma. Large cell and anaplastic lymphomas are reactive to lymphoid markers such as CD45. Metastatic melanoma is reactive for S-100 protein and HMB-45 antigen. Ultrastructural examination of large cell undifferentiated carcinoma may reveal glandular, squamous or neuroendocrine features which are not evident under light microscopy.

Prognosis

These are aggressive tumors that frequently metastasize. Tumors which are 4 cm or more in size have a very poor prognosis. Ten year survival rate varies from 0 to 35%.

Lymphoepithelial Carcinoma

(Lymphoepithelioma-like carcinoma, malignant lymphoepithelial lesion, undifferentiated carcinoma with lymphoid stroma or carcinoma ex-lymphoepithelial lesion)

Lymphoepithelial carcinoma is an undifferentiated tumor that is associated with a dense lymphoid stroma. There is a high prevalence of this tumor among Eskimos/Inuits and Southern Chinese and a strong association with EBV. These tumors are rare and comprise only about 0.4% of salivary gland neoplasms.

Clinical Features

Adults with a mean age of 40 years are affected and there is a slight female predilection. Pain is a frequent symptom followed by facial palsy and cervical lymphadenopathy (40%). Local recurrence and distant metastases (20%) to the lung, liver, bone and brain can occur. The tumor occurs most frequently in the parotid and submandibular glands; minor salivary glands may also be affected.

Microscopic Features

The infiltrative tumor grows in diffuse sheets, anastomosing islands, nests, cords, trabeculae and isolated cells which resemble those of large cell undifferentiated carcinoma. Focal squamous differentiation may occur. Few amyloid globules can occur among the tumor cells. Tumor necrosis and mitotic figures are present. These tumor cells are separated by a desmoplastic stroma and there is dense infiltration of lymphocytes and plasma cells with lymphoid follicle formation. Histiocytes may infiltrate the tumor cells producing a starry sky appearance. Non-caseating granulomas with or without giant cells are found in some cases. Perineural and vascular invasion may be present.

The tumor cells in lymphoepithelial carcinoma are positive for cytokeratin and EMA. Ultrastructural examination shows squamous features like desmosomal cell attachments and tonofilaments. *In situ* hybridization for EBV is positive in Eskimos and those of oriental origin.

Differential Diagnosis

The differential diagnosis includes metastatic nasopharyngeal undifferentiated carcinoma, benign lymphoepithelial lesion, large cell lymphocytic and histiocytic neoplasms and metastatic amelanotic melanoma. Lymph oepithelial carcinoma is histologically, immuno-histochemically and ultrastructurally indistinguishable from nasopharyngeal undifferentiated carcinoma. Hence the latter condition should be excluded by a thorough clinical and endoscopic examination before making a diagnosis of lymphoepithelial carcinoma of the salivary gland. Another condition to be excluded is benign lymphoepithelial lesion (BLEL). The epithelial cells of BLEL lack atypia and have excessive basement membrane material. The epithelial cells of BLEL are negative for EBV by *in situ* hybridization.

LeuM1 and Ki-1 and epithelial markers, help differentiate large cell lymphocytic and histiocytic neoplasms from lymphoepithelial carcinoma. Melanoma is differentiated by staining for S-100 protein and HMB-45.

Prognosis

Lymphoepithelial carcinoma has the best prognosis among the undifferentiated carcinomas. High mitotic rate, anaplasia, necrosis, features of BLEL, large size, and lymph node metastasis are indicators of poor prognosis. Survival rates vary from 17 to 86%.

HYALINIZING CLEAR CELL CARCINOMA

Hyalinizing clear cell carcinoma forms a distinct group among the clear cell carcinomas of the salivary glands. Most arise in the minor salivary glands of the oral cavity and have also been reported to occur in the parotid gland, larynx and as a primary intraosseous tumor of the jaws. Less than 20 cases have been reported in literature.

The tumor is hypocellular and is composed of nests, cords, trabeculae and columns of uniform clear cells separated by abundant hyalinized stroma resembling amyloid. The hyaline material is PAS positive and Congo red negative. There is infiltration into surrounding tissue. Immunoreactivity is seen for cytokeratin, EMA and focally for CEA. S-100 protein, calponin and smooth muscle actin are negative. Electron microscopy confirms the pure epithelial differentiation of this tumor.

Prognosis

Recurrence rate of 8 and 15% of metastasis to regional lymph nodes have been reported but no patients are known to have died from the disease.

SIALOBLASTOMA

(Embryoma, congenital carcinoma, congenital basal cell adenoma)

Sialoblastoma is a rare, congenital/perinatal, low grade malignant neoplasm composed of primitive appearing cells with occasional ductal formations, recapitulating the embryonic salivary tissue at various stages of development. Great variation has been reported in cytological atypia, mitotic rates, necrosis and infiltration in these tumors and it has been suggested that they may be separated into benign and malignant categories.

Clinical Presentation

Sialoblastoma presents at birth or soon thereafter as a firm asymptomatic mass. It may cause obstruction during labor. A case of sialoblastoma and an associated hepatoblastoma has been reported in the literature. Sialoblastoma has been reported to occur in the parotid (75%) and submandibular (25%) salivary glands.

Macroscopic Features

The tumor ranges in size from 1.5 to 15 cm.

Microscopic Features

The tumor may be circumscribed or infiltrative and is composed of many islands and sheets of primitive basaloid cells separated by a fibrous or fibromyxomatous stroma. Most of the tumor cells are primitive looking and have large ovoid vesicular nuclei and moderate cytoplasm with indistinct cell borders. Mild nuclear atypia and variable number of mitotic figures are present. A vague palisading of nuclei may be seen at the periphery of the tumor islands. Within these islands are seen small ducts lined by cuboidal or low columnar cells.

Immunohistochemistry

Staining for cytokeratin has shown accentuation of the ductal structures with positivity for vimentin, actin and S-100 protein in the outermost layer of the ducts. The solid nests have been shown to be focally reactive to S-100 protein and vimentin. In a case of sialoblastoma reported with evidence of increasing anaplasia, Her-2-neu protein showed moderate cytoplasmic staining, whereas p53 showed only occasional labeling of nuclei.

Ultrastructural examination has shown myoepithelial cells with replication of basement membrane material.

Differential Diagnosis

Sialoblastoma has more primitive cells, greater cytologic atypia and more mitotic activity than basal cell adenoma. The former often infiltrates surrounding tissues. Other basaloid neoplasms like adenoid cystic carcinoma and basal cell adenocarcinoma are extremely rare in the first decade of life.

Prognosis

Sialoblastoma is a tumor with low malignant potential. Local recurrence rate is about 27%. One case of regional lymph node metastasis has been reported. No distant metastases have been reported.

MESENCHYMAL TUMORS

The nonepithelial tumors of the salivary gland comprise about 10% of all tumors arising in the salivary glands with mesenchymal tumors and lymphoma sharing an equal incidence. Benign mesenchymal tumors are more common than malignant tumors with hemangioma being the most common childhood salivary gland tumor. In a review of 85 cases, the most frequent types of sarcoma of the salivary gland were found to be rhabdomyosarcoma and malignant fibrous histiocytoma. Most of these tumors arise in the major glands and histologically have the same morphologic features and behavior as those in other parts of the body.

LYMPHOMAS

Lymphomas form a significant portion of malignant salivary gland tumors. Their incidence is about 1.7 to 16% of all malignant tumors in this site. Most cases arise in the parotid (50–93%) and submandibular salivary glands. The tumors may arise in either intraglandular/juxtaglandular lymph nodes or salivary gland proper. In a study by Gleeson et al, 35% of these cases were reported to be large cell lymphomas, 35% were follicular lymphomas and 30% were small cell lymphomas. The majority of these are B-cell origin with rare reports of T-cell types.

Origin

Lymphomas Arising in Intraglandular or Juxtaglandular Lymph Nodes

The most common types are Hodgkin's lymphoma, follicular lymphoma and diffuse large B cell lymphoma. These tumors are similar to those occurring in lymph nodes at other sites.

Lymphomas Arising in the Salivary Gland Proper

The lymphomas that arise in the salivary gland parenchyma are low grade B-cell MALT lymphoma (extranodal marginal zone B-cell lymphoma), diffuse large B-cell lymphoma, peripheral T-cell lymphoma, anaplastic large cell lymphoma and NK/T cell lymphoma. There is an increased risk of high grade B-cell tumors in patients with acquired immunodeficiency Syndrome and some of these tumors are associated with Epstein-Barr virus infection.

LOW GRADE B-CELL MALT LYMPHOMA

(Extranodal marginal zone B-cell lymphoma of MALT type)

Low grade B-cell MALT lymphomas are the most common lymphomas of salivary gland origin. The predisposing factors are benign lympho-epithelial lesion (Mikulicz disease) or Sjogren's syndrome. This tumor may also arise *de novo*.

Clinical Presentation

Patients with low grade B-cell MALT lymphoma usually present with salivary gland swelling or rarely with cervical lymphadenopathy. The tumor is usually non-circumscribed, firm and tan colored. The cut surface may show cysts formed by dilation of ducts.

Histologically, the tumor is composed of a mixture of cell types, reactive follicles and numerous lymphoepithelial lesions. The salivary gland may either be extensively involved or the lobular architecture may still be preserved. The earliest evidence of MALT lymphoma is the presence of broad collars of clear cells around lymphoepithelial (LEL) lesions. The lymphoid cells in and around the ducts in the LEL resemble monocytoid B-cells and are large with oval to indented nuclei and abundant pale-staining to clear cytoplasm. Other lymphoid cells have folded nuclei or are like small lymphocytes. A variable number of plasma cells may be present showing mild atypia and containing Dutcher bodies. Large lymphoid cells with round nuclei and distinct nucleoli are commonly seen. Occasionally, wreaths of epithelioid histiocytes are seen surrounding the LELs.

Immunohistochemically the tumor cells are CD20+ with light chain restriction. Aberrant coexpression of CD43 may be present.

Prognosis

The prognosis of these tumors is excellent. Rare reports of regression of these tumors with anti-Helicobacter therapy have been reported.

DIFFUSE LARGE B-CELL LYMPHOMA

These tumors arise from transformation of a low grade MALT lymphoma. Unless a component of low grade MALT lymphoma is present, it is difficult to say if the diffuse large B-cell lymphoma is of salivary or nodal origin. Large B-cell lymphoma is diagnosed when there are dense sheets of large cells. When the large cells are intimately mixed with small cells the designation of low grade B-cell MALT lymphoma with increased large cells is given. Diffuse large B-cell lymphomas are more aggressive than low grade MALT lymphomas and have a worse prognosis.

PRIMARY T-CELL LYMPHOMA OF THE SALIVARY GLAND

Primary T-cell lymphoma of the salivary gland is rare, with only 14 cases described so far, all but two of which have been from Oriental countries. The parotid and submandibular glands are the most frequently involved salivary tissues, although occasional cases have been described in the sublingual glands. The most frequent histological type of this condition is a peripheral T-cell lymphoma, often of low grade morphology, although occasionally they may be pleomorphic. Staining for markers indicative of NK cell differentiation further identifies a few cases of angiocentric T/NK lymphomas and a similar number of cases of T-anaplastic large cell lymphoma are also described. Of the 11 cases where data have been recorded, seven of the cases, harbored EBV, with all of the previously reported T/NK lymphomas being positive for EBV, a background of autoimmune sialadenitis or enteropathy has been suggested as a predisposing factor to the development of this tumor. Chan et al suggest a variable outcome, with survival after diagnosis ranging from six weeks to more than four years.

METASTATIC TUMORS

Metastases occur in the intraparotid and submandibular lymph nodes. Tumors that have been reported to metastasize here are squamous cell carcinoma from any region of the upper aerodigestive tract and skin, malignant melanoma, tumors of the lung, kidney, breast, prostate, and large bowel. These tumors may mimic a primary salivary gland tumors and it should be remembered that the most common tumor of the submaxillary region is a metastatic carcinoma in the submandibular lymph node rather than a primary salivary gland neoplasm.

CK7/20 immunoprofile facilitate differentiation of primary salivary gland neoplasia from metastatic tumors and squamous carcinoma, and the diagnosis of metastatic salivary gland tumors.

OTHER ENTITIES

Hybrid Carcinomas

Hybrid carcinomas of the salivary gland are recently defined, rare tumors, consisting of two histologically distinct types of carcinoma within the same topographic area. They have been reported mainly in the parotid gland followed by the submandibular gland.

In one series of 1863 cases of parotid gland tumors, the prevalence of hybrid carcinomas was about 0.4%. They occur in both men and women with the age ranging from 40 to 81 years. Tumor size ranged from 2 to 10 cm (mean, 4.2 cm). The combinations of carcinomatous components in hybrid carcinomas were as follows: epithelial-myoepithelial carcinoma and basal cell adenocarcinoma in two cases, epithelial-myoepithelial carcinoma and squamous cell carcinoma in one case, salivary duct carcinoma and adenoid cystic carcinoma in two cases, myoepithelial carcinoma and salivary duct carcinoma in one, acinic cell carcinoma and salivary duct carcinoma in one, and squamous cell carcinoma and salivary duct carcinoma in two. Although the proportion of each carcinoma component in a tumor mass varied from case to case, the minor component always represented greater or equal to 10% of the area.

BIBLIOGRAPHY

1. Alaeddini M, Khalili M, Tirgary F, Etemad-Moghadam S. Argyrophilic proteins of nucleolar organizer regions (AgNORs) in salivary gland mucoepidermoid carcinoma and its relation to histological grade. Oral Surg Oral Med Oral Pathol Oral Radiol Endod 2008;105(6):758-62.
2. Albores-Saavedra J, Wu J, Uribe-Uribe N. The sclerosing variant of adenoid cystic carcinoma: a previously unrecognized neoplasm of major salivary glands. Ann Diagn Pathol 2006;10(1):1-7.
3. Alos L, Lujan B, Castillo M, Nadal A, Carreras M, Caballero M, de Bolos C, Cardesa A. Expression of membrane-bound mucins (MUC1 and MUC4) and secreted mucins (MUC2, MUC5AC, MUC5B, MUC6 and MUC7) in mucoepidermoid carcinomas of salivary glands. Am J Surg Pathol 2005;29(6): 806-13.
4. Andreadis D, Epivatianos A, Mireas G, Nomikos A, Poulopoulos A, Yiotakis J, Barbatis C. Immuno-histochemical detection of E-cadherin in certain types of salivary gland tumours. J Laryngol Otol 2006;120(4):298-304.
5. Araújo VC, Demasi AP, Furuse C, Altemani A, Alves VA, Freitas LL, Araújo NS. Collagen type I may influence the expression of E-cadherin and beta-catenin in carcinoma ex-pleomorphic adenoma. Appl Immunohistochem Mol Morphol 2009; 17(4):312-8.
6. Auclair PL, Ellis GL. Major salivary glands. In: Silverberg SG, DeLellis RA, Frable WJ (Eds). Principles and practice of surgical pathology and cytopathology. 3rd edn. New York: Churchill Livingstone; 1997. pp. 1463-1473, 1505-8.
7. Auclair PL, Ellis GL, Gnepp DR, Wenig BM, Janney CG. Salivary gland neoplasms: General considerations. In: Ellis GL, Auclair PL, Gnepp DR (Eds). Surgical pathology of the salivary glands. 1st edn. Philadelphia: WB Saunders Company; 1991. pp. 135-64.
8. Aygit AC, Top H, Cakir B, Yalcn O. Salivary duct carcinoma of the parotid gland metastasizing to the skin: A case report and review of the literature. Am J Dermatopathol 2005;27(1):48-50.
9. Barnes L, Brandwein M, Som PM. Surgical Pathology of the Head and Neck. 2nd edn. Marcel Dekker Inc: New York, 2001.
10. Barnes L, Eveson JW, Reichart P, Sidransky D. World Health Organization Classification of Tumours. Pathology and Genetics of Head and Neck Tumours. Salivary glands. Lyon, IARC Press, 2005;5.
11. Batsakis JG. Tumors of the head and neck: Clinical and pathological considerations, 2nd edn. Baltimore, MD: Williams and Wilkins, 1979.
12. Bell D, Luna MA, Weber RS, Kaye FJ, El-Naggar AK. CRTC1/MAML2 fusion transcript in Warthin's tumor and mucoepidermoid carcinoma: Evidence for a common genetic association. Genes Chromosomes Cancer 2008;47(4):309-14.
13. Brandewein MS, Huvos AG. Oncocytic tumours of major salivary glands. A study of 68 cases

with follow-up of 44 patients. Am J Surg Pathol 1991;15:514-28.

14. Brandwein MS, Ivanov K, Wallace DI, Hille JJ, Wang B, Fahmy A, Bodian C, Urken ML, Gnepp DR, Huvos A, Lumerman H, Mills SE. Mucoepidermoid carcinoma a clinicopathologic study of 80 patients with special reference to histological grading. Am J Surg Pathol 2001;25:835-45.

15. Calearo C, Pastore A. Parotid carcinoma. In: Hermarek P, Gospodarowicz M, Henson D, Hutter R, Sobin L (Eds). Prognostic factors in cancer. Berlin: Springer-Verlag; 1995. pp. 23-7.

16. Camilleri IG, Malata CM, McLean NR, Kelly CG. Malignant tumours of the submandibular salivary gland: A 15 year review. Br J Plast Surg 1998;51:181-5.

17. Cavaliéri Gomes C, da Silveira e Oliveira C, Santos Pimenta LG, De Marco L, Santiago Gomez R. Immunolocalization of DNMT1 and DNMT3a in salivary gland neoplasms. Pathobiology. 2009;76(3):136-40.

18. Cawson RA, Odell EW, Porter SR. Cawson's essentials of oral pathology and oral medicine, 7th edn. Churchill Livingstone, 2002.pp.255-74.

19. Chan JK, Yip TT, Tsang WY, Poon YF, Wong CS, Ma VW. Specific association of Epstein-Barr virus with lymphoepithelial carcinoma among tumours and tumorlike lesions of the salivary gland. Arch Pathol Lab Med 1994;118:994-7.

20. Chandana SR, Conley BA. Salivary gland cancers: current treatments, molecular characteristics and new therapies. Expert Rev Anticancer Ther 2008;8(4):645-52.

21. Chao TK, Tsai CC, Yeh SY, Teh JE. Hyalinizing clear cell carcinoma of the hard palate. J Laryngol Otol 2004;118:382-4.

22. Cheuk W, Chan JK, Ngan RK. Dedifferentiation in adenoid cystic carcinoma of salivary gland: An uncommon complication associated with an accelerated clinical course. Am J Surg Pathol 1999;23(4):465-72.

23. Cheuk W, Chan JKC. Advances in salivary gland pathology. Histopathol 2007;51:1-20.

24. Cheuk W, Chan JKC. Salivary gland tumours. In: Fletcher CDM (Ed), Diagnostic Histopathology of Tumours, 2/e (Vol 1), Churchill Livingstone, 2002.

25. Cheuk W, Milauskas JR, Chan JKC. Intraductal carcinoma of the oral cavity. A case report and a reappraisal of the concept of pure ductal carcinoma in situ in the salivary gland. Am J Surg Pathol 2004;28(2):266-70.

26. Cho NP, Han HS, Soh Y, Son HJ. Overexpression of cyclooxygenase-2 correlates with cytoplasmic HuR expression in salivary mucoepidermoid carcinoma but not in pleomorphic adenoma. J Oral Pathol Med 2007;36(5):297-303.

27. Choi S, Sano D, Cheung M, Zhao M, Jasser SA, Ryan AJ, Mao L, Chen WT, El-Naggar AK, Myers JN. Vandetanib inhibits growth of adenoid cystic carcinoma in an orthotopic nude mouse model. Clin Cancer Res 2008;14(16):5081-9.

28. Costa AF, Demasi AP, Bonfitto VL, Bonfitto JF, Furuse C, Araújo VC, Metze K, Altemani A. Angiogenesis in salivary carcinomas with and without myoepithelial differentiation. Virchows Arch 2008;453(4):359-67.

29. Croitoru CM, Mooney JE, Luna MA. Sebaceous lymphadenocarcinoma of salivary glands. Ann Diagn Pathol 2003;7(4):236-9.

30. Daa T, Kashima K, Kaku N, Suzuki M, Yokoyama S. Mutations in components of the Wnt signaling pathway in adenoid cystic carcinoma. Mod Pathol 2004;17(12):1475-82.

31. Dahse R, Driemel O, Schwarz S, Dahse J, Kromeyer-Hauschild K, Berndt A, Kosmehl H. Epidermal growth factor receptor kinase domain mutations are rare in salivary gland carcinomas. Br J Cancer 2009;100(4):623-5.

32. Dahse R, Kosmehl H. Detection of drug-sensitizing EGFR exon 19 deletion mutations in salivary gland carcinoma. Br J Cancer 2008;99(1):90-2.

33. Darling MR, Jackson-Boeters L, Daley TD, Diamandis EP. Human kallikrein 13 expression in salivary gland tumors. Int J Biol Markers 2006;21(2):106-10.

34. De Araujo VC, de Sousa SO, Carvalho YR, et al. Application of immunohistochemistry to the diagnosis of salivary gland tumors. Appl. Immunohistochem Mol Morph 2000;8:195-202.

35. De Araujo VC, de Sousa SO. Expression of different keratins in salivary gland tumours. Eur. J. Cancer B Oral Oncol 1996;32:14-8.

36. Delgado R, Vuitch F, Albores-Saavedra J. Salivary duct carcinoma. Cancer 1993;72(5):1503-12.

37. Demasi AP, Furuse C, Soares AB, Altemani A, Araújo VC. Peroxiredoxin I, platelet-derived growth factor A, and platelet-derived growth factor receptor alpha are overexpressed in carcinoma ex-pleomorphic adenoma: association with malignant transformation. Hum Pathol. 2009;40(3):390-7.

38. Di Palma S, Simpson RHW, Skalova A, Leivo I. Major and minor salivary glands. In: Cardesa A, Slootweg PJ (Eds)Pathology of the head and neck. Springer Verlag; 2006;5:132-7.

39. Drut R, Giménez PO. Acinic cell carcinoma of salivary gland with massive deposits of globular amyloid. Int J Surg Pathol 2008;16(2):202-7.

40. Ellis GL, Auclair PL, Gnepp DR. Surgical pathology of the salivary glands. 1st edn. WB Saunders: Philadelphia, Saunders, 1991.

41. Ellis GL, Auclair Pl. Major Salivary Glands. In: Silverberg SG, DeLellis RA, Frable WJ (Eds). Principles and Practice of Surgical Pathology and Cytopathology, 3/e (Vol 2), Churchill Livingstone, 1997.

42. Ellis GL, Auclair PL. Tumours of the salivary glands. 3rd edn. Armed Forces Institute of Pathology: Washington, 1996.

43. El-Naggar AK, Abdul-Karim FW, Hurr K, Callender D, Luna MA, Batsakis JG. Genetic alterations in acinic cell carcinoma of the parotid gland determined by microsatellite analysis. Cancer Genet Cytogenet 1998;102(1):19-24.

44. El-Naggar Ak, Callender D, Coombes MM, Hurr K, Luna MA, Batsakis JG. Molecular genetic alterations in carcinoma ex-pleomorphic adenoma: A putative progression model? Genes Chromosomes Cancer 2000;27:162-8.

45. El-Naggar AK, Hurr K, Kagan J, Gillenwater A, Callender D, Luna MA, Batsakis JG. Genotypic Alterations in Benign and Malignant Salivary Gland Tumors: Histogenetic and Clinical Implications. Am J Surg Pathol 1997;21:691-7.

46. Eneroth CM, Franzen S, Zajicek J. Aspiration biopsy of salivary gland tumors. A critical review of 910 biopsies. Acta Cytol 1967;11(6):470-2.

47. Ettl T, Schwarz S, Kleinsasser N, Hartmann A, Reichert TE, Driemel O. Overexpression of EGFR and absence of C-KIT expression correlate with poor prognosis in salivary gland carcinomas. Histopathology 2008;53(5):567-77.

48. Fadare O, Hileeto D, Gruddin YL, Mariappan MR. Sclerosing mucoepidermoid carcinoma of the parotid gland. Arch Pathol Lab Med 2004; 128(9):1046-9.

49. Felix A, Rosa JC, Nunes JF, Fonseca I, Cidadao A, Soares J. Hyalinizing clear cell carcinoma of salivary glands: A study of extracellular matrix. Oral Oncol 2002;38:364-8.

50. Fonseca I, Felix A, Soares J. Dedifferentiation in salivary gland carcinomas. Am J Surg Pathol 2000;24:469-71.

51. Foschini MP, Marucci G, Eusebi V. Low-grade mucoepidermoid carcinoma of salivary glands: Characteristic immunohistochemical profile and evidence of striated duct differentiation. Virchows Arch. 2002;440:536-42.

52. Frankenthaler RA, Luna MA, Lee SS, et al. Prognostic variables in parotid gland tumors. Arch Otolaryngol Head Neck Surg 1991;117:1251-6.

53. Fukuda M, Kusama K, Sakashita H. Cimetidine inhibits salivary gland tumor cell adhesion to neural cells and induces apoptosis by blocking NCAM expression. BMC Cancer 2008;8:376.

54. García de Marcos JA, Calderón-Polanco J, Poblet E, del Castillo-Pardo de Vera JL, Arroyo-Rodríguez S, Galdeano-Arenas M, Dean-Ferrer A. Primary adenoid cystic carcinoma of the mandible: Case report and review of the literature. J Oral Maxillofac Surg 2008;66(12):2609-15.

55. Ghannoum JE, Freedman PD. Signet-ring cell (mucin-producing) adenocarcinomas of minor salivary glands. Am J Surg Pathol 2004;28(1):89-93.

56. Gnepp DR, Brandenwein MS, Henley JD. Salivary and lacrimal glands. In: Gnepp DR (Ed). Diagnostic surgical pathology of the head and neck. WB Saunders, Philadelphia, 2001.

57. Gnepp DR. Diagnostic Surgical Pathology of the Head and Neck. WB Saunders: Philadelphia, 2001.

58. Gnepp DR. Sebaceous neoplasms of salivary gland origin: A review. Pathol Annu 1983;18:71-102.

59. Greene FL, Page DL, Fleming ID, Fritz AG, Balch CM, Haller DG, Morrow M. American Joint Committee on cancer. Cancer Staging Manual. Springer: New York, 2002.

60. Grisius MM, Fox PC. Salivary gland diseases. In: Greenberg MS, Glick M (Eds). Burket's Oral Medicine Diagnosis and Treatment. BC Decker Inc, Ontario, 2003.

61. Gürbüz Y, Yildiz K, Aydin O, Almaç A. Immuno-phenotypical profiles of salivary gland tumours: A new evidence for their histogenetic origin. Pathologica 2006;98(2):147-52.

62. Guo Y, Yang MC, Weissler JC, Yang YS. Modulation of PLAGL2 transactivation activity by Ubc9 co-activation not SUMOylation. Biochem Biophys Res Commun 2008;374(3):570-5.

63. Handra-Luca A, Lamas G, Bertrand JC, Fouret P. MUC1, MUC2, MUC4, and MUC5AC expression in salivary gland mucoepidermoid carcinoma: Diagnostic and prognostic implications. Am J Surg Pathol 2005;29(7):881-9.

64. Hannen EJM, J Bulten J, Festen J, Wienk SM, De Wilde PCM. Polymorphous low grade adeno-carcinoma with distant metastases and deletions on chromosome 6q23–qter and 11q23–qter: A case report . J Clin Pathol 2000;53:942-5.

65. Harry L, Evans HL, Luna MA. Polymorphous low-grade adenocarcinoma a study of 40 cases with long-term follow-up and an evaluation of the importance of papillary areas. Am J Surg Pathol 2000;24:1319-28.

66. Hellquist HB, Karlsson MG, Nilsson C. Salivary duct carcinoma: A highly aggressive salivary gland with overexpression of c-erbB-2. J Pathol 1994;172(1):35-44.

67. Henley JD, Geary WA, Jackson CL, Wu CD, Gnepp DR. Dedifferentiated acinic cell carcinoma of the parotid gland: A distinct rarely described entity. Hum Pathol 1997;28(7):869-73.

68. Henley JD, Seo IS, Dayan D, Gnepp DR. Sarcomatoid salivary duct carcinoma of the parotid gland. Hum Pathol 2000;31(2):208-13.

69. Hickman RE, Cawson RA, Duffy SW. The prognosis of specific type of salivary gland tumors. Cancer 1992;54:1620-54.

70. Hoch BL, Wu M, Lewis M, Gan L, Burstein DE. An immunohistochemical study of XIAP expression in pleomorphic adenoma and carcinoma ex pleomorphic adenoma. J Oral Pathol Med. 2008;37(10):634-8.

71. Huvos AG, Paulino AFG. Salivary glands. In: Sternberg SS, Antonioli DA, Carter D, Mills SE, Oberman HA (Eds). Diagnostic surgical pathology. 3rd edn. Philadelphia: Lippincott Williams and Wilkins; 1999. pp. 857-80.

72. Jamal AM, Sun ZJ, Chen XM, Zhao YF. Salivary duct carcinoma of the parotid gland: Case report and review of the literature. J Oral Maxillofac Surg. 2008;66(8):1708-13.

73. Jansisyanont P, Blanchaert Jr RH, Ord RA. Intraoral minor salivary gland neoplasm: A single institution experience of 80 cases. Int J Oral Maxillofac Surg 2002;31:257-61.

74. Jerome BT. Squamous carcinoma in a major salivary gland: A review of the diagnostic considerations. Arch Pathol Lab Med 2001;125(6): 740-5.

75. Jiang Li. Salivary adenocarcinoma, not otherwise specified: A collection of orphans. Arch Path Lab Med 2004;128:1385-94.

76. Kamio N. Coexpression of p53 and c-erbB-2 proteins is associated with histological type, stage, and cell proliferation in malignant salivary glands. Virchows Arch 1996;428(2):75-83.

77. Klijanienho J, Vielh P. Salivary gland tumours: Monographs in clinical cytology. Karger: Basel, 2000;15.

78. Kowalski PJ, Paulino AF. Perineural invasion in adenoid cystic carcinoma: Its causation/promotion by brain-derived neurotrophic factor. Hum Pathol 2002;33(9):933-6.

79. Krishnanand G, Kaur M, Rao RV, Monappa V. Oncocytic variant of mucoepidermoid carcinoma of submandibular gland: An unusual clinical and morphological entity. Indian J Pathol Microbiol 2007;50(3):538-40.

80. Kusafuka K, Takizawa Y, Ueno T, Ishiki H, Asano R, Kamijo T, Iida Y, Ebihara M, Ota Y, Onitsuka T, Kameya T. Dedifferentiated epithelial-myoepithelial carcinoma of the parotid gland: A rare case report of immunohistochemical analysis and review of the literature. Oral Surg Oral Med Oral Pathol Oral Radiol Endod 2008;106(1):85-91.

81. Lai G, Nemolato S, Lecca S, Parodo G, Medda C, Faa G. The role of immunohistochemistry in the diagnosis of hyalinizing clear cell carcinoma of the minor salivary gland: A case report. Eur J Histochem 2008;52(4):251-4.

82. Lee DJ, Ahn HK, Koh ES, Rho YS, Chu HR. Necrotizing sialometaplasia accompanied by adenoid cystic carcinoma on the soft palate. Clin Exp Otorhinolaryngol 2009;2(1):48-51.

83. Lewis JE, Olsen KD, Sebo TJ. Carcinoma ex-pleomorphic adenoma: Pathologic analysis of 73 cases. Hum Pathol 2001;32(6):596-604.

84. Li Y, Li LJ, Huang J, Han B, Pan J. Central malignant salivary gland tumors of the jaw: Retrospective clinical analysis of 22 cases. J Oral Maxillofac Surg 2008;66(11):2247-53.

85. Liu T, Zhu E, Wang L, Okada T, Yamaguchi A, Okada N. Abnormal expression of Rb pathway-related proteins in salivary gland acinic cell carcinoma. Hum Pathol 2005;36(9):962-70.

86. Locati LD, Bossi P, Perrone F, Potepan P, Crippa F, Mariani L, Casieri P, Orsenigo M, Losa M, Bergamini C, Liberatoscioli C, Quattrone P, Calderone RG, Rinaldi G, Pilotti S, Licitra L. Cetuximab in recurrent

and/or metastatic salivary gland carcinomas: A phase II study. Oral Oncol 2009;45(7):574-8.

87. Loh KS, Barker E, Bruch G, O'Sullivan B, Brown DH, Goldstein DP, Gilbert RW, Gullane PJ, Irish JC. Prognostic factors in malignancy of the minor salivary glands. Head Neck 2009;31(1):58-63.

88. Lopes MA, de Abreu Alves F, Levy BA, de Almeida OP, Kowalski LP. Intraoral salivary duct carcinoma: Case report with immunohistochemical observations. Oral Surg Oral Med Oral Pathol Oral Radiol Endod 2001;91(6):689-92.

89. Lopes MA, Kowalski LP, da Cunha Santos G, Paes de Almeida O. A clinicopathologic study of 196 intraoral minor salivary gland tumours. J Oral Pathol Med 1999;28:264-7.

90. Losito NS, Botti G, Ionna F, Pasquinelli G, Minenna P, Bisceglia M. Clear-cell myoepithelial carcinoma of the salivary glands: A clinicopathologic, immunohistochemical, and ultrastructural study of two cases involving the submandibular gland with review of the literature. Pathol Res Pract 2008;204(5):335-44.

91. Lueck NE, Robinson RA. High levels of expression of cytokeratin 5 are strongly correlated with poor survival in higher grades of mucoepidermoid carcinoma. J Clin Pathol 2008;61(7):837-40.

92. Luukkaa H, Klemi P, Hirsimäki P, Vahlberg T, Kivisaari A, Kähäri VM, Grénman R. Matrix metalloproteinase (MMP)-1, -9 and -13 as prognostic factors in salivary gland cancer. Acta Otolaryngol 2008;128(4):482-90.

93. Mahomed F, Altini M, Meer S, Rikhotso E, Pearl C. Central adenoid cystic carcinoma of the mandible with odontogenic features: Report of a case. Head Neck 2009;31(7):975-80.

94. Maiorano E, Favia G, Pece S, Resta L, Maisonneuve P, Di Fiore PP, Capodiferro S, Urbani U, Viale G. Prognostic implications of NUMB immuno-reactivity in salivary gland carcinomas. Int J Immunopathol Pharmacol 2007;20(4):779-89.

95. Manoharan M, Othman NH, Samsudin AR. Hyalinizing clear cell carcinoma of minor salivary gland: Case report. Braz Dent J 2002;13:66-9.

96. Mantravadi J, Roth L, Kafrawy A. Vascular neoplasms of the parotid gland. Parotid vascular tumors. Oral Surg Oral Med Oral Pathol 1993;75:70-5.

97. Marioni G, Marino F, Stramare R, Marchese-Ragona R, Stsaffieri A. Benign metastasizing pleomorphic adenoma of the parotid gland: A clinicopathologic puzzle. Head Neck 2003;25(12):1071-6.

98. Martinez-Barba E, Cortes-Guardiola JA, Minguela-Puras A, Torroba-Caron A, Mendez-Trujillo S, Bermejo-Lopez J. Salivary duct carcinoma: clinicopathological and immunohistochemical studies. J Craniomaxillofac Surg 1997;25(6):328-34.

99. Maruya S, Kurotaki H, Wada R, Saku T, Shinkawa H, Yagihashi S. Promoter methylation and protein expression of the E-cadherin gene in the clinicopathologic assessment of adenoid cystic carcinoma. Mod Pathol 2004;17(6):637-45.

100. Maruya S, Shirasaki T, Nagaki T, Kakehata S, Kurotaki H, Mizukami H, Shinkawa H. Differential expression of topoisomerase IIalpha protein in salivary gland carcinomas: Histogenetic and prognostic implications. BMC Cancer 2009;9:72.

101. Meer S, Altini M. CK7+/CK20- immunoexpression profile is typical of salivary gland neoplasia. Histopathology 2007;51(1):26-32.

102. Milchgrub S, Gnepp DR, Vuitch F, Delgado R, Albores-Saavedra J. Hyalinizing clear cell carcinoma of salivary gland. Am J Surg Pathol 1994;18:74-82.

103. Minamiguchi S, Iwasa Y, Shoji K, Higuchi K, Watanabe C, Haga H, Nakashima Y, Yamabe H. Salivary duct carcinoma: A clinicopathologic study of three cases with a review of the literature. Pathol Int 1996;46(8):614-22.

104. Mino M, Pilch BZ, Faquin WC. Expression of KIT (CD117) in neoplasms of the head and neck: An ancillary marker for adenoid cystic carcinoma. Mod Pathol 2003;16(12):1224-31.

105. Mukunyadzi P, Ai L, Portilla D, Barnes EL, Fan CY. Expression of peroxisome proliferator-activated receptor gamma in salivary duct carcinoma: Immunohistochemical analysis of 15 cases. Mod Pathol 2003;16(12):1218-23.

106. Nagao T, Gaffey TA, Olsen KD, Serizawa H, Lewis JE. Small cell carcinoma of the major salivary glands: Clinicopathologic study with emphasis on cytokeratin 20 immunoreactivity and clinical outcome. Am J Surg Pathol 2004;28(6):762-70.

107. Nagao T, Gaffey TA, Serizawa H, Sugano I, Ishida Y, Yamazaki K, Tokashiki R, Yoshida T, Minato H, Kay PA, Lewis JE. Dedifferentiated adenoid cystic carcinoma: A clinicopathologic study of 6 cases. Mod Pathol 2003;16(12):1265-72.

108. Nagao T, Sugano I, Ishida Y, et al. Salivary gland malignant myoepithelioma: A clinicopathologic and immunohistochemical study of ten cases. Cancer 1998;93:1292-9.

109. Nagao T, Sugano I, Ishida Y, Asoh A, Munakata S, Yamazaki K, Konno A, Iwaya K, Shimizu T, Serizawa H, Ebihara Y. Hybrid carcinomas of the salivary glands: Report of nine cases with a clinicopathologic, immunohistochemical, and p53 gene alteration analysis. Mod Pathol 2002;15(7): 724-33.

110. Nagao T, Sugano I, Ishida Y, Tajima Y, Matsuzaki O, Konno A, Kondo Y, Nagao K. Salivary gland malignant myoepithelioma: A clinicopathologic and immunohistochemical study of ten cases. Cancer 1998;83(7):1292-9.

111. Nagao T. Sarcomatoid variant of salivary duct carcinoma. clinicopathologic and immunohistochemical study of eight cases with review of the literature. Am J Clin Pathol 2003;122:222-31.

112. Nagarkar NM, Bansal S, Dass A, Singhal SK, Mohan H. Salivary gland tumours-Our experience. Indian J Otolaryngol Head Neck Surg 2004;56:31-4.

113. Nagler RM, Ben-Izhak O, Ostrovsky D, Golz A, Hershko DD. The expression and prognostic significance of Cks1 in salivary cancer. Cancer Invest 2009;27(5):512-20.

114. Navarro Rde L, Martins MT, de Araujo VC. Maspin expression in normal and neoplastic salivary gland. J Oral Pathol Med 2004;33:435-40.

115. Negri T, Tamborini E, Dagrada GP, Greco A, Staurengo S, Guzzo M, Locati LD, Carbone A, Pierotti MA, Licitra L, Pilotti S. TRK-A, HER-2/neu, and KIT Expression/Activation Profiles in Salivary Gland Carcinoma. Transl Oncol 2008;1(3):121-8.

116. Neville BW, Damm DD, Allen CM, Bouquot JE. Oral and Maxillofacial Pathology, 2nd edn. WB Saunders Co., 2002.

117. Nikitakis NG, Tosios KI, Papanikolaou VS, Rivera H, Papanicolaou SI, Ioffe OB. Immunohistochemical expression of cytokeratins 7 and 20 in malignant salivary gland tumors. Mod Pathol 2004;17:407-15.

118. Nordkvist A, Roijer E, Bang G, Gustafsson H, Behrendt M, Ryd W, Thoresen S, Donath K, Stenman G. Expression and mutation patterns of p53 in benign and malignant salivary gland tumours. Int J Oncol 2000;16(3):477-83.

119. Okabe M, Inagaki H, Murase, Inoue M, Nagai N, Eimoto T. Prognostic significance of p27 and Ki-67 expression in mucoepidermoid carcinoma of the intraoral minor salivary gland. Mod Pathol 2001;14:1008-14.

120. O'Neill ID. (11;19) translocation and CRTC1-MAML2 fusion oncogene in mucoepidermoid carcinoma. Oral Oncol 2009;45(1):2-9.

121. O'Neill ID. The expression and prognostic significance of Cks1 in salivary cancer. New insights into the nature of Warthin's tumour. J Oral Pathol Med 2009;38(1):145-9.

122. Penner CR, Folpe AL, Budnick SD. C-kit expression distinguishes salivary gland adenoid cystic carcinoma from polymorphous low-grade adenocarcinoma. Mod Pathol 2002;15(7):687-91.

123. Persson F, Andrén Y, Winnes M, Wedell B, Nordkvist A, Gudnadottir G, Dahlenfors R, Sjögren H, Mark J, Stenman G. High-resolution genomic profiling of adenomas and carcinomas of the salivary glands reveals amplification, rearrangement, and fusion of HMGA2. Genes Chromosomes Cancer 2009;48(1):69-82.

124. Perzin KH. A systematic approach to the diagnosis of salivary gland tumours. In: Fenoglio CM, Wolff M (Eds). Progress in surgical pathology. New York: Masson; 1982;4:137-80.

125. Phucareon J, Ohta Y, Woo JM, Eisele DW, Tetsu O. Genetic profiling reveals cross-contamination and misidentification of 6 adenoid cystic carcinoma cell lines: ACC2, ACC3, ACCM, ACCNS, ACCS and CAC2. PLoS One. 2009;4(6):e6040.

126. Pinkston JA, Cole P. Incidence rates of salivary gland tumours: Results from a population-based study. Otolaryngol Head Neck Surg 1999;120(6): 834-40.

127. Ponniah I, SureshKumar P, Karunakaran K. Clear Cell Carcinoma of Minor Salivary Gland – Case Report. Ann Acad Med Singapore 2007;36:857-60.

128. Prabhu S, Kaveri H, Rekha K. Benign and malignant salivary gland tumors: Comparison of immunohistochemical expression of e-cadherin. Oral Oncol 2009;45(7):594-9.

129. Pujary K, Rangarajan S, Nayak DR, Balakrishnan R, Ramakrishnan V. Hyalinizing clear cell carcinoma of the base of tongue. Int J Oral Maxillofac Surg 2008;37(1):93-6.

130. Quddus MR, Henley JD, Affify AM, Dardick I, Gnepp DR. Basal cell adenocarcinoma of the salivary gland: An ultrastructural and immuno-histochemical study. Oral Surg Oral Med Oral Pathol Oral Radiol Endod 1999;87(4):485-92.

131. Queimado L, Obeso D, Hatfield MD, Yang Y, Thompson DM, Reis AM. Dysregulation of Wnt pathway components in human salivary gland tumors. Arch Otolaryngol Head Neck Surg 2008;134(1):94-101.

132. Qureshi A, Barakzai A, Sahar NU, Gulzar R, Ahmad Z, Hassan SH. Spectrum of malignancy in mixed tumors of salivary gland: A morphological and immunohistochemical review of 23 cases. Indian J Pathol Microbiol 2009;52(2):150-4.

133. Rajendran R, Sivapathasundharam B. Diseases of salivary gland. In: Shafer's textbook of oral pathology, 5th edn. Elsevier, 2005.

134. Rao PH, Roberts D, Zhao YJ, Bell D, Harris CP, Weber RS, El-Naggar AK. Deletion of 1p32-p36 is the most frequent genetic change and poor prognostic marker in adenoid cystic carcinoma of the salivary glands. Clin Cancer Res 2008;14(16): 5181-7.

135. Rezende RB, Drachenberg CB, Kumar D, Blanchaert R, Ord RA, Ioffe OB, et al. Differential diagnosis between monomorphic clear cell adenocarcinoma of salivary glands and renal (clear) cell carcinoma. Am J Surg Pathol 1999;23:1532-8.

136. Riedel G, Coy JF, Spahn V, Hormann K. Salivary gland carcinosarcoma: Immunohistochemical, molecular genetic and electron microscopic findings. Oral Oncol 2000;36(4):360-4.

137. Roijer E, Nordkvist A, Strom AK. Translocation, deletion/amplification and expression of HMGIC and MDM2 in a carcinoma ex-pleomorphic adenoma. Am J Pathol 2002;160(2):433-40.

138. Sakamoto K, Ono T, Nakamura Y, Harada H, Nakashima T. Expression of cluster of differentiation 9 glycoprotein in benign and malignant parotid gland tumours. J Laryngol Otol 2009;123(31):58-63.

139. Schwarz S, Ettl T, Kleinsasser N, Hartmann A, Reichert TE, Driemel O. Loss of Maspin expression is a negative prognostic factor in common salivary gland tumors. Oral Oncol. 2008;44(6):563-70.

140. Seifert G, Miehlke A, Haubrich J, Chillar R. Disease of the salivary glands. Stuttgart: George Thieme; 1986.

141. Sequeiros-Santiago G, García-Carracedo D, Fresno MF, Suarez C, Rodrigo JP, Gonzalez MV. Oncogene amplification pattern in adenoid cystic carcinoma of the salivary glands. Oncol Rep 2009;21(5): 1215-22.

142. Shet T, Ghodke R, Kane S, Chinoy RN. Cytomorphologic patterns in papillary cystic variant of acinic cell carcinoma of the salivary gland. Acta Cytol 2006;50(4):388-92.

143. Shi L, Chen XM, Wang L, Zhang L, Chen Z. Expression of caveolin-1 in mucoepidermoid carcinoma of the salivary glands: Correlation with vascular endothelial growth factor, microvessel density, and clinical outcome. Cancer 2007;109(8): 1523-31.

144. Shigeishi H, Ohta K, Hiraoka M, Fujimoto S, Minami M, Higashikawa K, Kamata N. Expression of TPX2 in salivary gland carcinomas. Oncol Rep. 2009;21(2):341-4.

145. Shigeishi H, Yoneda S, Taki M, Nobumori T, Ohta K, Higashikawa K, Yasui W, Kamata N. Correlation of human Bub1 expression with tumor-proliferating activity in salivary gland tumors. Oncol Rep 2006;15(4):933-8.

146. Shintaku M, Honda T. Identification of oncocytic lesions of salivary glands by antimitochondrial immunohistochemistry. Histopathology 1997;31: 408-11.

147. Shirasaki T, Maruya S, Mizukami H, Kakehata S, Kurotaki H, Yagihashi S, Shinkawa H. Effects of small interfering RNA targeting thymidylate synthase on survival of ACC3 cells from salivary adenoid cystic carcinoma. BMC Cancer 2008; 8:348.

148. Simpson RH, Prasad AR, Lewis JE, Skalova A, David L. Mucin-rich variant of salivary duct carcinoma: A clinicopathologic and immuno-histochemical study of four cases. Am J Surg Pathol 2003;27(8):1070-9.

149. Simpson RH, Sarsfield PT, Clarke T, Babajews AV. Clear cell carcinoma of minor salivary glands. Histopathology 1990;17:433-8.

150. Skalova A, Simpson RH, Lehtonen H, Leivo I. Assessment of proliferative activity using the MIB1 antibody helps to distinguish polymorphous low adenocarcinoma from adenoid cystic carcinoma of salivary glands. Pathol Res Pract 1997;193:695-703.

151. Solar AA, Schmidt BL, Jordan RC. Hyalinizing clear cell carcinoma: Case series and comprehensive review of the literature. Cancer 2009;115(1):75-83.

152. Speight PM, Barrett AW: Salivary gland tumours. Oral Dis 2002;8(5):229-40.

153. Spiro RH. Salivary neoplasms: overview of a 35-year experience with 2,802 patients. Head Neck Surg 1986;8:177-84.

154. Strick MJ, Kelly C, Soames JV, McLean NR. Malignant tumours of the minor salivary glands – a 20 year review. Br J Plast Surg 2004;57:624–31.

155. Subhashraj K. Salivary gland tumors: A single institution experience in India. Br J Oral Maxillofac Surg 2008;46:635–8.

156. Suzuki H, Hashimoto K. Salivary duct carcinoma in the mandible: Report of a case with immuno-histochemical studies. Br J Oral Maxillofac Surg 1999;37(1):67-9.

157. Toida M, Shimokawa K, Makita1 H, et al. Intraoral minor salivary gland tumors: A clinicopathological study of 82 cases. Int J Oral Maxillofac Surg 2005;34:528-32.

158. Toshitaka N, Gaffey TA, Visscher DW, Kay PA, Hiroshi M, Hiromi S, Lewis JE. Invasive micro-papillary salivary duct carcinoma: A distinct histologic variant with biologic significance. Am J Surg Path 2004;28(3):319-26.

159. Tsang YT, Chang YM, LuX. Amplification of MGC2177, PLAG1, PSMC6P AND LYN in a malignant mixed tumour of salivary gland detected by cDNA microarray with tyramide signal amplification. Cancer Genet Cytogenet 2004; 152(2):124-8.

160. Urano M, Abe M, Horibe Y, Kuroda M, Mizoguchi Y, Sakurai K, Naito K. Sclerosing mucoepidermoid carcinoma with eosinophilia of the salivary glands. Pathol Res Pract 2002;198(4):305-10.

161. Vargas H, Sudilovsky D, Kaplan MJ, Regezi J, Weidner N. Mixed tumor, polymorphous low grade adenocarcinoma, and adenoid cystic carcinoma of the salivary gland: Pathogenic implications and differential diagnosis by Ki67, MIB1, Bcl2, and S100 immunohistochemistry. Appl Immunohistochem 1997;5:8-16.

162. Vargas PA, Cheng Y, Barrett AW, Craig GT, Speight PM. Expression of Mcm-2, Ki-67 and geminin in benign and malignant salivary gland tumours. J Oral Pathol Med 2008;37:309-18.

163. Vargas PA, Speight PM, Bingle CD, Barrett AW, Bingle L. Expression of PLUNC family members in benign and malignant salivary gland tumours. Oral Dis 2008;14(7):613-9.

164. Vargas PA, Torres-Rendon A, Speight PM. DNA ploidy analysis in salivary gland tumours by image cytometry. J Oral Pathol Med 2007;36(6):371-6.

165. Wah C, John RM, John KC. Intraductal carcinoma of the oral cavity: A case report and a reappraisal of the concept of pure ductal carcinoma in situ in salivary duct carcinoma. Am J Surg Path 2004;28(2):266-70.

166. Wang B, Brandwein M, Gordon R, Robinson R, Urken M, Zarbo RJ. Primary salivary clear cell tumors – A diagnostic approach. Arch Pathol Lab Med 2002;26:676-85.

167. Wang D, Li Y, He H, Liu L, Wo L, He Z. Intraoral minor salivary gland tumors in a Chinese population: A retrospective study on 737 cases. Oral Surg Oral Med Oral Pathol Oral Radiol Endod 2007;104:94-100.

168. Wen DS, Zhu XL, Guan SM, Wu YM, Yu LL, Wu JZ. Silencing of CXCR4 inhibits the proliferation, adhesion, chemotaxis and invasion of salivary gland mucoepidermoid carcinoma Mc3 cells in vitro. Oral Oncol 2008;44(6):545-54.

169. Wenghoefer M, Pantelis A, Dommisch H, Götz W, Reich R, Bergé S, Martini M, Allam JP, Jepsen S, Merkelbach-Bruse S, Fischer HP, Novak N, Winter J. Nuclear hBD-1 accumulation in malignant salivary gland tumours. BMC Cancer. 2008;8:290.

170. Williams SB, Ellis GL, Auclair PL. Immuno-histochemical analysis of basal cell adenocarcinoma. Oral Surg Oral Med Oral Pathol 1993;75(1):64-9.

171. Xin W, Paulino AF. Prognostic factors in malignant mixed tumours of the salivary gland: Correlation of immunohistochemical markers with histologic classification. Ann Diagn Pathol 2002;6(4):205-10.

172. Yamamoto Y, Kishimoto Y, Virmani AK, Smith A, Vuitch F, Albores-Saavedra J, Gazdar AF. Mutations associated with carcinomas arising from pleomorphic adenomas of the salivary glands. Hum Pathol 1996;27(8):782-6.

173. Yang S, Zhang J, Chen X, Wang L, Xie F. Clear cell carcinoma, not otherwise specified, of salivary glands: A clinicopathologic study of 4 cases and review of the literature. Oral Surg Oral Med Oral Pathol Oral Radiol Endod 2008;106(5):712-20.

174. Zhang J, Peng B. NF-kappaB promotes iNOS and VEGF expression in salivary gland adenoid cystic carcinoma cells and enhances endothelial cell motility in vitro. Cell Prolif 2009;42(2):150-61.

175. Zushi Y, Noguchi K, Hashitani S, Sakurai K, Segawa E, Takaoka K, Toyohara Y, Tanaka N, Kishimoto H, Urade M. Relations among expression of CXCR4, histological patterns, and metastatic potential in adenoid cystic carcinoma of the head and neck. Int J Oncol 2008;33(6):1133-9.

9

Investigations of Salivary Glands

Harsha Vardhan BG

INTRODUCTION

Thorough knowledge of salivary gland disorders and a variety of applicable investigations are an essential element of the clinician's armamentarium. Both major and minor salivary glands can be involved in a disease process, however primary importance is attached to major salivary glands. These paired glands secrete saliva through a branching duct system.

Patients with salivary gland disease most often present with symptoms of oral dryness, pain, swelling or a mass in the gland. Though saliva is not a popular bodily fluid, a growing number of physicians and dentists are finding that saliva provides an easily available, non-invasive diagnostic medium for a wide range of disease and clinical conditions.

Down the memory lane in ancient Egypt, Thoth is said to have spit into the empty eye socket of Horus, the sun god to restore his vision. The New Testament (MARK 8:23-25) tells us that Jesus took the blind man by the hand and led him out of town, and when he had spit on his eyes, and put his hands upon him, he was restored and saw every man clearly.

The people, who really appreciate the miracle of saliva, however are not the blind, but those who suffer from xerostomia (dry mouth) due to a variety of causes. They recognize belatedly that saliva is a natural resource with multiple functions such as antimicrobial, buffering, cleansing, digestive, lubricating, maintaining the mucosal integrity and remineralization. One function not bestowed by nature is the use of saliva for diagnostic purposes. Historically, this diagnostic value was first recognized by the ancient judicial community who employed salivary flow (or its absence) as the basis for a primitive lie detection test. The accused was given a handful of dry rice. If anxiety and presumably guilt, inhibited salivation that he or she could not form an adequate bolus to chew and swallow, then off with their head.

CLINICAL SIGNS AND SYMPTOMS

Diseases of the salivary glands may have single or multiple clinical features. Unilateral or bilateral swellings in the areas of the parotid and submandibular glands should create a clinical suspicion of salivary gland disease. Oral dryness, altered flow, metallic taste, burning sensation and pain are the usual features. As the duration and severity of symptoms play an important role in the differential diagnosis, a review of the medical histories and physical conditions of patients may provide vital information. A history of skin disease or endocrine abnormality may suggest a systemic collagen disease or metabolic disorder which may be the cause of the salivary gland disease (Table 9.1).

DIAGNOSTIC APPROACH OF A PATIENT WITH SALIVARY GLAND DISEASE

Evaluation of Xerostomia

The subjective feeling of oral dryness is termed xerostomia. Xerostomia is a symptom, not a disease or diagnosis. While oral dryness is most commonly the result of salivary gland dysfunction,

Table 9.1: Common symptoms and their possible etiology	
Symptoms	*Etiology*
Acute intermittent generalized swelling	Sialolithiasis, strictures, fibrosis and/or stenosis of the duct, usually secondary to surgery or foreign bodies.
Acute generalized swelling	Viral infection, e.g. mumps, bacterial sialadenitis
Chronic generalized swelling	Sjögren's syndrome, sialosis cystic fibrosis
Discrete swelling	Cysts, intrinsic tumor or extrinsic tumor, enlarged regional lymph nodes
Xerostomia	Sjögren's syndrome, post-radiation, mouth breathing Dehydration drugs: Tricyclic antidepressants, anxiety/depression/stress
Excess salivation	Psychological (false ptyalism), local stimulation, heavy metal poisoning

it may have other causes. So patients complaining of dry mouth cannot automatically be assumed to have salivary dysfunction. Evaluation of the patient should include careful history taking, assessment of medical status and thorough clinical examination to identify the basis of their problem. Determining the extent of altered salivary gland function is essential, since individuals with salivary gland dysfunction can be at risk for a variety of oral and systemic complications due to alterations in normal salivary function. This is followed by investigative techniques such as hematology, salivary imaging and biopsy that will aid in arriving at a correct diagnosis.

Dehydration is also considered as a causative factor for oral dryness. Although dehydration is considered to have a secondary effect on salivary gland output, changes in body water content can affect mucosal hydration, which may lead to changes in the perception of wetness in the oral cavity.

Saliva Collection and Sampling

Salivary flow rate provides vital information for diagnostic and research purposes. Salivary flow rates can be calculated from the individual major salivary glands or from mixed sample of the oral fluids, termed "whole saliva". Whole saliva is mixed fluid content of the mouth from all major and minor glands. The methods of whole saliva collection include the draining, spitting, suction and absorbent methods.

- The draining method is passive and requires the patient to allow saliva to flow from the mouth into a pre-weighed test tube or graduated cylinder for a specific time period.

- In the spitting method, the patient allows saliva to accumulate in the mouth and then expectorates into a pre-weighed graduated cylinder, usually every 60 seconds for 2 to 5 minutes.

- The suction method uses aspirator or saliva ejector to draw saliva from the mouth into a test tube for a defined time period.

- The absorbent method uses a preweighed gauze sponge that is placed in the patient's mouth for a set amount of time. After collection, the sponge is weighed again, and the volume of saliva is determined.

Of these four methods, the draining and the spitting methods are more reliable and reproducible for unstimulated whole saliva collection. It is difficult to determine a normal value for salivary output, as there is a large amount of variability resulting in a large range of normal values. Unstimulated whole saliva flow rates of less than 0.1 ml/min and stimulated whole saliva rates of less than 1.0 ml/min are considered abnormally low and indicative of marked salivary hypofunction.

Carlson-Crittenden collectors perform individual parotid gland saliva collection. The collectors are placed over the stensen's duct orifices and are held in place with gentle suction. Saliva from individual submandibular and sublingual glands is collected with an aspirating device or an alginate-held collector called a segregator. When using the suction device, gauze is placed sublingually to dry and isolate the sublingual region; the gauze and tongue are gently retracted away from the duct orifice. Gentle suction is used to collect the saliva that is secreted. The segregator is positioned over Wharton's duct and is then held in place by alginate. As saliva is produced, it flows through tubing and is collected in a preweighed vessel.

Stimulated saliva from individual glands is obtained by applying a sialagogue such as citric acid to the dorsal surface of the tongue. Pre-weighed tubes are used for individual salivary gland collections and for some of the whole saliva collection techniques, and flow rates are determined gravimetrically in millimeters per minute per gland, assuming that the specific gravity of saliva is 1 (i.e., 1 g equals 1 mL of saliva).

Salivary flow rates can be influenced by many factors. Patient position, hydration, diurnal variation, and time since stimulation can affect salivary flow. It is always preferred to collect saliva using a well-defined, standardized, and clearly documented procedure. It is best to collect saliva during morning hours. To ensure that an unstimulated sample is collected, patients should refrain from eating, drinking, or smoking for 90 minutes prior to the procedure. For a general assessment of salivary function, unstimulated whole saliva collection is preferred the most.

Sialometry

Salivary flow rate is denoted as ml/min/gland. Under resting conditions the flow rate of the parotid amounts to 0 to 0.1 ml/min. Following stimulation, it ranges from 0.5 to 1.5 ml/min. Stimulated values below 0.3 ml/min are considered pathological. Elevated flow rates are seen in conditions such as gingivitis, denture prosthesis, Parkinson's disease (due to increase in cholinergic activity), and intoxication. Low values are found with the use of tricyclic anti depressants, radical surgical treatment and irradiation.

Sialochemistry—A Diagnostic Tool

Saliva has proven to be an indicator in acute diseases of salivary glands, a promising probe for drug trial and monitoring, and invaluable factor in forensic applications. With the advent of highly sensitive immunochemical assays, the compositional profile of saliva has expanded widely. The establishment of a range of normal values for a variety of "intrinsic" and "extrinsic" components is the initial step to use saliva as a diagnostic tool for oral health status. A number of cross-sectional studies conducted in this regard have shown that there is a wide variation in the salivary composition in healthy population. This is possible as a result of wide functional versatility of salivary molecules. For instance, in addition to the digestive properties of salivary amylase, it recognized recently that it can also modulate bacterial colonizations. Low levels of already known antimicrobial salivary molecules (e.g. lactoferrin, lysozyme) is compensated with higher concentrations of other molecules such as amylase. This explains the possible reason for variation in the composition among the healthy individuals.

Sialochemistry could Provide Valuable Information Regarding

- Differentiation between normal and abnormal gland function.
- Effect of dysfunction on oral environment—Mucosa and periodontal tissues.
- Homeostatic fluctuations as a result of circulatory, innervatory and/or hormonal imbalances.

Routine Laboratory Investigations

Investigation using sialochemistry is based on relationships with intraglandular transport processes (sodium), intracellular synthesis (protein, amylase) and diffusion by plasma constituents (urea). Routine laboratory investigations include estimation of potassium, calcium, sodium, chloride, bicarbonate, urea, total protein, amylase, and osmolarity.

Sodium: A number of membrane processes facilitate sodium and water transport from the interstitial tissues into the acinar lumen. Following cholinergic and sympathetic stimulation, plasma values are found in the primary fluid for sodium, chloride, and bicarbonate. Potassium is slightly elevated. The variable sodium concentrations at different flow rates depend on changes that take place during duct passage. Within the ductules, the striated ducts are responsible for sodium, chloride and bicarbonate reabsorption. The sodium concentration is proportional to flow rates from 0.1 to 2.5 ml/min. Damage of any kind to the striated duct leads to decreased sodium reabsorption.

Bicarbonate: It plays an important role in the salivary buffer system. Reabsorption mainly takes place during passage through the intralobular duct. Usually, low concentrations of bicarbonate are present along with low sodium levels. In inflammatory conditions or irradiation, the concentration of bicarbonate remains low, even when sodium concentrations are high.

Urea: Urea provides another buffer system in the oral cavity. A number of characteristics such as its central production in the liver, low molecular weight and electric neutrality make this substance a useful tool in sialochemistry. These properties allow a quantitative assessment of the reabsorption of water within the gland. Laboratory findings show a steady state of urea concentration in saliva at 30% below the plasma value, when salivary flow rates exceed 1ml/min. The mean salivary urea approaches plasma urea values at flow rates of about 0.3 mL/min. It surpasses the plasma value at rates beneath 0.3 ml/min.

Potassium: The salivary concentration shows a constant level of 20 to 25 mmol/L. High values up to 60 mmol/L are reached. Active potassium secretion takes place mainly in the striated duct. Hence low level values of less than 10 mmol/L are seen following destruction of this ductal segment. The estimation of active potassium may allow differentiation between destruction by inflammation and irradiation.

Protein: The salivary glands play an active role in the synthesis of numerous proteins. Abnormal proteins are also produced in some tumors and nutritional deficiency states. The exocrine secretion is dominated by amylase. Other products are proline-rich proteins, immunoproteins and growth factors. The glycoproteins (mucins), which play an important role, originate mainly from the sublingual and minor glands. Mucin disturbances are known to occur in case of cystic fibrosis. The functions of producing, storing and discharging secretory protein are mainly under the influence of sympathetic nervous system. Any disturbance may lead to derangement, abnormal storage and acinar swelling. The clinical effect is bilateral swelling in the parotid and submandibular regions. Low amylase concentrations are seen in cases of starvation and acinar destruction. Elevated levels are expected in conditions leading to abnormal ductal water loss.

Acute inflammation of glands will result in a rise of plasma and urine amylase due to gross glandular leakage. This may be encountered in mumps and sialolithiasis.

Sialochemistry in Salivary Gland Disease

Etiological Factors

Inflammatory conditions of the salivary glands caused by different etiological factors will show some changes in their sialochemistry. It is a useful means of chronologically, monitoring quantitative changes.

Inflammation: Inflammation of salivary glands is characterized by accumulation of B-lymphocytes around the ducts and acinar cells, causing destruction and /or proliferation. Atrophy of the acini may follow ductal obstruction. This results in decreased sodium reabsorption and potassium secretion in the duct.

Mumps: Mumps or epidemic parotitis is one of the most common salivary gland diseases. In about 50% of cases, clinical changes in the glands are absent. Where swelling is prominent, edema and dense accumulation of lymphocytes and plasma cells compress the salivary duct, result in almost complete asialism.

The diagnosis is made by detection of a rise in antibody titer by complement fixation test. Elevated values for serum and urine amylase are consistently found. Differentiation of the isoamylases distinguishes between a rise due to parotid as opposed to pancreatic pathology. In mumps, the saliva shows a sharp increase in the sodium concentration and an exceptionally low potassium concentration, which approaches its plasma equivalents. Sodium values rise to 90 to 120 mmol/L while potassium values fall below 10 mmol/L.

Recurrent obstructive parotitis: Histological, ductal damage by lymphatic invasion is observed in recurrent obstructive parotitis. As lymphatic tissue gradually disappears by puberty, attacks fade away in most patients. During the acute phase, flow rates of saliva are reduced and areas of purulent necrotic discharge are found from which physiologic oral flora can be cultivated. Sialochemistry demonstrates all the signs of inflammation.

Sarcoidosis (Heerfordt's disease): As a part of systemic sarcoidosis, granulomatous foci may be seen in the salivary glands, which may even cause bilateral swelling of the parotid gland. This epithelioid sialadenitis does not lead to serious functional glandular disorders. The flow is elevated as a result of slight tissue compression. Sialochemistry fails to reveal inflammatory changes. Angiotensin converting enzyme (ACE) will be elevated in the plasma, it is not known whether ACE is present in the saliva.

Sjögren's Syndrome: This includes kerato-conjunctivitis sicca, xerostomia and rheumatoid arthritis, probably depends on the presence of activated T-lymphocytes and hyper-reactive B-lymphocytes in exocrine organs. The autoimmune behavior of these lymphocytes expresses itself by producing a large number of non-specific antibodies, which can be demonstrated by investigations. The parenchyma of all the salivary glands reveals destruction of the ductules, creating myoepithelial islands. The acini are gradually lost. There is swelling of the major glands, at times with redness and pain. In cases of purulent flow, *Streptococcus viridans*, *Klebsiella* or Enterobacteriaceae can be cultured. While the 'primary'type of Sjögren's is seen in all the salivary glands, a biopsy, from the lower lip confirms the diagnosis if accumulation of IgM and IgG are demonstrated. The multiple foci of gland destruction and the degeneration of acinar cells results in decreased flow. This is more pronounced in resting secretion. High sodium concentrations ranging from 60 to 100 mmol/L are found at any given flow rate. The potassium concentration lies between 10 and 20 mmol/L. The total protein production is lower during the disease while concentrations of protein persist at an elevated level. Further laboratory investigations, including electrophoresis, immunochemistry, and blood counts, should always be performed. While erythrocyte sedimentation rates above 60 mm and globulins more than 18 g alone are not pathognomic, their appearance in combination with the described sialochemistry is highly suggestive of Sjögren's syndrome.

Irradiation: Radiotherapy causes rapid and severe destruction of the parenchyma of the glands. A loss of function of up to 50% is measured within the first week. In the most susceptible serous glands, cell enlargement, formation of vacuoles with degranulation, and finally necrosis develops. Capillary walls are thickened and atrophy of the nerves follows after several months.

Sialochemistry immediately reveals inflammatory changes. Salivary flow rates fall to zero while the rise in sodium level is steep (80–120 mmol/L) potassium values are stable, while amylase diminishes both in concentration and production. These alterations indicate decisive acinar destruction and relative radio resistance in the ductal segments there will never be a return to pre-therapy values. While the effects of radiotherapy are generally described as quantitative, the subjective sensations and experiences are not. Complaints of intense oral dryness and sticky saliva are the rule. A shift in oral flora towards the gram-negative will also be responsible for superficial mucositis and distorted oral perception.

Sodium retention dysfunction syndrome: The normal proportional relationship between salivary flow and sodium concentration is absent in a number of persons. Not only are smaller flow rates measured but also the sodium concentration is relatively low and fluctuates around a steady state of 2.5 mmol/L while most other substances are slightly raised. In some cases, the saliva has a milky appearance. These indications of sodium retention dysfunction syndrome are fairly typical and may be found at all ages, although they are more prevalent in later life. Prominent clinical signs are the sensation of a dry mouth and incidental unilateral painless swelling of the parotid gland for a few hours, e.g. during breakfast with some exceptions, the dysfunction persists through life. Risk factors can be listed in subgroups such as both hyper- and hypotension, cardiac failure, local and systemic edema from other causes, and dehydration. A sudden onset of sodium retention is seen after arteriovenous shunt in hemodialysis. This phenomenon is not related to the time at which dialysis was actually performed. Increased sodium reabsorption may be due to hormonal effects on the sodium/potassium exchange rate or even to elongation of the striated duct. The reduced flow with sodium retention and low bicarbonate values accompanying the sodium retention dysfunction syndrome may have a profound impact in the oral environment. This kind of gland dysfunction is, in fact, a common

finding in periodontal disease, superficial glossitis, glossodynia, and taste disorders.

Sialadenosis: Painless, bilateral non-inflammatory swelling of the major glands particularly the parotid is called sialadenosis. Though this condition is seen in various disorders, namely nutritional and metabolic defects, obesity, starvation, alcoholism, diabetes mellitus, heavy metal intoxication and the like, no characteristic pattern is seen sialochemistry. Increased salivary flow rate may be present due to pressure effects. Low amylase concentration reflects the failure of exhausted acinar cells.

Drugs: Most anticholinergics, including the majority of antihistaminics, tricyclic anti-depressants, and anti-Parkinson's drugs, suppress the pulse frequency of the salivatory nucleus. Apart from age dependent changes during prolonged drug administration, these effects are reversible. In sialochemistry, the stimulated saliva values in this group come very close to those of the resting saliva. There is a small risk of obstructive edematous swelling of the parotid gland on waking up, probably due to adhesion of the duct orifice lining. Accelerated flows are seen after administration of cholinergics, with sodium and bicarbonate concentrations corresponding to the flow rates. The output and concentration of total protein amylase and calcium are increased while potassium is diminished. The immunosuppressive, myelo-suppressive and cytotoxic effects of chemo-therapeutic agents profoundly influence salivary gland function. Reduced flow rate and inflammatory changes dominate in sialochemistry.

Digitalis and the other cardiac glycosides produce their effect on the heart by altering the activity of the sodium/potassium pump and by mobilizing cell calcium. The margin for safe usage of digitalis is small, and toxic effects are seen with even slight over dosage. The drug causes an increase in salivary concentrations of potassium and calcium. Over dosage rapidly produces a noticeable change in these concentrations.

There are two recent applications of salivary analysis. The first of these relates to thiocyanate ions. Maliszewski and Bass (1955) postulated that thiocyanate concentrations are higher in the saliva of smokers than in that of non-smokers. This observation has proved to be of value in the confirmation or rejection of self-reports of cigarette usage among children and adolescents. Gillies et al (1982) found that exposure to cigarette smoke, the so-called passive smoking, could raise salivary thiocyanate levels so that children from homes where heavy smoking occurred might have elevated thiocyanate levels without necessarily themselves being smokers. Nicotine-containing chewing gums, on the other hand, do not change salivary thiocyanate levels. The other ion, which has been the subject of much interest, is nitrate. Salivary nitrate levels parallel blood nitrate levels, which in turn are directly related to nitrate intake. Nitrate in saliva is important in that the ion is converted by oral bacteria into nitrite (Goaz and Biswell 1961) and nitrite has been shown to be converted to nitrosamines in the stomach. High levels of nitrate in the saliva might be associated with carcinoma of the digestive tract, and there is evidence of increased incidence of gastric and hepatic carcinoma with high nitrate intakes and high salivary concentrations of nitrate. Hence saliva can certainly be used as an index of nitrate intake, and this may be an early warning of the possibility of cancer of the digestive tract.

Saliva and Hepatitis

Hepatitis is one of the common infectious diseases affecting the world population. The major means of transmission include blood, saliva and body fluids. A virus that belongs to the picornaviridae family, genus Hepatovirus, causes it.

The term viral hepatitis refers to a primary infection of the liver that may be caused by hepatitis A virus or hepatitis B virus (HAV, HBV). Other viruses that have been associated with hepatitis include Herpes simplex, Varicella Zoster, Cytomegalovirus, Rubella, and coxsackie viruses. Patients who have the following history may also be suspected for the virus. Leukemia, blood transfusions, immunosuppression, organ transplantation, renal dialysis, Down's syndrome, drug addicts, homosexuals, and tattooing/body piercing.

HAV and HBV are distinct both clinically and immunologically. HAV have an incubation period of 15 to 40 days, whereas HBV has a much longer incubation period of 60 to 160 days. HAV is often called as infection hepatitis because it is more commonly transmitted by oral intestinal route. HBV is thought to be transmitted via parenteral means from infected blood. It can be also contracted by infected saliva.

Currently, viral antigens and antibodies against hepatitis are detected by traditional serological and molecular tests such as enzyme immunoassay and polymerase chain reaction. In comparison with the venepuncture, the collection of oral fluids is non-invasive, painless, economical and safe from needle prick injuries. Large samples can be collected easily for epidemiological and prevalence studies. (Parry et al, 1989). The collection of oral fluids introduces an effective means for population surveillance, monitoring and screening. Serum testing can then be used for confirmation of positive results obtained from saliva.

Various studies (Archibald et al 1986, Parry et al 1989, Thieme et al 1992, Laufer et al 1995, De cock et al 2004) proved that oral fluid test has sensitivity accounting to 90.7% and 100% specificity. Nevertheless, the serum test remains more accurate with a sensitivity of 95% and a specificity of 100%. Saliva can be a good alternative for serum, in study groups such as small children, intravenous drug users, and obese persons who are difficult to bleed.

SALIVARY GLAND IMAGING

The choice of which imaging modality one should use to investigate a patient with major salivary gland disease, has changed over the recent years from one that primarily relied on plain films and sailograms to one that relies on computed tomography (CT), magnetic resonance imaging (MRI), and ultrasound. There is still some confusion regarding which modality should be the first choice in certain clinical situations.

However, the choice can also be influenced by user preference and familiarity with a specific modality, as well as the clinical presentation of the patient.

If the patient's history is one of an acute, painful, primarily diffuse swelling of the parotid or the submandibular gland, the primary clinical diagnostic consideration is that of an inflammatory process. Similarly, recurrent subacute episodes of mildly painful and tender parotid or submandibular swelling usually indicates an inflammatory related process, either infectious or noninfectious. Such inflammatory disease is usually initially best studied by either ultrasound or CT.

If the clinical finding is of a mass, whether it is slightly tender or non-tender, solitary or multiple, discrete or diffuse, the initial imaging evaluation is usually by MRI. However CT can be an acceptable alternative to MRI, while ultrasound may be utilized as a complementary study.

In children and adolescents, it has been suggested that ultrasound be used for inflammatory and superficially located disease, while MRI is utilized for more deeply positioned masses.

If a minor salivary gland tumor is clinically suspected, either MRI or CT performed as the examination of choice. For major salivary glands use of intravenous contrast agent with CT is well established and such contrast should be used whenever possible to improve tumor conspicuity.

Plain Films

Plain films are used almost exclusively as a survey examination to detect gross pathoses. It can be obtained quickly and relatively is inexpensive, but are of limited clinical value. It is considered as a fundamental part of the examination of the salivary gland and may provide sufficient information to preclude the use of more sophisticated imaging techniques. It has the potential to identify unrelated pathoses in the areas of the salivary gland that may be mistakenly identified as salivary gland disease, such as resorptive or osteoblastic changes in adjacent bone causing preauricular swelling mimicking a parotid tumor. By using panoramic and conventional posteroanterior (PA) radiographs one can demonstrate bony lesions

Table 9.2: Common radiographic projection for the parotid and submandibular gland

Salivary gland	Radiographic projections
Parotid	Dental panoramic tomograph
	Oblique lateral
	Rotated PA or AP
	Intraoral view of the cheek
Submandibular	Dental panoramic tomograph
	Oblique lateral
	Lower 90 occlusal (to show the duct)
	Lower oblique occlusal (to show the duct)
	Lateral skull with the tongue depressed

in the area, thus eliminating salivary pathoses from the differential diagnosis. Unilateral or bilateral, functional or congenital hypertrophy of the masseter may clinically mimic a salivary tumor. A plain film extraoral radiograph may demonstrate a deep antegonial notch, overdeveloped mandibular angle, and exostosis on the outer surface of the angle in cases of masseter hypertrophy.

Plain film radiographs are most useful when the clinical impression suggests the presence of sialoliths. Such an examination should include both intraoral and extraoral images to demonstrate the entire region of the gland, since sialoliths may be present at different locations (Table 9.2).

Intraoral Radiography

This investigative modality is usually employed to visualize calculi in the parotid and submandibular glands. Sialoliths in the anterior two thirds of the submandibular duct are typically imaged with a mandibular occlusal projection (Figs 9.1A to C). The posterior part of the duct is demonstrated with a posterior oblique view, wherein the head of the patient is tilted back and maximally inclined toward the unaffected side. The central ray is directed parallel with the mandible in the area of the submandibular fossa and into the posterior part of the floor of the mouth.

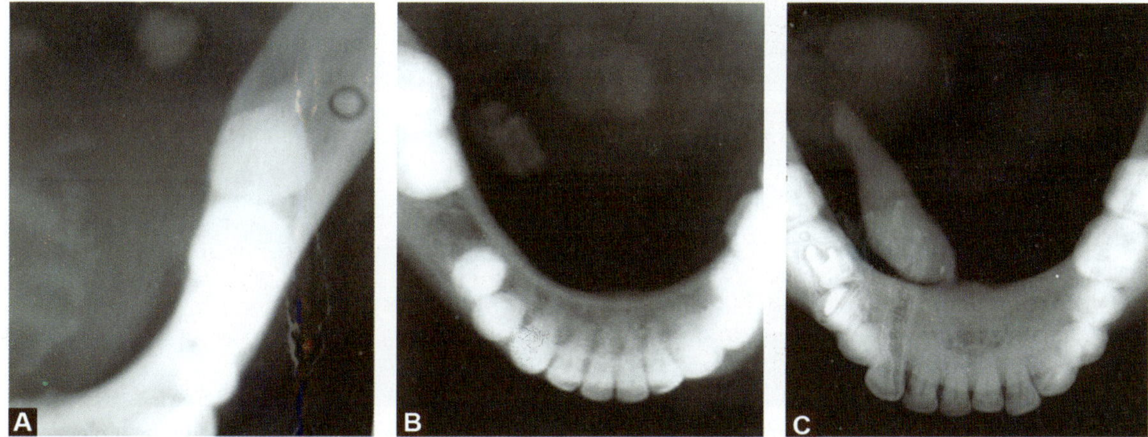

Figures 9.1A to C: Sialolith of submandibular duct: Mandibular occlusal view shows sialolith in the submandibular duct as a radiopaque mass (*Courtesy:* Dr S Karthiga Kannan, Sree Mookambika Institute of Dental Sciences, Kanyakumari District)

Parotid stones are more difficult to demonstrate as a result of the tortuous course of Stensen's duct around the anterior border of the masseter and through the buccinator muscle. Only sialoliths present in the anterior part of the duct, anterior to the masseter muscle, can be imaged on an intraoral film. To demonstrate sialoliths in the anterior part of the duct, an intraoral film is held with a hemostat against the cheek, as high as possible in the buccal sulcus and over the parotid papilla. The central ray is directed perpendicular to the center of the film.

Extraoral Radiography

A panoramic projection is used to demonstrate sialolith in the posterior duct or reveals intraglandular sialoliths in the submandibular gland (Fig. 9.2A). The image of most parotid calculi superimposed over the ramus and body of the mandible, making lateral radiographs of limited value. In order to demonstrate sialoliths in the submandibular gland, the lateral projection is modified by opening the mouth, extending the chin, and depressing the tongue with the index finger. This usually moves the image of the sialoliths inferior to the mandibular border, where its image is more apparent (Fig. 9.2B).

Sialoliths in the distal portion of the parotid gland are usually difficult to demonstrate by intraoral or lateral extraoral views. A PA projection with the cheeks puffed out may move the image of the sialoliths free of the bone, rendering it visible on the projected image (Fig. 9.3). This technique may also demonstrate intraglandular sialoliths. Less mineralized sialoliths may also be obscured by heavy soft tissue shadows in the PA view.

Sialography

First performed by Carpy in 1902, it was described as a diagnostic tool by Barsony and Uslenghi in 1925. Sialography is an imaging examination that uses positive contrast media to radiographically demonstrate the ductal anatomy of either the parotid gland or submandibular gland. Since the minor salivary glands cannot be cannulated and the sublingual gland duct rarely can be cannulated, the sublingual and minor salivary glands are not studied by this technique.

Sialography remains the only imaging modality for examining the fine anatomy of the salivary

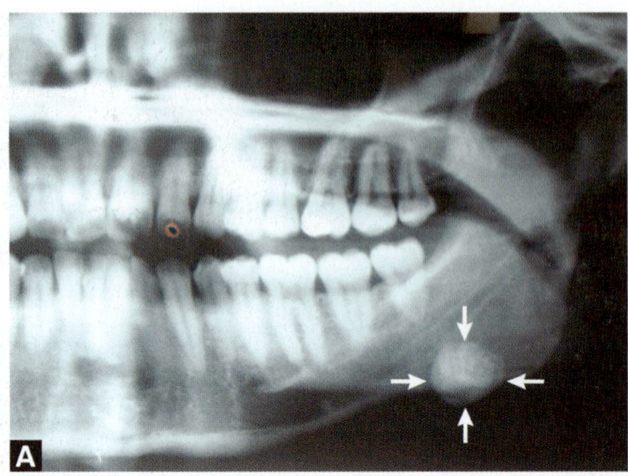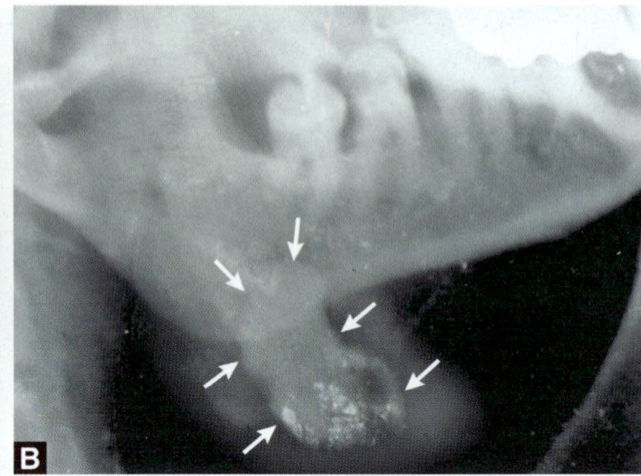

Figures 9.2A and B: Sialolith of submandibular duct: (A) Panoramic radiograph; (B) Lateral oblique projection (*Courtesy to:* Dr S Karthiga Kannan, Sree Mookambika Institute of Dental sciences, Kanyakumari District)

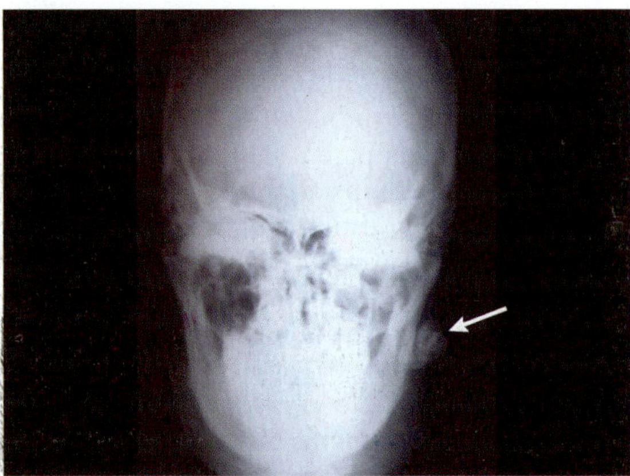

Figure 9.3: Sialolith of parotid duct

gland ductal system. On CT and MRI, only gross pathologic ductal detail can be imaged, and small to moderate degrees of functional anatomic alteration cannot be identified. Thus in clinical situations that require such analysis of ductal morphology sialography is the examination of choice.

Differentiating between certain cases of subacute and chronic sialadenitis, autoimmune related disease, and sialosis often relied on the sialographic finding, which are distinctive for each of these diseases.

Sialography is an invasive procedure in which radiopaque contrast material is injected into the gland's ductal system through the intraoral opening of Wharton's or Stensen's duct. If the patient has a clinically active infection, the procedure is contraindicated because the injection drives the infection back into the gland. In addition, because of the pain present with an acute sialadenitis, the patient will not tolerate the retrograde pressure injection required to perform a sialogram, and a technically adequate study is not possible.

If the patient has had a recent acute sialadenitis, although the gland may have returned to an apparently normal clinical state, when a follow-up sialogram is performed, this examination can reactivate a clinically quiescent infection. In such cases antibiotic administration immediately after the study, is advised to avoid a reinfection. The other major deterrent to performing a sialogram is history of allergic sensitivity to contrast materials.

Indications

- The detection or confirmation of small parotid or submandibular gland sialoliths or foreign bodies.

- The evaluation of the extent of irreversible ductal damage present as a result of infection.
- The differentiation of disease such as chronic sialadenitis, Sjögren's syndrome, and sialosis.
- The evaluation of fistulae, stricture, diverticula, communicating cysts and ductal trauma.
- Rarely, as a dilating procedure for mild ductal stenosis.

Contrast Media

The original sialographic contrast agents used were fat-soluble materials because they were viscid, had high iodine concentration, and produced sharp boundaries with the salivary secretion. There were instances of salivary parenchymal foreign body reaction due to perforation of the ductal system with agent such as Lipiodol or Pantopaque. When water-soluble agents became available, they did not initially have high iodine content. They were too watery to remain within the ductal system long enough to produce a good study, and their boundary with saliva was unsharp. When Ethiodol was clinically introduced, it became the agent of choice because it had all of the benefits of the fat-soluble material and a very low reported incidence of foreign body reactions.

Over the recent years, the water-soluble agents have improved, but in general they remain less viscid and more miscible with saliva than the fat-soluble agent. Water-soluble Sinografin has an iodine content of 38% to Ethiodol with 37% and a workable viscosity that makes injection easy, while not being so watery that it rapidly empties from the main ductal system. In addition, there is no reported incidence of any foreign body reaction subsequent to perforation. If radiographs are taken, before admixture of Sinografin and saliva occurs, the study demonstrates clear and sharp ductal anatomy, equivalent to that seen on an Ethiodol study. Therefore water-soluble agents such as Sinografin have replaced the fat-soluble agents.

Armamentarium

- Sialographic cannulas: The most commonly used are the Rabinov-type cannulas with tips ranging form 0.012 to 0.033. Variations such as the Manashil modifications of the Rabinov cannulas designed by Lowman and Belleza are also commercially available. Modifications of butterfly needles also can be used for parotid cannulation. The larger diameter cannulas are used for the parotid gland, the smaller ones for the submandibular gland. A polyethylene connecting tube is used, which allows the examiner to work outside of the patient's mouth and therefore has greater mobility during the procedure.
- A set of Lacrimal dilators ranging from 0000 through 0 caliber.
- 5 or 10 ml syringes.
- 4 x 4 inch gauze sponge pads.
- Sinografin (or equivalent contrast agent).
- Secretogogue such as fresh lemon, lemon extract, or lemon concentrate.
- Adequate lighting.
- High-powered magnifying glass.

Once the salivary duct is cannulated, the injection is usually made with hand pressure. The patient may complain of local pressure or mild pain during the injection; a slow, constant injection technique usually can accomplish complete ductal filling without much patient discomfort. This is best done when monitored by fluoroscopy. The patient sensation of glandular fullness and pressure usually abates within minutes after the study. The patient should be informed that there should be no residual discomfort by 24 hours after the procedure. If local pain increases and becomes more intense 24 to 36 hours after the examination, a post sialogram infection is present and antibiotic therapy should be started immediately. This will avoid or reduce the severity of an iatrogenic acute sialadenitis and abscess formation.

Parotid Gland Study (Fig. 9.4)

The intraoral opening of Stensen's duct is opposite the second upper molar tooth. In some patients this opening is clinically seen; however in others it may be very difficult to identify, especially in individual who have a dry, obstructed gland or a mucosal bite ridge across the region. After drying the mucosa with gauze, milking of the gland and Stensen's duct may produce a drop of saliva that allows identification of the duct opening. The use of a secretogogue (lemon) may be of help in identification. Once the opening is identified, the dilators can be used to widen the opening for easier cannula placement. Slight abduction of the cheek with the thumb and index finger provides a better exposure and angulation for cannula insertion. The cannula is then gently inserted, and 0.5 to 1.5 ml of contrast material is slowly injected. The injection is best monitored under fluoroscopy so that optimum ductal filling and gland positioning can be achieved. Spot-filming can be performed to document the procedure. Stensen's duct is approximately 6 cm long and has a small C - shaped curve anteriorly as it bends around the buccal fat pad and pierces the buccinator muscle to open opposite the second upper molar tooth. The duct's normal luminal caliber. The duct usually lies within 15 to 18 mm of the lateral mandibular cortex. If the duct is more laterally placed, there is either hypertrophy of the masseter muscle or there is a space occupying mass in or near the masseter muscle. There is no specific parotid ductal branching pattern, and variation is noted from right side to left side within the same person as well as among different individuals. There are main upper and lower hilar – intraglandular ducts, and it is from these that the glandular arborization pattern takes form. The overall appearance is that of a leafless tree. As the ducts arch behind the ramus of the mandible, they may appear slightly stretched on frontal films. This appearance should not be misinterpreted for a mass/lesion; on lateral films, no mass effect will be seen. Physiologically, the ducts do not lie parallel to one another in any plane. If this is evident, it usually indicates the presence of a mass displacing some of the ducts away from their normal arborization configuration and causing them to appear parallel to one another.

Acinar filling can be accomplished with a normal effect of slight overfilling of the ductal system. It can be a useful technique to help identify small masses; however, the acinar filling should be carefully limited so that it does not obscure the ductal anatomy.

Following sialography, the evacuation film should reveal complete and rapid ductal emptying. A complete evacuation can be achieved if a secretogogue is given. Any delayed ductal emptying or trapping of the contrast material indicates the presence of a functional obstruction.

Multiple or solitary accessory parotid glands may be present and are usually situated above Stensen's duct, anterior to the main parotid gland with a normal branching ductal pattern. These accessory glands are routinely filled in a retrograde manner as the contrast material courses through Stensen's duct.

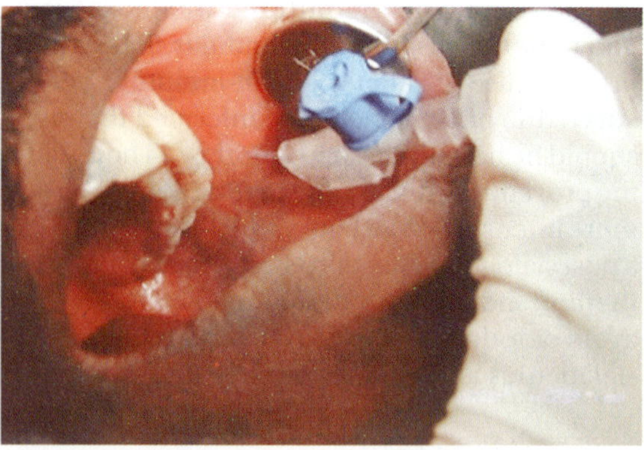

Figure 9.4: Cannulation of parotid duct (*Courtesy:* Dr S Karthiga Kannan, Sree Mookambika Institute of Dental Sciences, Kanyakumari District

Submandibular Gland Study

The orifice of Wharton's duct lies in the floor of the mouth on or near the sublingual papilla. The opening is smaller than that of Stensen's duct, and thus it is usually more difficult to cannulate.

To visualize the orifice of Wharton's duct, the area should be dried with gauze and the tongue pushed upward and backward to put some tension on the papilla. Milking of the gland or using a secretogogue can aid in identifying the orifice by producing a drop of saliva. Once the duct is cannulated, care must be taken to gently advance the cannula, because painless perforation into the floor of the mouth can occur. Only 0.2 to 0.5 ml of contrast material should be injected. The volume injected only reflects the fact that the submandibular gland is smaller than the parotid gland, and the ductal walls of the submandibular gland are more easily perforated than are those of the parotid gland. If extensive perforation should occur as a result of the administration of too much contrast material, ductal detail can be completely obscured on the sialographic study, rendering the examination non diagnostic.

Wharton's duct is seen to run downward and laterally at about a 45° angle to both the sagittal and horizontal planes. It is about 5 cm long and has a luminal caliber of 1 to 3 mm. Just before the duct enters the submandibular gland, it may curve caudally over the back of the mylohyoid muscle. The intraglandular ducts are short and taper more abruptly than those in the parotid gland.

Occasionally, Bartholin's duct will be filled, extending from Wharton's duct. In some cases the sublingual gland may be visualized.

Systematic Approach for Viewing Sialographs

1. Assess the degree of filling of the duct structure
2. Assess the main duct:
   - Diameter of the duct
   - Course and direction of the duct
   - Presence and position of any filling defects
3. Assess the duct structure within the gland:
   - The branching and gradual tapering of the minor ducts towards the periphery of the gland
   - Overall pattern and shape of the ducts
   - Degree of overall glandular filling
   - Presence and position of any filling defects
4. Assess the degree of emptying

Sialographic Appearance of Normal Salivary Gland

Parotid Gland

- The main duct has an even diameter of 1–2 mm width.
- The duct structure within the gland branches regularly and tapers gradually towards the periphery of the gland, the so—called ***tree in winter*** appearance.

Submandibular Gland

- The main duct has a even diameter of 3–4 mm width
- Smaller than the parotid, the overall appearance is similar with the branching duct structure tapering gradually towards the periphery—the so—called ***bush in winter*** appearance

Sialographic Appearance in Salivary Gland Diseases

Calculi

- Filling defect(s) in the main duct
- Ductal dilatation caused by associated sialodochitis
- The emptying film usually shows contrast medium retained behind the stone.

Sialodochitis

- Segmented sacculation or dilatation and stricture of the main duct, called ***sausage link appearance***.
- Associated with calculi or ductal stenosis
- Sialographic appearance of sialadenitis: Dots or blobs of contrast medium within the gland, an appearance known as sialectasis caused by the inflammation of the glandular tissue producing saccular dilatation of the acini.

Sjögren's Syndrome

- Widespread dots or blobs of contrast medium within the gland, an appearance known as ***Punctate sialectasis*** or ***snowstorm***. This is caused by weakening of the epithelial lining of the intercalated ducts, allowing the escape of the contrast medium out of the ducts
- Considerable retention of the contrast medium during the emptying phase

Intrinsic Tumors

- An area of under filling within the gland, due to ductal compression by the tumor

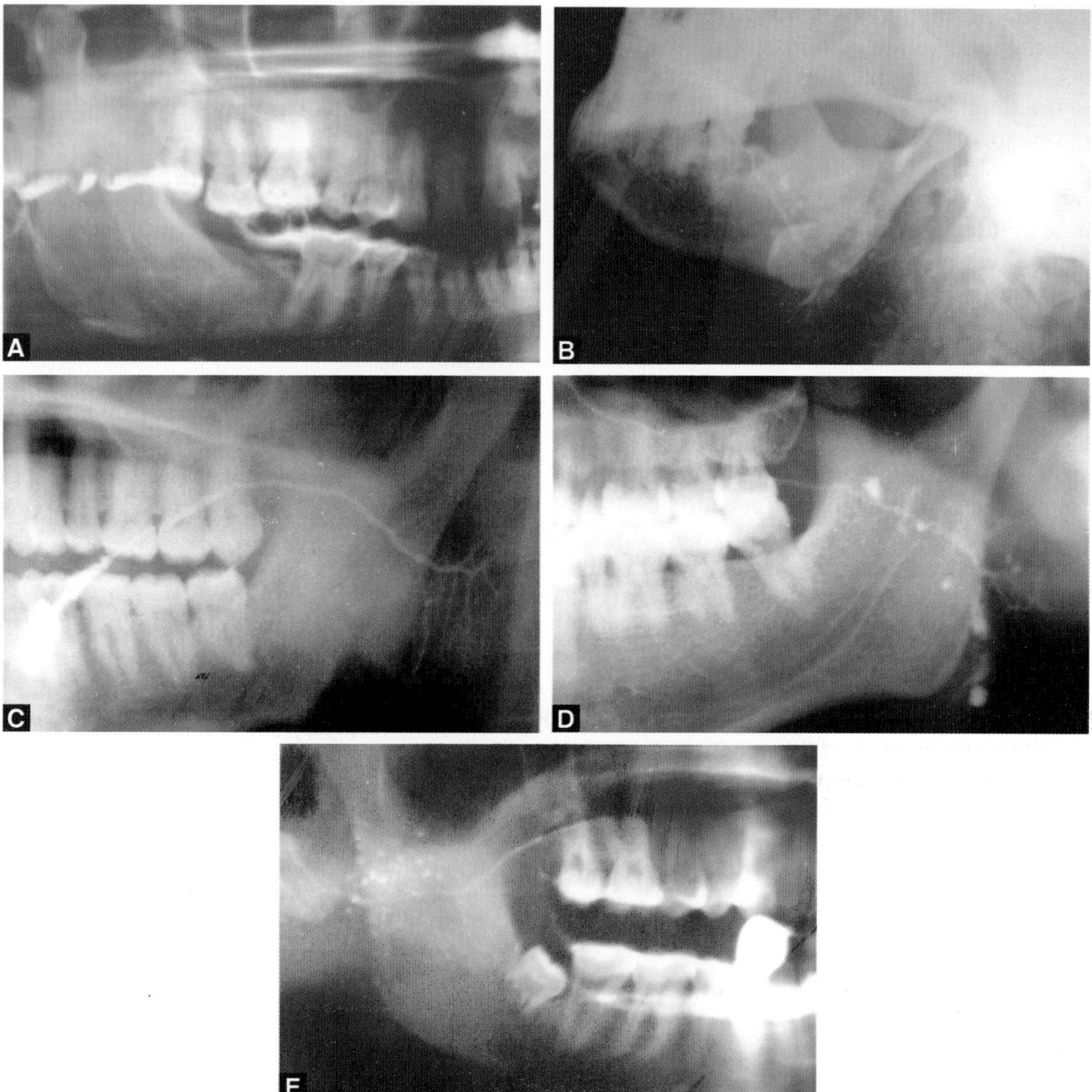

Figures 9.5A to E: Sialographs of various salivary gland lesions (*Courtesy:* Dr S Karthiga Kannan, Sree Mookambika Institute of Dental Sciences, Kanyakumari District

- Ductal displacement—the duct adjacent to the tumors are usually stretched around it, an appearance known as ***ball in hand***
- Retention of contrast medium in the displaced ducts during the emptying phase (Figs 9.5A to E).

Digital Subtraction Sialography

This is a variant of conventional sialography reported by Gullotta and Schekatz, and Lightfoote, et al.

Table 9.3: Advantages and disadvantages of oil and aqueous based contrast agents

Contrast medium	Advantages	Disadvantages
Oil based	• Densely radiopaque, thus has good contrast • High viscosity, thus slows excretion from the gland	• Extravasated contrast may remain in the soft tissues for many months, and may produce a foreign body reaction • High viscosity means considerable pressure needed to introduce the contrast, calculi may be forced down the main duct
Aqueous	• Low viscosity, thus easily introduced, easily and rapidly removed from the gland • Easily absorbed and excreted if extravasated	• Less radiopaque, thus has reduced contrast • Excretion from the gland is very rapid unless used in a closed system

Advantages and disadvantages of oil and aqueous based contrast agents shown in Table 9.3.

Advantages

- Minimal amount of contrast medium required because of digital enhancement and lack of overlapping skeletal structure.
- Precise delineation of the size of the gland
- Accessory glands are recognized.
- Fine changes of the intraglandular ducts can be better appreciated.
- Post processing with variable mask setting as well as manipulation of window level and window width offer the best possible images.

Disadvantages

- Patients must keep their head absolutely motionless, hold their breath and not swallow during the exposure.
- A repeated injection of contrast is required for each additional view unless using a continuous infusion technique.

Summary of Sialography

Indications

- Sialoliths: Radiopaque/ Radiolucent
- Duct strictures and diverticula
- Chronic inflammation
- Autoimmune disorders like Sjögren's syndrome

- Space filling tumors within or adjacent to the gland
- To identify inflammatory and fibrotic changes following chemotherapy and radiograph

Contraindications

- Acute inflammation
- Allergy to Iodine
- Known case of tumors of salivary gland
- Improper equipment

Advantages

- High resolution of duct system
- Controlled and localized radiation dose
- Information on appearance of specific disease states that is already present

Disadvantages

- Parenchymal changes are not obtained. It has to be inferred by observing the changes in ductal morphology and function.
- Medical contraindications
- Pain on injection
- Extravasation into adjacent tissues causing irritation or possible necrosis.

Failure

- Restricted mouth opening
- Failure to locate and cannulate the salivary duct
- Perforation of the duct either into the cheek or the floor of the mouth
- Suboptimum filling of the ductal system so that areas of the gland are not visualized
- Complete acinarization of the gland so that all ductal detail is obscured.

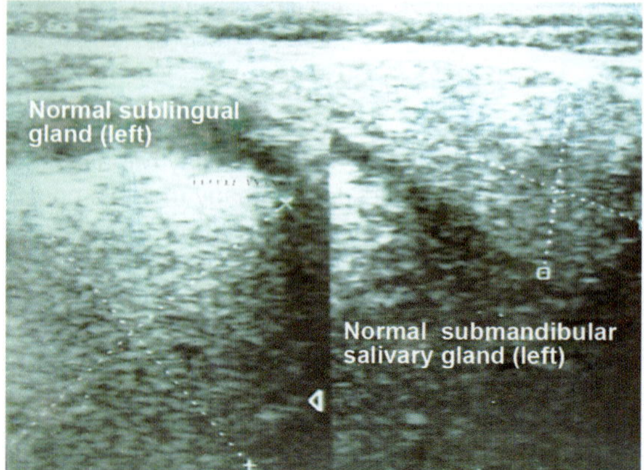

Figure 9.6: Ultrasonography of normal submandibular and sublingual salivary glands, seen as homogeneous echogenicity (*Courtesy:* Dr S Karthiga Kannan, Sree Mookambika Institute of Dental Sciences, Kanyakumari District)

ULTRASONOGRAPHY

Due to their superficial locations, the parotid and submandibular glands are easily visualized by ultrasonography although the deep portion of the parotid gland is difficult to visualize because the mandibular ramus lies over the deep lobe (Fig. 9.6). This modality is best at differentiating between intra- and extra-glandular masses as well as between cystic and solid lesions. In general, solid benign lesions present as well circumscribed hypoechoic intraglandular masses. It can also demonstrate the presence of an abscess in an acutely inflamed gland, as well as the presence of sialoliths, which appear as echogenic densities that exhibit acoustic shadowing. Studies conducted in a group of patients with Sjögren's syndrome have reported the appearance of parenchymal inhomogeneity. The diagnosis of multiple parotid cysts in HIV positive patients can also be made by ultrasound. Optimal ultrasound requires appropriate equipment with high resolution small parts transducers. Ultrasound sequences between 5 and 20 MHz are used (most commonly 7.5–10 MHz). This allows an axial resolution of 0.5 mm or less and a lateral resolution of 1 mm or less. The spatial resolution

improves when high frequencies (15–20 MHz) are used, which provide nearly microscopic resolution of small areas. Ultrasound, because of its low cost, lack of ionizing radiation and avoidance of the use of contrast, has a definite place in the investigation of salivary gland disorders.

Acute and Chronic Sialadenitis

Acute bacterial sialadenitis occurs predominantly in elderly and debilitated patients. The salivary glands can also be involved in viral infections, including epidemic parotitis. In about 50% of cases with stones there is associated sialadenitis. In acute or chronic sialadenitis sonography demonstrates inhomogeneous hypoechogenicity of the glandular parenchyma. In acute inflammation hypoechogenicity is often more dominant than in chronic inflammation. Sonographic findings occur in 18 of patients with chronic recurrent inflammation. These consist of inhomogeneous, patchy changes with ductal ectasia in the parenchyma.

Sjögren's Syndrome

In advanced cases of autoimmune disorders, sonography visualizes multiple cystic lesions caused by parenchymal destruction along with dilatation of the intraglandular ducts. The remaining parenchyma is inhomogeneous and hypoechoic. With color Doppler sonography, hypervascularization of the gland parenchyma can be demonstrated in 50% of patients. Increased vascularization of the involved gland correlates with the severity of the parenchymal changes.

Sarcoidosis

The extrapulmonary manifestations of sarcoidosis affect the parotid glands in 1 to 6% of cases and may be associated with uveitis and facial paralysis. Sonography demonstrates well defined, painless enlargement of the parotid glands with few or multiple small hypoechogenic granulomatous nodules, which are diffusely distributed throughout the glands.

Sialolithiasis

Salivary stones cause painful, intermittent swelling and pain during eating. The submandibular gland is the most common site of involvement (83%), followed by the parotid (13%) and, rarely, the sublingual gland (4%). Eighty percent of the stones are calcified and can be detected by conventional radiographs. Sonography has the capability to localize non-opaque stones that cannot be visualized by pain film examination. The accuracy of sonography in sialolithiasis ranges from 80 to 94%, the typical sonographic appearance of a salivary stone reveals an echogenic complex with sound shadowing. Stones smaller than 2 mm in diameter may not show a shadow. Error in diagnosis can occur in case of very small stones in the intraglandular ducts without ductal dilatation. Increasing salivary flow with the administration of a lemon stick, which leads to duct ectasia, demonstrates the stones more clearly.

Sialadenosis

The sonographic examination shows enlarged glands, with homogeneous, echogenic parenchyma excluding enlargement of the glands secondary to tumor or adjoining lymph node enlargement (Figs 9.7A and B) in sialadenosis.

Pleomorphic Adenoma

It is the most frequent tumor of the salivary glands (24–71%). The adenoma is localized in the superficial lobe of the gland in 90% and deep lobe in about 10% of cases. The tumor is composed histologically of epithelial, myoepithelial, and mesenchymal tissues. Because of its mixed and variable composition, the sonographic appearance is also varied. The tumor is well circumscribed and reveals a homogeneous ultrasonic pattern with decreased echogenicity and a smooth or polycystic border. Occasionally, the tumor is hyperechoic and cystic areas or calcifications may be seen (Figs 9.8A and B). Malignant transformation of a pleomorphic adenoma occurs in 1.5 to 4.5%, which is characterized by an irregular border and an inhomogeneous, hypoechoic, or nonechoic imaging pattern.

Cystadenolymphoma (Warthin's Tumor)

It is the most frequent monomorphic adenoma of the salivary glands. It is composed histologically of epithelial and lymphoid components. This tumor represents 2 to 24% of all tumors of the salivary glands. About 90% of Warthin's tumors are located in the superficial lobe of the parotid gland, and in 8 to 30% they occur bilaterally.

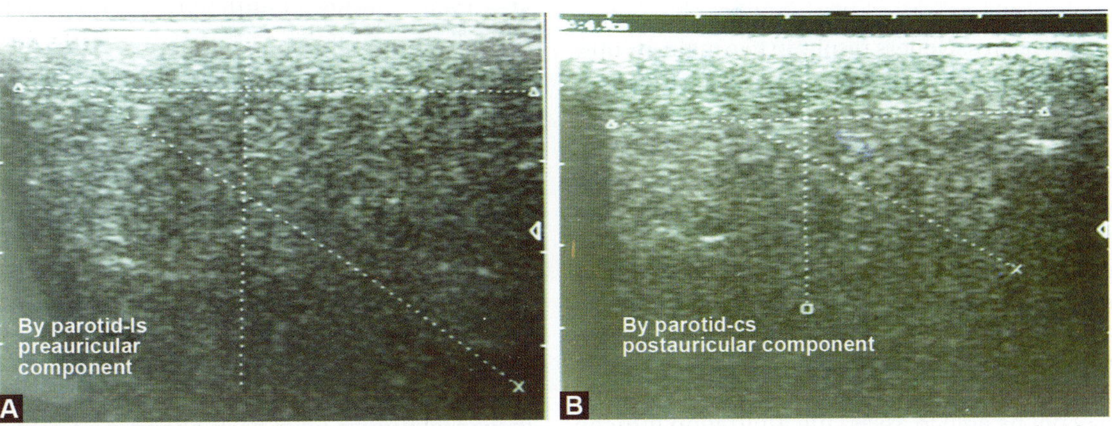

Figures 9.7A and B: Sialadenosis: Ultrasonography of parotid gland shows enlargement of the parotid with homogeneous, echogenic parenchyma

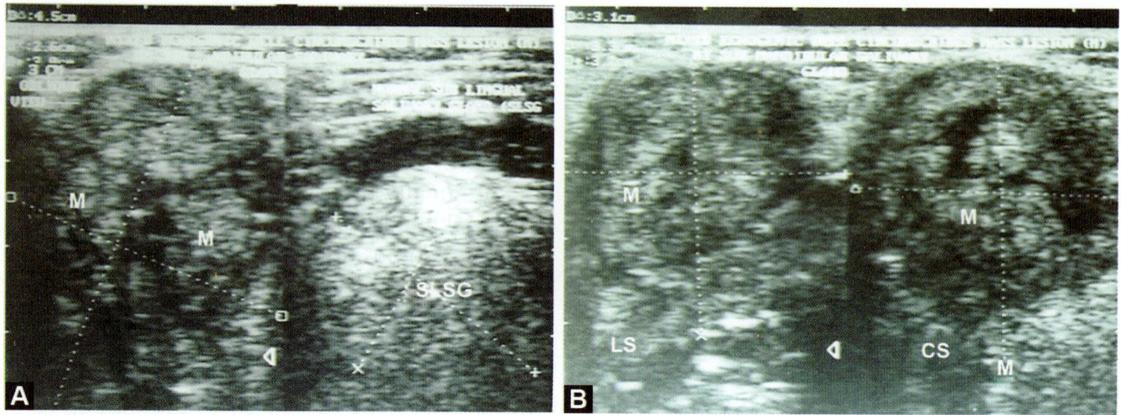

Figures 9.8A and B: Pleomorphic adenoma: Ultrasonography of parotid gland showing well circumscribed, mixed echogenic lobulated mass within the parenchyma of parotid (*Courtesy:* Dr S Karthiga Kannan, Sree Mookambika Institute of Dental Sciences, Kanyakumari District)

Sonographically, the Warthin's tumor has a smooth border, is hypoechogenic, and homogeneous or inhomogeneous with cystic areas with multiple septae. Larger cysts appear nonechoic with posterior acoustic enhancement.

MALIGNANT TUMORS OF THE SALIVARY GLANDS

The most frequent malignant tumors of the salivary glands are mucoepidermoid carcinoma followed by adenoid cystic carcinoma, squamous cell carcinoma, acinic cell tumor, and adenocarcinoma. The histologic differentiation according to their aggressiveness results in two main groups:

1. Tumors with high grade malignancy
2. Tumors with low grade malignancy.

Malignant tumors of small size (less than 2 cm) and tumors of low-grade malignancy usually have a homogeneous sonographic pattern and smooth borders and are assessed incorrectly as benign. Tumors of high grade malignancy and larger than 2 cm in diameter show mostly irregular border and an internal heterogeneous echo pattern with irregular, fluid filled necrotic areas. If the tumor is very large, sonography may not be able to assess the infiltration into the deeper structures, including the base of skull and mandible. Color Doppler sonography may demonstrate hypervascularity in carcinomas of the salivary glands and reveal multiple irregular vessels within the tumor.

THERMOGRAPHY

This investigative procedure permits the recording of the heat gradients between superficial areas by detecting the infrared radiation emitted through the skin and which can be represented on a video screen (Dynamic telethermography). It has also been combined with Tc – pertechnetate scanning to give thermoscintigraphy. Using these techniques it has been reported that inflammatory processes in the parotid are demonstrable as either hot or cold areas depending on the chronicity of the lesion. Acute inflammatory processes showing up as hyperthermia and in some cases chronic inflammation results in the functional death of the parotid gland, which appears on the thermogram as a hypothermal area. Benign masses can be demonstrated as either hyperthermic or hypothermic areas, while malignant lesions are characterized by hyperthermal values. At present, these techniques have been abandoned as they lack sensitivity and specificity.

COMPUTED TOMOGRAPHY

This modality is useful in evaluating structures in and adjacent to salivary gland and can distinguish both soft and hard tissues as well as minute differences in soft tissue densities. Glandular tissues can be differentiated from surrounding fat and muscle. Parotid glands are more radiopaque than the surrounding fat and less opaque than adjacent muscles. The submandibular and sublingual glands have a similar density to that of the adjacent muscles and can be identified on the basis of shape and location.

Indications

- Identification of tumors within or adjacent to the glands.
- Specific identification of tumors of adipose tissue (lipoma and liposarcoma) and vasculature (hemangioma).
- Identification cysts, abscess, diffuse inflammation, necrosis, and hematoma.
- Demonstration of abnormal glands with diffuse inflammatory reaction due to sialadenitis, radiation fibrosis.
- Deciding between the various therapeutic modalities in complicated cases.
- Planning the most effective radiotherapy portal.
- Following patients to determine effectiveness of radiotherapy and chemotherapy.
- Demonstrating recurrent disease.

Advantages

- Completely eliminates superimposition of images of structures superficial or deep to the area of interest.
- Differentiates tissues that differ in physical density by less than 1%.
- Data from a single imaging procedure consists of images in axial, coronal and axial planes. This is referred to as Multiplanar Reformatted Imaging.

Computed tomography (CT) has been used in an attempt to assess whether a lesion is benign or malignant. Benign lesions characteristically appear as discrete, sharply marginated, high density masses embedded in an otherwise normal gland. Malignant lesions usually present as poorly defined, relatively dense lesions, which obliterate and/or transgress adjacent fat and facial planes. However, this distinction is not completely reliable and malignant lesions may have a benign radiographic appearance.

The CT has been used to determine the relationship of a tumor to the facial nerve, which could be of particular surgical importance. Tumors that lie superficial to the nerve are usually treated by superficial parotidectomy. A deep lesion, a superficial parotidectomy is performed first, the facial nerve is retracted and then the deep lobe is removed. The course of the facial nerve has been described in terms of its relationship to the adjacent anatomical structures such as posterior belly of digastric, the sternomastoid muscle, the styloid process, the lateral border of mandible and the retromandibular vein. However, the variability of these landmarks was difficult in their visualization at different levels to examine the relationship between the facial nerve and parotid gland. It is suggested that the plane of the facial nerve can be reliably represented on a CT by measuring an arc of radius 8.5 mm centered on the most posterior point of the ramus of the mandibular angle.

Previous evaluation of a mass in or around the major salivary glands was limited to plain films and sialography, prior to the introduction of this modality. These earlier methods relied on secondary changes such as bone erosion or ductal displacement to suggest the presence of a mass.

Sialography has limited value for detecting masses less than 2 cm especially when they are superficially located, and this is where CT offers a considerable advantage. Even today conventional sialography is still the method of choice for a clinically suspected inflammatory disease. In all other cases of salivary gland enlargement, CT with or without sialography has emerged as the preferred radiological examination. The main drawback of CT is its high cost and availability when compared to sialography. The first detailed report of CT with sialography was done in 1978 and still considerable debate about its value exists. Initial reports suggested there was the significant advantage with the combined use leading to a decreased false negative rate for tumor detection. Some workers have expressed the need of intravenous contrast to perform a CT – sialography.

Computed tomography (CT) images of salivary glands should be obtained by using continuous fine cuts through the involved gland. Axial plane cuts should include the superior aspect of the gland, continuing till the hyoid bone. Non-enhanced and enhanced CT images are the routinely followed imaging protocol. The non-enhanced images are used for viewing the presence of salivary calculi, masses, glandular enlargements and nodular involvement. Glandular damage can cause alteration in the density of the salivary gland. Contrast enhanced images are used to view tumors, abscesses and inflamed lymph nodes as they have abnormal enhancement.

Ultrafast CT has been reported to be an effective method for visualizing masses that are poorly defined on MRI. It is also advocated for patients who are unable to tolerate the long imaging sequence on MRI (pediatric, geriatric, mentally or physically challenged and claustrophobic patients). CT has the ability to detect calcium deposits with ten-fold sensitivity over plain films. Thus in elusive clinical cases in which a small calculus is suspected, a thin section (1.5–3 mm contiguous scans) non-contrast CT scans may be used to localize the calculus.

In general, CT is the modality of choice to image a patient with a history suggestive of inflammatory disease and has reported over all sensitivity that approaches 100%.

MAGNETIC RESONANCE IMAGING

Magnetic resonance imaging (MRI) offers another relatively a new method of imaging of major salivary glands. It has become the modality of choice for pre-operative evaluation because of its ability to differentiate soft tissue. It provides images of salivary gland pathology, adjacent structures and proximity of the facial nerve. In T1 - weighted images, the normal parotid gland has higher intensity than muscle, lower intensity than fat or subcutaneous tissue. In T2-weighted images, the parotid has greater intensity than the adjacent muscle and a lower intensity than fat. The use of intravenous contrast agents can improve imaging and aid in better identification of neoplastic process.

MRI offers the advantage of being able to obtain section in any anatomical plane, which is of benefit in determining the relationship of pathology to the great vessels of the neck. The facial nerve can be visualized on T1-weighted sequence as an intermediate signal linear structure surrounded by a high fat signal. On further sectioning, the fat begins to disappear and facial nerve can be visualized as a slightly lower signal than the surrounding parotid tissue, which appears bright.

Recent development in the field of MRI contrast agents has been the introduction of intravenous agent such as Gadolinium Diethylene Triamine Pent Acetic Acid (DTPA). This agent acts paramagnetically having a magnetic moment 1000 times greater than the hydrogen nucleus and has been successfully used to give better delineation in soft tissue tumor.

Advantages of MRI

- No ionizing radiation
- Fewer artifacts from dense bone and metal clips
- Imaging possible in several planes without moving the patient.
- Superior anatomic details of soft tissue.

Disadvantages of MRI

- High initial cost of the scanner
- Special site for installation
- Patient claustrophobia in magnet Inferior images of bone.

Absolute Contraindications to MRI

- Patients with aneurysm clips
- Patients with cardiac pace makers

Relative Contraindications to MRI
- Ferro-magnetic foreign bodies in critical location (Eyes)
- Metallic prosthetic heart valves
- Claustrophobic (or) Un-cooperative patients. Implanted stimulator wires.

MRI not Contraindicated
- Metallic dental prostheses
- Orthodontic fixed appliances

3D Magnetic Resonance Imaging

3D MR imaging has been proposed as a good investigative tool when describing pathology to clinicians who have difficulty in assimilating serial images to display pathology. The use of MR contrast has been proposed to improve the identification of salivary tumors on such 3D images. As technology advances, the CT and MR data can be incorporated to produce a 3D image, the use of this approach may soon become popular.

Magnetic Resonance Spectroscopy

Magnetic Resonance Spectroscopy (MRS) is recently introduced into clinical practice where it offers a great potential as a research tool for investigation of normal and abnormal tissue metabolic pathways. MRS requires a magnet, which is considerably stronger than the one used for conventional MRI. Studies have shown that 31-phosphorus spectroscopy of salivary malignancy has a significant increase in the concentration of phosphomonoesters, phosphodiesters, and inorganic phosphates when compared to normal patients. This early work may lead the way to more pathologic and diagnostic information in the coming years.

ANGIOGRAPHY

Interventional vascular investigation plays a little role in the diagnosis and management of salivary gland disorders with the rare exception of the embolization of an unusually large vascular lesion.

RADIONUCLIDE SALIVARY STUDIES

Over two decades ago salivary gland scintigraphy was introduced in clinical practice with the use of technetium pertechnetate (^{99}Tc). The advantage of scintigraphy is that the salivary gland dynamics can be visualized and quantified by the uptake and excretion of pertechnetate by the glandular parenchyma. This modality provides valuable information on the functional aspect and, to a lesser extent, the morphology and topographical the status of the glands involved in the disease process.

A variety of radioisotopes have been used in investigation of salivary glands disorders, including Iodine (^{131}I), Technetium (^{99}Tc), Gallium (^{67}Ga), Selenium (^{75}Se), and Indium (^{111}In). Both iodine and technetium share a common transport system in the salivary glands, being transported from the peritubular capillaries, which surround ductal epithelium and across the intratubular duct into the saliva. Gallium citrate has also been used in the investigation of sarcoidosis, Sjögren's syndrome, inflammatory diseases, postradiation sialadenitis, acute sialadenitis, and salivary gland tumors. Lymphomas that occasionally involved the salivary glands have been investigated with indium and iodine.

This modality has been utilized effectively in the examination of salivary gland aplasia. Sequential images of the salivary gland are obtained following administration of the agent, which demonstrate distinct physiological faces of vascularity, concentration, secretion, and drainage of the isotope.

Scintigraphy is an adjunctive, non-invasive technique to demonstrate a tumor mass and occasionally aids in the diagnosis of specific tumor types. It assesses the physiological activity of tumors by demonstrating their ability to concentrate the isotope. About half the lesions are cold when comparing with the surrounding gland and the remainder are equivalent to the surrounding gland or appear hot. This scanning modality does not permit differentiation between benign and malignant tumors, both of which may be vascular. Of particular interest, Wharthin's tumors (adenolymphoma) and oncocytoma with their retained function being demonstrable as a hot spot on the scan. This tumor is able to concentrate the isotope often at a higher level than the parotid tissue. Lesions which are not clinically palpable (less than 1 cm diameter) are not demonstrated on the scan and therefore radionuclide scanning is not useful in search of occult salivary tumors.

Positron Emission Computed Tomography and Single Photon Emission Computed Tomography Scanning

Recent developments in the field of nuclear medicine include the development of Positron Emission Computed Tomography (PET) and Single Photon Emission Computed Tomography (SPECT). PET relies on positron emitting agents like 2-[F-18] Fluoro-2-deoxy-D-glucose generated in a cyclotron. These scans have been utilized extensively in research programs; particularly to examine the resolution of cerebral blood flow. While PET imaging of the brain and perhaps of other parts of the body is capable of providing unique metabolic information, its high cost limits its utilization.

Single photon emission computed tomography (SPECT) can be performed with radio isotopes without the complexity of a cyclotron. Gamma cameras have been used in this technique, which rotate around the patient. It has shown its worthiness in assessing cerebral ischemia and infarction, showing changes and abnormalities much before CT or MRI picks them up. To date, this technology has not been applied to the study of salivary glands but it does offer considerable promise in the near future.

Catheter Dilation and Endoscopy

Sialendoscopy is a new procedure, aiming to visualize the lumen of the salivary duct and their pathologies. The first reported attempts to visualize the ducts were conducted in early 1990s. This technique can be performed in most cases as an ambulatory, out-patient procedure. The most frequent ductal pathology being sialolithiasis, interventional sialendoscopy aims to retrieve salivary stones by fragmentation.

Indications

All salivary glands swellings of unclear origin are indicated for this procedure. Even children and elderly patient can benefit from this technique, which is performed under local anesthesia. Despite its apparent simplicity, interventional sialendoscopy is a technically challenging procedure. Operating the rigid sialendoscope is delicate, requires experience and has the risk of perforation and vascular or neural damage. Iatrogenic perforations can lead to diffuse swellings of the floor of the mouth, with potential risks of life-threatening swelling.

Limitations

The course of the ductal system puts certain limitations on semi-rigid endoscopy, especially in cases of sharply bent curvatures. Also, maneuvering within the small salivary ducts has to be absolutely atraumatic because of possible ductal perforation of yet uncertain consequences. Significant trauma to the ductal wall could result in stenosis.

SALIVARY HORMONE PROFILE

Endocrine hormones are secreted within the glands and from there they move into extracellular spaces, including formed saliva stored in the salivary glands. Once a hormone is bound to its receptor, the transduction of the signal may initiate a wide range of intracellular events including protein synthesis and secretion. Hormones act over a range of distances and many of their functions are integrative and aimed at coordinating the wide variety of functions required to maintain overall good health.

Salivary Hormone Testing

Saliva testing is the most reliable method to measure free bioavailable hormone activity at cellular level. Free steroid hormones passively traverse into the cells in the salivary gland and flow with the fluid that passively accompanies Na+ that is pumped by the sodium/potassium ATPase mechanism. Bound steroids are too large to diffuse freely through the salivary cells into the salivary gland lumen as they have a large molecular weight. Saliva testing can help to identify hormonal imbalances that may be causing chronic health problems. Testing can also be used to monitor the effects of bio-identical/natural hormone replacement therapy.

Benefits of Salivary Hormone Testing

- Determine free, bioavailable hormone levels
- Baseline hormone levels can be assessed and hormone replacement therapy can be monitored and adjusted
- Painless, noninvasive and economical
- Specimens can be sent directly to the laboratory without any special care (storage and handling)
- Multiple saliva samples can be collected on a single day or over a number of weeks
- Salivary hormones are stable at room temperature.

Hormones Tested in Saliva

- Cortisol
- Melatonin
- Progesterone
- Testosterone
- Estradiol (E2)
- DHEA (Androgens in both men and women).

FINE NEEDLE ASPIRATION CYTOLOGY

This is a simple and effective technique that aids the diagnosis of solid/cystic lesions. A syringe is used to aspirate cells from the lesion for cytological examination. Microscopic examination of the individual cells will offer a diagnosis based on the cellular characteristics of different lesions. It may also suggest if a lesion is benign or malignant. By knowing the aggressiveness of the tumor, it is helpful for an appropriate surgical management.

SALIVARY GLAND BIOPSY

Definitive diagnosis of a salivary pathology may require a tissue examination. When major salivary gland biopsy is indicated, it usually requires an extraoral approach. In cases of suspected lymphoma, immunophenotyping of the tissue is required for a definite diagnosis. Biopsies of minor salivary glands are performed to diagnose conditions such as Sjögrens syndrome and amyloidosis with limited morbidity using appropriate techniques.

CONCLUSION

Salivary gland investigations can aid the clinician in a wide variety of disorders. Often more than one investigative modalities is utilized in a particular clinical situation. The individual choice of examination will depend upon the availability as well as appropriateness of each investigation in a particular area.

At present, high resolution CT scanning is the method of choice in the investigation of salivary gland neoplasm. In a few conditions, MRI may prove as an alternative. When functional aspect of the salivary gland is under investigation, Scintigraphy appears to offer the most suitable option. Sialography is the method of choice in case of obstructive lesions. Ultrasound has a role in investigating inflamed glands to assess abscess formation and it also provides an economic alternative to specialized radiographic techniques.

MRS, PET and SPECT offers existing prospects for future research in both normal and abnormal salivary glands study. Giant leaps have been made in investigative modalities during the recent years and it remains for these to be applied extensively.

BIBLIOGRAPHY

1. Auclair PL, Ellis GL. Major salivary glands. In: Silverberg SG, DeLellis RA, Frable WJ (Eds). Principles and practice of surgical pathology and cytopathology. 3rd edn. New York: Churchill Livingstone; 1997.pp.1463-73,1505-8.
2. Batsakis JG. Tumors of the head and neck: Clinical and pathological considerations, 2nd edn. Baltimore, MD: Williams and Wilkins, 1979.

3. Breeze J, Andi A, Williams MD, Howlett DC. The use of fine needle core biopsy under ultrasound guidance in the diagnosis of a parotid mass. Br J Oral Maxillofac Surg 2009;47(1):78-9.

4. Carlson AV, Crittenden AL. The relation of ptyalin concentration to the diet and to the rate of secretion of saliva. Am J Physiol 1910;26:169-77.

5. Chan JK, Tang SK, Tsang WY, Lee KC, Batsakis JG. Histologic changes induced by fine- needle aspiration. Adv Ana Pathol 1996;3:71-90.

6. Cheuk W, Chan JKC. Salivary gland tumours. In: Fletcher CDM (Ed), Diagnostic Histopathology of Tumours. 2/e (Vol 1), Churchill Livingstone, 2002.

7. Daneshbod Y, Daneshbod K, Khademi B. Diagnostic difficulties in the interpretation of fine needle aspirate samples in salivary lesions: Diagnostic pitfalls revisited. Acta Cytol 2009; 53(1):53-70.

8. Di Palma S, Simpson RHW, Skalova A, Leivo I. Major and minor salivary glands. In: Cardesa A, Slootweg PJ (Eds). Pathology of the head and neck. Springer Verlag, 2006;5:132-7.

9. Ellis GL, Auclair PL, Gnepp DR. Surgical pathology of the salivary glands. 1st edn. WB Saunders: Philadelphia, Saunders, 1991.

10. Ellis GL, Auclair Pl. Major Salivary Glands. In: Silverberg SG, DeLellis RA, Frable WJ (Eds). Principles and Practice of Surgical Pathology and Cytopathology, 3/e (Vol 2), Churchill Livingstone, 1997.

11. Ellis GL, Auclair PL. Tumours of the salivary glands. 3rd edn. Armed Forces Institute of Pathology: Washington, 1996.

12. Eneroth CM, Franzen S, Zajicek J. Aspiration biopsy of salivary gland tumors. A critical review of 910 biopsies. Acta Cytol 1967;11(6):470-2.

13. Gnepp DR, Brandenwein MS, Henley JD. Salivary and lacrimal glands. In: Gnepp DR (Ed). Diagnostic surgical pathology of the head and neck. WB Saunders, Philadelphia, 2001.

14. Gnepp DR. Diagnostic Surgical Pathology of the Head and Neck. WB Saunders: Philadelphia, 2001.

15. Graamans K, Vanden Akker. In: Diagnosis of salivary gland disorders 1st edn. Kluwer Academic, 1991.

16. Handa U, Dhingra N, Chopra R, Mohan H. Pleomorphic adenoma: Cytologic variations and potential diagnostic pitfalls. Diagn Cytopathol 2009;37(1):11-5.

17. Harring JL. Diagnosing salivary stones. J Am Dent Assoc 1991.pp.122-75.

18. Jafari A, Royer B, Lefevre M, Corlieu P, Périé S, St Guily JL. Value of the cytological diagnosis in the treatment of parotid tumors. Otolaryngol Head Neck Surg 2009;140(3):381-5.

19. Klijanienho J, Vielh P. Salivary gland tumours: Monographs in clinical cytology. Karger: Basel, 2000;15.

20. Kohn WG, Ship JA, Atkinson JC, et al. Salivary gland Tcscintigraphy: A grading scale correlation with major salivary gland flow rates. J Oral Pathol Med 1992;21:70-4.

21. Lee YY, Wong KT, King AD, Ahuja AT. Imaging of salivary gland tumours. Eur J Radiol 2008;66(3): 419-36.

22. Mandel ID. Sialochemistry in diseases and clinical situations affecting salivary glands. Crit Rev Clin Lab Sci 1980;12:321-66.

23. Metzger ED, Levine JM, McArdle CR,Wolfe BE, Jimerson DC. Salivary gland enlargement and elevated serum amylase in bulimia nervosa. Biol Psychiatry 1999;45:1520-2.

24. Navazesh M. Methods for collecting saliva. Ann N Y Acad Sci 1993;694:72–4.

25. Perzin KH. A systematic approach to the diagnosis of salivary gland tumours. In: Fenoglio CM, Wolff M (Eds). Progress in surgical pathology. New York: Masson; 1982;4:137-80.

26. Valdez IH, Fox PC. Diagnosis and management of salivary dysfunction. Crit Rev Oral Biol Med 1993;4:271–7.

27. Walsh BT, Lo ES, Cooper T, Lindy DC, Roose SP, Gladis M, et al. Dexamethasone suppression test and plasma dexamethasone levels in bulimia. Arch Gen Psychiatry 1987;44:797-800.

10

Management of Salivary Gland Diseases

Vinod Narayanan

INFECTIOUS AND INFLAMMATORY DISEASES

Acute Sialadenitis

Parotid gland is most commonly affected due to ascending infection and is commonly seen in dehydrated patients, elderly, malnourished, chronically ill, Sjögren's syndrome and patients who have undergone radiotherapy to the head and neck.

The commonly implicated organism is Staphylococcus aureus followed by Streptococcus viridans. Pus should be sent for culture and sensitivity. Management includes intravenous beta lactamase resistant antibiotics such as flucloxacillin, cloxacillin, methicillin, amoxicillin with clavulanate or cephalosporins. aggressive rehydration of dehydrated and post- operative patients must be ensured. Surgical drainage by the parotidectomy approach must be carried out if an abscess is present.

Chronic Sialadenitis

Usually affects the parotid salivary gland and is the sequellae of inadequate treatment of acute sialadenitis due to any of the previously mentioned causes. Initial treatment should include systemic antibiotics followed by ductal irrigation with antibiotics. If these measures do not resolve the infection, then excision of the gland should be considered.

Necrotizing Sialometaplasia

It is a benign disease of unknown etiology which usually presents in males at the junction of hard and soft palate as a painless, deep and demarcated ulcer. The disease is self-limiting and heals in 6 to 8 weeks.

Mumps

It is the most common cause for infective parotid swelling and it mainly affects children. Mumps is caused by RNA paramyxovirus. Management is usually symptomatic and involves providing pain relief, adequate hydration and reduction of fever.

Tuberculosis

Although pulmonary tuberculosis is the main form of tuberculosis, salivary gland involvement is not uncommon. It affects the parotid gland more often than the other major glands. Clinical manifestations include swelling of the gland which may be painful. Diagnosis is usually by FNAB and subsequent AFB staining, culture, PCR and histological examination of the aspirate for epithelioid granulomas. Treatment is mainly by multi-drug anti-tuberculous antibiotics for several months. Surgery may later be considered for limited excision of residual nodules or swelling.

Sarcoidosis

Sarcoidosis is a chronic granulomatous disease associated with pulmonary problems and bilateral hilar lymphadenopathy. Parotid gland is the most common site of salivary gland enlargement. A positive skin test (Kveim) is diagnostic but biopsy of positive the lesion will confirm the diagnosis.

IMMUNOLOGIC INFLAMMATORY DISORDERS

Sjögren's Syndrome

It is an autoimmune disease mediated by intense T lymphocyte reaction leading to destruction of salivary, lacrimal and other exocrine glands. Salivary, mucous and lacrimal gland replacement by a lymphocytic infiltrate is responsible for the triad of symptoms namely-dry mouth, dry eyes and parotid swelling.

Management of Sjögren's syndrome (SS) involves supportive care with artificial tears and saliva along with treatment of the underlying autoimmune condition. Plaque control and fluoride therapy should be used to decrease caries susceptibility. The increasing popularity of systemic cholinergics like pilocarpine to stimulate salivary secretion is however tempered by the associated side effects like bradycardia.

Management of Sjögren's syndrome involves supportive care and symptomatic relief of oral and ocular symptoms.

Management of Oral Disease

Management of the oral consequences of salivary dysfunction in SS is similar to that in xerostomia. Symptomatic therapy is targeted towards use of saliva substitutes, stimulation of saliva secretion, and prevention of dental caries and infections. In patients with remaining salivary function, salivary flow can be stimulated by chewing sugarfree gum or by sucking on sugarfree candies.

Saliva substitutes can be used for patients with severe dryness and no residual salivary function. Dental care should include frequent dental examinations and fluoride application. Intraoral candidiasis can be managed with nystatin. Because the oral suspension of nystatin that is commonly used contains a significant amount of sucrose, which is not appropriate for patients with SS, an alternative is nystatin vaginal tablets dissolved orally. In addition, clotrimazole lozenges, taken 5 times daily for 14 days, may also be used. Nystatin or clotrimazole cream can also be used to treat angular cheilitis. Patients with SS should, if possible, avoid diuretics, antihypertensive drugs, antidepressants, and antihistamines, all of which may worsen salivary hypofunction.

Management of Ocular Disease

Frequent use of tear substitutes will help to replace moisture. Corticosteroid-containing ophthalmic solutions should be avoided because they may induce corneal lesions or promote infection. Blepharitis, or inflammation of the meibomian glands, is a possible complication of dry eyes and can be treated with warm compresses, cleansing of the eyelids, and a topical antibiotic, if needed.

Temporary occlusion of the puncta through the insertion of plugs (collagen or silicone) or permanent occlusion by electrocautery can be used to block tear drainage and thus retain existing tears. Existing moisture can also be preserved by goggles.

For patients whose eye dryness is not adequately controlled by moisture preservation or replacement methods, secretagogues are a potential treatment. Secretagogues (pilocarpine and cevimeline) can enhance secretion through the stimulation of the muscarinic receptors of the salivary glands and other organs. Because of this stimulation, however, caution is advised in administering secretagogues to patients with asthma, narrow-angle glaucoma, acute iritis, severe cardiovascular disease, gastritis, biliary disease, nephrolithiasis, or diarrhea.

FUNCTIONAL DISORDERS

Xerostomia

Xerostomia or oral dryness results from decreased salivary flow. The management starts with evaluating the patients to find out the cause. Some of the causes can be corrected and this will aid therapy. Palliative treatment can be used but does not cure the condition.

Symptomatic treatment of xerostomia includes sipping water and artificial saliva. Some patients find relief by chewing sugar free chewing gum. Special food preparations—blended and moist foods are easier to swallow. Use of water and glycerin mixed in a small aerosol spray bottle. The symptomatic treatments are often not completely successful and thus interest in the possibility of treatment that systemically stimulate salivary flow evolved.

Drugs used to increase salivary flow can be classified as medications that alter the disease process, or sialogogues. When xerostomia is secondary to an underlying autoimmune disorder, medications that are used to treat the autoimmune process may have beneficial effects on salivary gland tissue. Sialogogues stimulate salivary flow through their cholinergic effects on functional salivary acinar cells. A large number of agents have been described as systemic sialogogues to treat salivary gland dysfunction. It has been determined that the principal control of salivary secretion is mediated by sympathetic and parasympathetic innervation. The adrenergic receptors are regulated by the sympathetic nervous system and the muscarinic receptors by the parasympathetic nervous system. Transmission of a neural signal to a salivary gland acinar cell occurs chemically through neurotransmitters that bind to specific cell surface proteins. Once bound, the neurotransmitter activates specific signals inside the cell that initiate saliva secretion. The different adrenergic receptors vary in activity depending on what agonist or antagonist binds with the receptor. It is now accepted that parasympathetic nerve stimulation leads to an increased volume of saliva secretion, whereas sympathetic stimulation has a greater effect on protein content and salivary composition.

Sialogogues

Pilocarpine hydrochloride: It is a parasympathetic agent that functions as a muscarinic agonist with mild adrenergic activity. This alkaloid causes pharmacologic stimulation of exocrine glands in human beings. Because pilocarpine acts by stimulating functioning salivary gland tissue, patients with little remaining functional salivary gland may not demonstrate a dramatic improvement in symptoms. However, patients with severe salivary gland destruction often report some improvement of symptoms and relief, with a modest increase in flow.

Fox et al reported a double-blind, placebo-controlled, crossover trial in a well characterized primary Sjögren's syndrome (SS) population with gustatory function. The patients were given pilocarpine; they subsequently reported subjective improvement of their xerostomia. More importantly, parotid and submandibular salivary flow rates demonstrated improvement after separate assessment of each gland. This study was the first controlled pilocarpine trial published.

The usual oral dosage for pilocarpine is 5 to 10 mg 1 hour before eating. The onset of action is 30 minutes and duration of action is approximately 2 to 3 hours. Common side effects include those of other cholinergic medications, including gastrointestinal upset, sweating, tachycardia, bradycardia. Contraindications include gallbladder disease, glaucoma, acute iritis, and renal colic.

Cevimeline hydrochloride: This medication, like pilocarpine, is a cholinergic agonist that binds to muscarinic receptors and stimulates remaining functional salivary gland tissue. Cevimeline reportedly has a 40-fold greater affinity for M3 receptors than does pilocarpine. The recommended dosage is 30 mg 3 times daily. In theory, cevimeline would more specifically target the salivary glands and possibly lead to side effects that are less severe; the effects would be similar to those seen with pilocarpine, including sweating, gastrointestinal upset, urinary frequency, and visual disturbances. It has been suggested that medically compromised individuals, such as patients with controlled hypertension, may tolerate cevimeline better, but the same precautions and contraindications for pilocarpine apply to cevimeline.

Bethanechol chloride: The rationale for using bethanechol as a sialogogue is that it stimulates the parasympathetic nervous system, which causes the release of acetylcholine at the nerve endings, triggering saliva production. Bethanechol is given 4 times a day in doses ranging from 10 to 50 mg.

Tissue Engineering

Tissue engineering of functional salivary gland tissue has been described by Sullivan CA et al. as a potential physiologic solution for xerostomia. They hypothesized that autologous human engineered salivary cells seeded on polymers could form functional tissues when implanted *in vivo*.

Drooling

Drooling is the unintentional loss of saliva from the oral cavity. It is a significant disability for a large number of pediatric and adult patients with cerebral palsy and for a smaller number of patients with other types of neurologic or cognitive impairment.

Patients often experience repeated perioral skin breakdown and infections. Clothing becomes soiled and need frequent changing, which can become very laborious. Severe cases may lead to dehydration.

Medical Therapy

Treatment of patients with drooling problems has been successful at some centers using a team approach, including dentists, oral and maxillofacial surgeons, pediatric dentist and speech therapist. Medical management prior to considering surgical intervention is a logical approach. Direct treatment aims at correcting the oral motor dysfunction and decreasing the secretory volume of salivary glands.

Oral motor trainings for patients with cerebral palsy are aimed at exercises to normalize muscle tone, stabilize body and head position, promote jaw stability and lip closure, decrease tongue thrust, increase oral sensation, and promote swallowing. Oral motor training is time consuming. The therapy requires a minimal level of cognitive function and motivation on the part of the patient and caregiver. Very few data are available to confirm the effectiveness of these therapies. However, because of the noninvasive nature and the varied response of individual patients, all the patients capable of the therapy should undergo at least a 6-month trial of oral motor training.

Behavioral Training

Verbal and auditory cues are used to attempt to increase the frequency and efficiency of swallowing. Methods including reward, overcorrection, and punishment are used by caregivers to initiate swallowing. The success of therapy is dependent on the patient's cognitive level of function and ability to concentrate. Repeat therapy is often required.

Pharmacological Therapy

Anticholinergics inhibit activation at muscarinic receptors and decrease the volume of drooling. The doses tolerated have not caused drooling to completely cease. Adverse effects experienced secondary to the lack of selectivity of the muscarinic receptors affected often limit treatment. Adverse effects include irritability, restlessness, sedation, and delirium from central effects of the drugs. Also, the inhibition of sweat glands has caused significant inhibition of temperature regulation. Inhibition of GI motility has resulted in worsening constipation in a population already plagued with such difficulties. Transdermal scopolamine has been used with success for short periods.

Radiotherapy

Radiotherapy to the major salivary glands has been used in an attempt to decrease the rate of saliva secretion. Success has been variable, and the adverse effect profile is extensive. This therapy is to be used with caution because of the risk of late malignancy in the irradiated field.

Surgical Therapy

In most cases, surgical intervention should be instituted following the failure of at least 6 months of more conservative therapy. Surgery is best delayed until the patient is aged 6 years or older in order to allow time for complete maturation of oral motor function and coordination.

Three surgical approaches can help decrease salivary flow, including removing the salivary glands, ligating the salivary ducts, or sectioning the nerves involved in salivary production. Most commonly, gland excision involves the submandibular glands. A large percentage of resting salivary production comes from the submandibular glands and their removal is associated with minimal morbidity and risk. The sublingual glands make only a very small contribution to the volume of saliva, and parotid gland excision is a more hazardous procedure associated with greater risk. Excision of submandibular glands with bilateral parotid duct ligation has also been done with 85 to 100% success rate.

Transtympanic neurectomy: In this procedure, the parasympathetic nerve supply to the parotid, submandibular, and sublingual glands is interrupted as the nerves traverse the middle ear along the medial wall with a success rate of 50 to 80%. This procedure may be used to complement another drooling procedure or after other procedures fail to control dro*oling.*

Procedures to redirect salivary flow: Rerouting procedures have the positive effect of preserving salivary production and taste. Many authors have described transposition of the submandibular ducts. The procedure is accomplished by making an elliptical incision around the ducts to form a mucosa island and dissecting the ducts for a length of 3 to 4 cm. A submucosal tunnel is then developed between the incision and the tonsillar fossa just behind the anterior pillar. The ducts are then passed posteriorly in the submucosal plane, and the mucosal islands are secured with 2 to 3 sutures. The success rate reported in the literature is 80 to 100%.

OBSTRUCTIVE DISEASES

Sialolithiasis

It is the most common cause of salivary gland obstruction and is usually caused by a calculus and rarely due to strictures and tumors. It can be complete or partial and may show recurrence. The retained saliva applies retrograde pressure on the salivary gland and the ductal system leading to painful and intermittent swelling particularly at mealtimes.

The accepted treatment is to postpone sialolithectomy in the acute stage, particularly in those cases in which removal of the sialolith is surgically difficult. In such cases, antibiotic treatment is essential until the swelling and pain subsides and surgery becomes possible.

Successful treatment of sialolithiasis depends on accurate diagnosis on the location of the obstruction. It is useful to remember that 40 to 50 percent (particularly parotid) of calculi may be radiolucent. Hence diagnostic modalities like sialography, ultrasound and computerized tomography (CT) scanning may be needed if the calculus is not demonstrable on plain radiographs.

The surgical treatment for obstructive diseases of salivary gland has been divided into two following categories on the basis of location:

1. Obstructions that can be reached by an intraoral route (i.e. up to the curvature above the lingual nerve in the Wharton's duct and anterior to the curvature around the masseter muscle in the Stensen's duct) (Figs 10.1A and B).
2. All other sialoliths that could not be reached intraorally are removed during sialadenectomy or through an external approach.

More recently there have been advancements in the field of minimally invasive surgery in the major salivary glands, including **endoscopy**, owing partly to the advancement in technology and to new surgical techniques. Interventional **sialoendoscopy** can be divided into an intraductal approach that is a pure endoscopic technique and an extraductal approach that is an endoscopic assistance technique. The indications for sialoendoscopy are screening the ductal system for any residual calculi after sialolith removal, and determining the status of the major duct lumens. The intraductal approach is used for: endoscopic mechanical retrieval and endoscopic energy-induced lithotripsy.

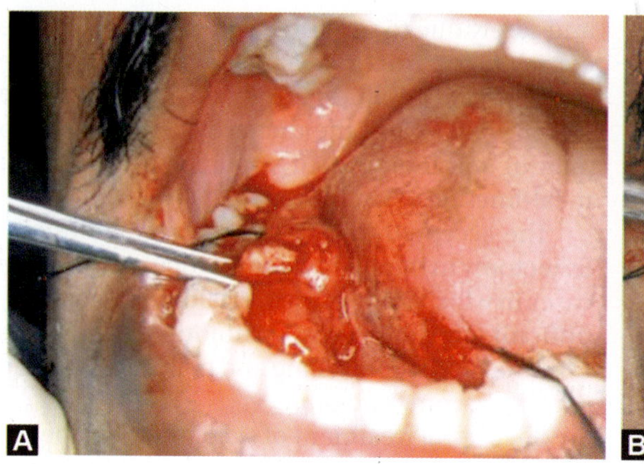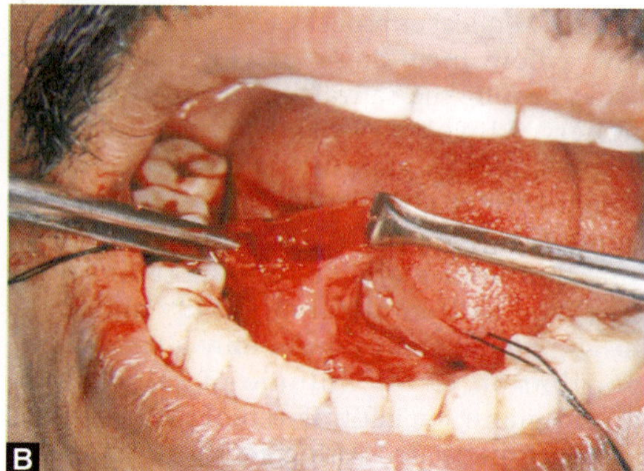

Figures 10.1A and B: Surgical removal of sialolith of the submandibular duct

Lithotripsy, both endoscopically controlled intracorporeal and extracorporeal piezoelectric shock wave have been used effectively as a noninvasive therapy for sialolithiasis. However, its use has been associated with salivary tissue damage.

Mucous Retention Phenomenon

Collectively, the **mucocele, the ranula, and the cervical or plunging ranula** are clinical terms for a pseudocyst that is associated with mucus extravasation into the surrounding soft tissues. These lesions occur as the result of trauma to the salivary gland excretory duct, although obstruction of salivary flow is implicated in some instances. Mucoceles and ranulas tend to be relatively painless or asymptomatic lesions with little or no associated morbidity or mortality.

Besides ductal disruption, partial or total excretory duct obstruction is involved in the pathogenesis of ranulas in some instances. The duct may become occluded by a sialolith, congenital malformation, stenosis, periductal fibrosis, periductal scarring due to prior trauma, excretory duct agenesis, or even a tumor. Although most oral ranulas originate from the secretions of the sublingual gland, they may develop from the secretions of the submandibular gland duct or the minor salivary glands on the floor of the mouth.

The mucus extravasation of the sublingual gland almost exclusively causes cervical ranulas. The mucus escapes through openings or dehiscence in the underlying mylohyoid muscle. Plunging ranulas are associated with a discontinuity of the mylohyoid muscle. Oral and plunging ranulas, if large, may affect swallowing, speech, mastication, or respiratory function.

Surgical excision of the mucocele along with the adjacent associated minor salivary glands is recommended. The risk for recurrence is minimal when appropriate surgical excision has been performed. Aspiration of the mucocele contents often results in recurrence and is not appropriate therapy, except to exclude other entities prior to surgical excision. Large lesions may be marsupialized to prevent significant loss of tissue or to decrease the risk for significantly traumatizing the labial branch of the mental nerve. If the fibrous wall is thick, moderate-sized lesions may be treated by dissection. If this surgical approach is used, the adjacent minor salivary glands must be removed.

Laser ablation with CO_2 laser, cryosurgery, and electrocautery are approaches that have also been used for the treatment of the conventional mucocele with variable success.

With most oral ranulas, surgical management is preferred. The first attempt at management may be marsupialization of the ranula with packing of the entire pseudocyst with gauze for 7 to 10 days.

The more traditional method of surgery for an oral ranula is complete excision of the ranula and associated major salivary gland. Laser ablation and cryosurgery, either alone or after marsupialization, have been used for some patients with oral ranula. Isolated reports have demonstrated that oral ranulas have been successfully treated with intracystic injection of the streptococcal preparation, OK-432. Resolution or marked reduction in size have been documented following this sclerotherapy. But, local pain at the injection site and fever are reported in almost 50% of the cases. Currently, the use of this sclerosing agent for the treatment of oral ranulas is considered experimental.

Inadequate surgical therapy for oral ranulas may result in the creation of plunging ranulas. As noted previously, almost one-half of cervical ranulas are those occurring after surgical attempts to eliminate oral ranulas. When these lesions are managed by marsupialization alone, the recurrence rate is high, and the lesions usually develop 6 to 8 weeks after surgery.

TUMORS OF SALIVARY GLAND

Salivary gland tumors present significant diagnostic and management challenges. The ubiquitous deposition of the minor salivary glands complicates the diagnosis and management of these neoplasms.

Benign Tumors

The standard treatment for benign tumors of salivary gland is excision of the involved gland (superficial or deep parotidectomy, total submandibular excision, etc.) with a margin of 10 mm of clinically uninvolved tissue. However contemporary literature suggests a more conservative approach to benign tumors such as *limited parotidectomy* and recommending margins as little as 1 mm. In the hard palate the excision plane is subperiosteal and down to bone, which is burnished with burs. With the appropriate treatment of benign neoplasms, the outcome is excellent and the recurrence rate is very low.

Malignant Tumors

A widely used but little reported guide to the management of salivary gland cancers is the 4 cm rule. Tumors that are less than 4 cm (T1 or T2) do well regardless of histological type or grade. It has also been shown that adjuvant radiotherapy has a distinct survival advantage for patients with tumors over 4 cm, but has little benefit for smaller tumors.

The minimum therapy for low-grade malignancies of the superficial portion of the parotid gland is a superficial parotidectomy. For all other lesions, a total parotidectomy is often indicated. The facial nerve or its branches should be resected if involved by tumor; repair can be done simultaneously. Growing evidence suggests that postoperative radiation therapy augments surgical resection, particularly for the high-grade neoplasms, or when margins are close or involved. Clinical trials, which have been completed in the United States and United Kingdom, indicate that fast neutron-beam radiation improves disease-free and overall survival in patients with unresectable tumors or for patients with recurrent neoplasms. Accelerated hyperfractionated photon-beam radiation therapy has also resulted in high rates of long-term local regional controls. The use of chemotherapy for malignant salivary gland tumors remains under evaluation. Chemotherapy using doxorubicin, cisplatin, cyclophosphamide, and fluorouracil as single agents or in various combinations is associated with modest response rates.

Stage I Major Salivary Gland Cancer

Low-grade stage I tumors of the salivary gland are curable with surgery alone. Surgery may be either local excision of the gland with or without a neck dissection depending on demonstrability of neck nodes clinically or radiologically. Radiation therapy may be used for tumors for which resection involves a significant cosmetic or functional deficit or as an adjuvant to surgery when positive margins are present. Neutron-beam therapy is effective in the treatment of poor-prognosis malignant salivary gland tumors. High-grade stage I salivary gland tumors that are confined to the gland in which they arise may be cured by surgery alone, though adjuvant radiation therapy may be used, especially with the presence of positive margins or perineural invasion.

The role of chemotherapy remains under evaluation, though data suggest that some salivary gland tumors may be responsive to chemotherapy.

Stage II Major Salivary Gland Cancer

Low-grade stage II tumors of the salivary gland may be cured with surgery alone. Radiation therapy as primary treatment may be used for tumors for which resection involves a significant cosmetic or functional deficit or as an adjuvant to surgery when positive margins are present. Neutron-beam therapy may also be effective in the treatment of tumors that have spread to lymph nodes. Chemotherapy is usually considered in situations such as when radiation therapy or surgery is refused.

High-grade stage II salivary gland tumors that are confined to the gland in which they arise may be cured by surgery alone, though adjuvant radiation therapy may be used, especially if positive margins are present. Primary radiation therapy may be given for tumors that are inoperable, unresectable, or recurrent. Fast neutron-beam radiation has been shown to improve disease-free and overall survival in this clinical situation.

Stage III Major Salivary Gland Cancer

Patients with low-grade stage III tumors of the salivary gland may be cured with surgery alone. Radiation therapy as primary treatment is not often required but may be used for tumors for which resection involves a significant cosmetic or functional deficit, or as an adjuvant to surgery when positive margins are present. Patients with low-grade tumors that have spread to lymph nodes may be cured with resection of the primary tumor and the involved lymph nodes, with or without radiation therapy. Neutron-beam therapy is effective in the treatment of tumors that have spread to local lymph nodes.

Patients with high-grade stage III salivary gland tumors that are confined to the gland in which they arise may be cured by surgery alone, though adjuvant postoperative radiation therapy may be used, especially if positive margins are present. Primary conventional X-ray radiation therapy may provide palliation for patients with unresectable tumors. Fast neutron beams, however, have been reported to improve disease-free and overall survival in this clinical situation. Patients with tumors that have spread to regional lymph nodes should have a regional lymphadenectomy as part of the initial surgical procedure. Adjuvant radiation therapy for these tumors may reduce the local recurrence rate.

Fast neutron-beam radiation or accelerated hyperfractionated photon beam schedules have been reported to be more effective than conventional radiation therapy in the treatment of inoperable, unresectable or recurrent malignant salivary gland tumors.

Stage IV Major Salivary Gland Cancer

Standard therapy for patients with tumors that have spread to distant sites is not curative includes fast neutron-beam radiation or accelerated hyperfractionated photon beam schedules along with chemotherapy.

Surgical Anatomy

The parotid gland is situated in the musculo-skeletal recess formed by portions of the temporal bone, atlas and mandible, and their related muscles. The gland has a superficial and deep lobe, between which runs the extratemporal portion of the facial nerve. The deep lobe is in contact with the parapharyngeal space. The deep cervical fascia surrounds the parotid gland. This fascia has an anteroinferior portion that becomes the stylomandibular ligament, separating the parotid gland from the submandibular gland.

The facial nerve exits the stylomastoid foramen just posterior to the base of the styloid, gives off small branches to the postauricular and posterior belly of the digastric muscles, and then turns anterolaterally. The main trunk then becomes embedded in parotid tissue and divides into temporofacial and cervicofacial branches just superficial to the retromandibular vein and external carotid artery. Beyond this point, the nerve anatomy varies some; however, 5 general peripheral nerve branches exist: frontal, zygomatic, buccal, marginal mandibular, and cervical (Figs 10.2A to C). Surgical landmarks for the main trunk of the facial nerve include the tragal pointer and the tympanomastoid suture line.

The submandibular gland encompasses most of the submandibular or digastric triangle. Similar to the parotid gland, the submandibular gland can be divided into a superficial and deep lobe based on the relationship to the mylohyoid muscle. The marginal mandibular branch of the facial nerve courses between the deep surface of the platysma and the superficial aspect of the fascia that lies over the submandibular gland. The facial artery and vein are located just deep to this nerve, and ligation and superior traction of these vascular structures can prevent nerve injury. Along the posterior border of the mylohyoid are located the lingual nerve and submandibular duct (Wharton duct). The hypoglossal nerve courses deep to the tendon of the digastric and then lies medial to the deep cervical fascia.

The sublingual gland occupies the same anatomical space as the submandibular gland, located between the mylohyoid and hyoglossus muscles. The gland can often be palpated in the floor of mouth, as it is rather superficial, covered by only a thin layer of oral mucosa.

The minor salivary glands are widely dispersed throughout the upper respiratory tract, including the palate, lip, pharynx, nasopharynx, larynx, and parapharyngeal space. The greatest densities of glands are located in the hard (250 glands) and soft (150 glands) palates.

Parotidectomy

The cornerstone of this procedure is to localize the facial nerve at the main trunk proximal to the gland safely. One has to include the possibility of total parotidectomy in the preoperative plan. The patient has to be informed about the potential need to sacrifice the facial nerve, with immediate grafting, neck dissections, and mandibulectomy.

Superficial parotidectomy remains the initial procedure of choice for benign parotid gland tumors. The incision usually starts just anterior to the ear helix, extends inferiorly below the ear lobe, and then moves anteriorly to parallel the angle of the jaw within a 2 cm distance (Figs 10.2A to C)

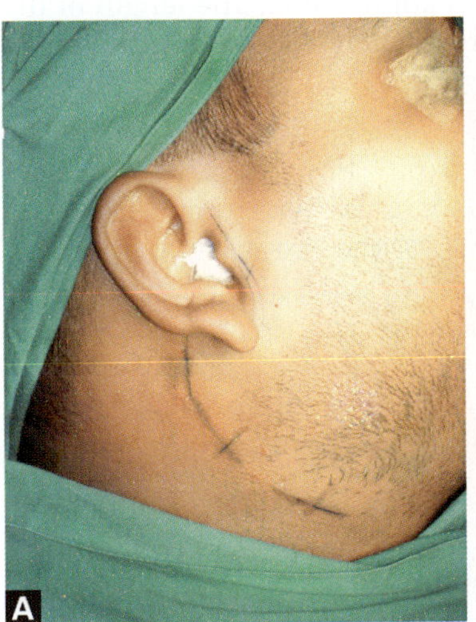
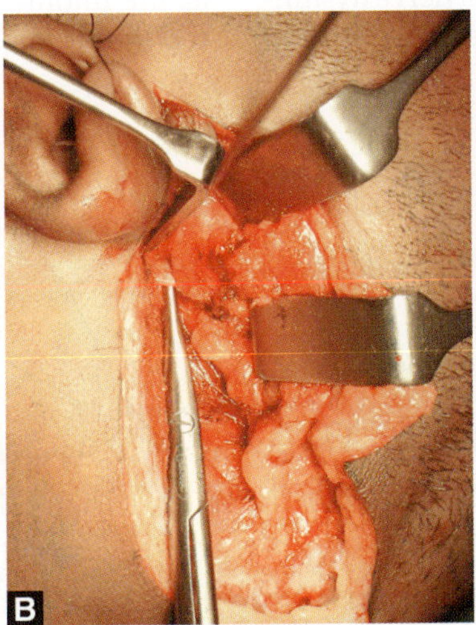
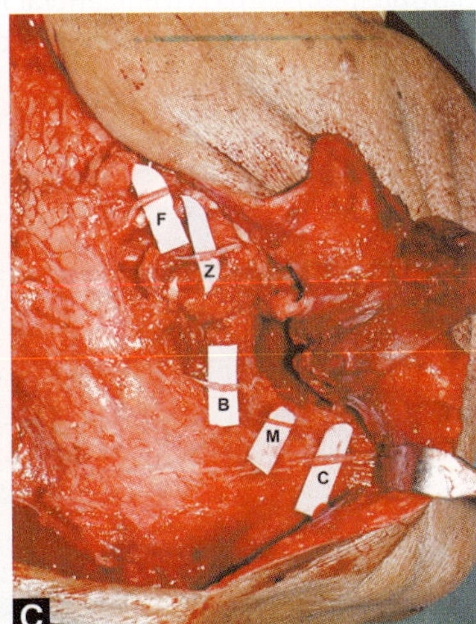

Figures 10.2A to C: (A) Parotidectomy incision; (B) Exposure of facial nerve trunk; (C) Exposure of branches of facial nerve. Abbreviations: F: Frontal; Z: Zygomatic; B: Buccal; M: Marginal mandibular; C: Cervical

Dissection is usually performed sharply down to the superficial parotid fascia. Then, the skin flap is sutured and retracted from the surgical field. Dissection is continued to expose the remainder of the gland anteriorly and the anterior border of the sternocleidomastoid muscle. At this location, the greater auricular nerve is identified and preserved because it carries sensation to the ear lobule and provides the best option for nerve grafting, if needed. Access to deep lobe of parotid is facilitated by access osteotomies of the mandibular ramus, angle and body (Figs 10.3A and B). Occasionally, deeper-lobe parotid tumors may displace the facial nerve to a more superficial location, where it is easily injured. Limited parotidectomy, a concept gaining popularity is used primarily for excising benign tumors with a margin as close as 1 mm of clinically unaffected tissue.

If a facial nerve stimulator is used, testing it on the muscle and setting it at 0.5 mA before use is recommended. If the facial nerve is sacrificed because of direct tumor involvement, immediate grafting (using the greater auricular nerve or sural nerve) is required.

Complications of Parotidectomy

A common complication of surgical treatment for parotid neoplasms is transient facial nerve dysfunction. Transient facial nerve paralysis (paresis) takes a few weeks to resolve spontaneously but can last as long as 6 months. Direct trauma to the nerve, devascularization, or postoperative nerve inflammation is believed to be a cause for paresis.

Other complications include Frey's syndrome also known as gustatory flushing and sweating and the auriculotemporal syndrome. The manifestations range from erythema related to eating to copious gustatory sweating. The cause is believed to be an abnormal connection of the parasympathetic fibers to the sweat gland of the overlying flap of skin. Frey's syndrome has been successfully treated with injections of botulinum toxin A and by interposition of muscle flaps like pedicled sternomastoid into the dead space following parotidectomy. Another measure is to raise a thick parotid flap just above the parotid fascia. Salivary fistulae after complete wound healing are rare.

Submandibular Gland Surgery

Submandibular gland surgery is performed with the patient under general anesthesia with endotracheal intubation. Head rotation is to the opposite side of the tumor (Fig. 10.4).

An incision is made at the mastoid process and curved along the inferior aspect of the mandible as the midline is approached. The length of the incision is approximately 4-6 cm. The incision is

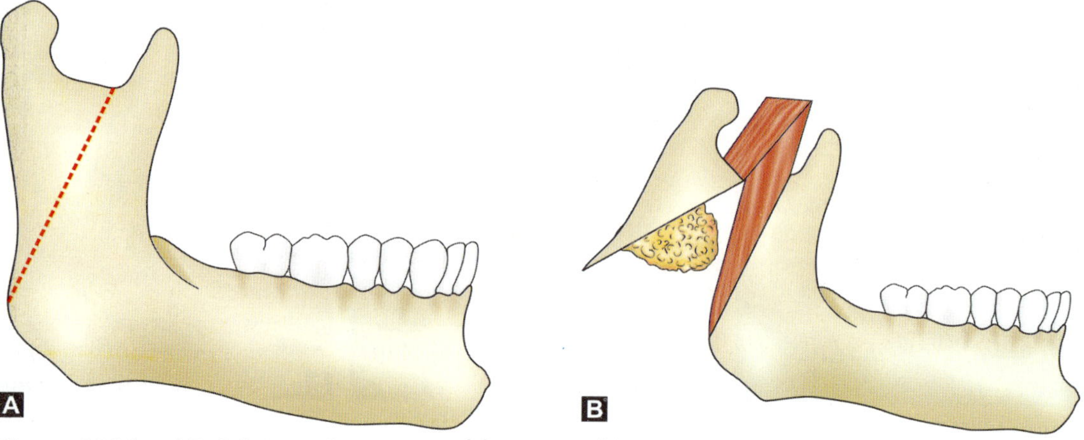

Figures 10.3A and B: Subsigmoid osteotomy of the ramus of the mandible for access to deep lobe of parotid

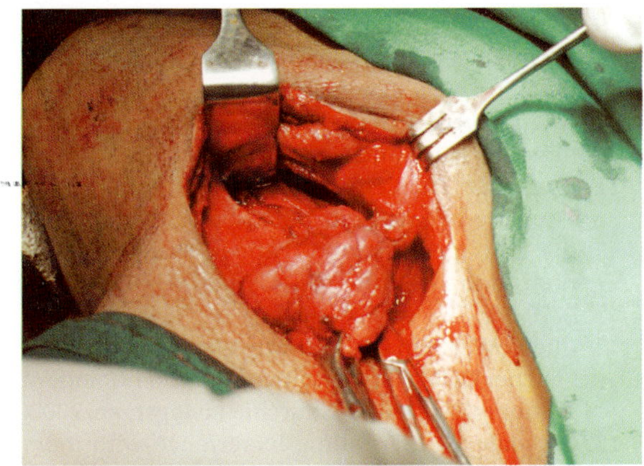

Figure 10.4: Excision of submandibular gland

taken down through the platysma muscle, leaving the muscle attached to the skin as a musculocutaneous flap. At this point, the marginal branch of the facial nerve is identified and preserved unless it is directly involved with the tumor. The nerve is located just below the muscle and superficial to the facial vessels. The safest technique is to divide the inferior aspect of the posterior facial vein and to raise the flap to the depth of the vessels and nerve.

Start the dissection of the gland at the level of the hyoid bone and the lower aspect of the gland. Identifying the digastric muscle is the next step and is important because the hypoglossal nerve with the vessels runs in between the gland and the digastric muscle. Dissection continues on the posterior aspect of the gland, superiorly to where the facial artery is located. Now, the blood supply to the gland is ligated. The lingual nerve is visualized by anterior retraction of the mylohyoid muscle, and the pedicle of the gland is then carefully ligated, with attention to the main trunk of the lingual nerve. Next, the duct is identified and ligated to conclude the resection. Layered closure with suction drain completes the procedure.

Minor Salivary Gland Resection

Surgical treatment of minor salivary glands depends on the site of origin and the extent of disease. For tumors of the lip or palate, this may simply involve a wide local excision (hemi maxillectomy, extended maxillectomy) with primary closure. Larger tumors of the parapharyngeal space may require a more complex surgical procedure, as intraoral resection is not recommended. The options for external approaches to the parapharyngeal space include a cervical-parotid approach (parotid incision with cervical extension) or a cervical-parotid approach with mandibulotomy.

Often, an attempt is made to avoid a mandibulotomy when treating benign lesions that arise from the minor salivary glands. Although this procedure does not require a full facial nerve dissection, the inferior division must be located and preserved. By retracting the sternocleidomastoid muscle laterally, the surgeon can identify the internal jugular vein, external and internal carotid arteries, and cranial nerves IX-XII. In order to access the space, the posterior belly of the digastric and stylohyoid muscles must be divided, followed by the external carotid artery and stylomandibular ligament. In addition, the styloid process may be resected for delivery of larger tumors and greater visualization.

Prognosis

The prognosis for salivary gland malignancies depends on the following:
- Gland in which they arise.
- Histopathology.
- Grade (i.e. degree of malignancy).
- Extent of primary tumor (i.e. the stage).
- Whether the tumor involves the facial nerve, has fixation to the skin or deep structures, or has spread to lymph nodes or distant sites.

Early stage low-grade malignant salivary gland tumors are usually curable by adequate surgical resection alone. The prognosis is more favorable when the tumor is in a major salivary gland; the parotid gland is most favorable, then the submandibular gland; the least favorable primary sites are the sublingual and minor salivary glands. Large bulky tumors or high-grade tumors carry a poorer prognosis and may best be treated by surgical resection combined with postoperative radiation therapy.

The 10-year disease-specific survival was 97% for stage I, 81% for stage II, 56% for stage III, and 20% for stage IV. Cure is expected in almost all cases when a complete resection with clear margins is performed. Recurrence is usually caused by inadequate excision spillage or inoculation. The recurrence rate, as reported after a mean follow-up period of 11.8 years, is as high as 25%.

Overall, clinical stage, particularly tumor size, may be the crucial factor to determine the outcome of salivary gland cancer and may be more important than histologic grade. The size of tumor at presentation is a strong predictor of prognosis and the 4 cm rule has proved to be a useful clinical guide to behavior and outcome.

Perineural invasion can also occur, particularly in high-grade adenoid cystic carcinoma, and should be specifically identified and treated.

BIBLIOGRAPHY

1. Aidan P, de Kerviler E, Le Duc A, Monteil JP. Treatment of salivary stones by extracorporeal lithotripsy. Am J Otolaryngol 1996;17:246-50.
2. Anjum K, Revington PJ, Irvine GH. Superficial parotidectomy: Antegrade compared with modified retrograde dissections of the facial nerve. Br J Oral Maxillofac Surg 2008;46(6):433-4.
3. Bailey CM, Wadsworth PV. Treatment of the drooling child by submandibular duct transposition. J Laryngol Otol 1985;99(11):1111-7.
4. Barnes L, Brandwein M, Som PM. Surgical Pathology of the Head and Neck. 2nd edn. Marcel Dekker Inc: New York, 2001.
5. Batsakis JG. Tumors of the head and neck: Clinical and pathological considerations, 2nd edn. Baltimore, MD: Williams and Wilkins, 1979.
6. Baurmash HD. Mucoceles and ranulas. J Oral Maxillofac Surg 2003;61:369-78.
7. Beahrs OH, Adson MA. The surgical anatomy and technique of parotidectomy. Am J Surg 1958;95(6):885-96.
8. Blitzer A. Inflammatory and obstructive disorders of salivary glands. J Dent Res 1987;66:675-81.
9. Borg M, Hirst F. The role of radiation therapy in the management of sialorrhea. Int J Radiat Oncol Biol Phys 1998;41:1113-9.
10. Brein. Current management of benign parotid tumours. Head and Neck 2003;25:946-52.
11. Buchholz TA, Laramore GE, Griffin BR, et al. The role of fast neutron radiation therapy in the management of advanced salivary gland malignant neoplasms. Cancer 1992;69(11): 2779-88.
12. Cheuk W, Chan JKC. Salivary gland tumours. In: Fletcher CDM (Ed). Diagnostic Histopathology of Tumours 2/e (Vol 1), Churchill Livingstone, 2002.
13. Crysdale WS. Drooling. Experience with team assessment and management. Clin Pediatr 1992;31:77-80.
14. Di Palma S, Simpson RHW, Skalova A, Leivo I. Major and minor salivary glands. In: Cardesa A, Slootweg PJ (Eds). Pathology of the head and neck. Springer Verlag, 2006;5:132-7.
15. Ellis GL, Auclair PL, Gnepp DR. Surgical pathology of the salivary glands. 1st edn. WB Saunders: Philadelphia, Saunders, 1991.
16. Ellis GL, Auclair Pl. Major Salivary Glands. In: Silverberg SG, DeLellis RA, Frable WJ (Eds). Principles and Practice of Surgical Pathology and Cytopathology, 3/e (Vol 2), Churchill Livingstone, 1997.
17. Ellis GL, Auclair PL. Tumours of the salivary glands. 3rd edn. Armed Forces Institute of Pathology: Washington, 1996.
18. Epstein JB, Stevenson-Moore P, Scully C. Management of xerostomia. J Can Dent Assoc 1992;58:140-3.
19. Escudier MP, Brown JE, Drage NA, McGurk M. Extracorporeal shockwave lithotripsy in the management of salivary calculi. Br J Surg 2003;90:482-5.
20. Ethunandan M, Macpherson DW. Persistent drooling: Treatment by bilateral submandibular duct transposition and simultaneous sublingual gland excision. Ann R Coll Surg Engl 1998;80:279-82.
21. Fox PC, van der Ven PF, Baum BJ, Mandel ID. Pilocarpine for the treatment of xerostomia associated with salivary gland dysfunction. Oral Surg Oral Med Oral Pathol 1986;61:243-8.
22. Gnepp DR, Brandenwein MS, Henley JD. Salivary and lacrimal glands. In: Gnepp DR (Ed). Diagnostic surgical pathology of the head and neck. WB Saunders, Philadelphia, 2001.

23. Gnepp DR. Diagnostic Surgical Pathology of the Head and Neck. WB Saunders: Philadelphia, 2001.

24. Granick MS, Solomon MP, Hanna DC. Management of benign and malignant salivary gland tumors. In: Georgiade GS, Riefkohl R, Levin LS (Eds). Plastic, maxillofacial, and reconstructive surgery. 3rd edn. Baltimore, Md: Williams and Wilkins; 1997.pp.155-65.

25. Han S, Isaacson G. Recurrent pneumoparotid: Cause and treatment. Otolaryngol Head Neck Surg 2004;131(5):758-61.

26. Hickman RE, Cawson RA, Duffy SW. The prognosis of specific type of salivary gland tumors. Cancer 1992;54:1620-54.

27. Inga CJ, Reddy AK, Richardson SA, Sanders B. Appliance for chronic drooling in cerebral palsy patients. Pediatr Dent 2001;23:241-2.

28. Iro H, Zenk J, Benzel W. Laser lithotripsy of salivary duct stones. Adv Otorhinolaryngol 1995;49:148-52.

29. Jafari A, Royer B, Lefevre M, Corlieu P, Périé S, St Guily JL. Value of the cytological diagnosis in the treatment of parotid tumors. Otolaryngol Head Neck Surg 2009;140(3):381-5.

30. Johnson JT, Ferretti GA, Nethery WJ, Valdez IH, Fox PC, Ng D. Oral pilocarpine for post-irradiation xerostomia in patients with head and neck cancer. N Engl J Med 1993;329:390-5.

31. Kater W, Meyer WW, Wehrmann T, et al. Efficacy, risks and limits of extracorporeal shock wave lithotripsy for salivary gland stones. J Endourol 1994;8(1):21-4.

32. Lohuis PJ, Tan ML, Bonte K, van den Brekel MW, Balm AJ, Vermeersch HB. Superficial parotidectomy via facelift incision. Ann Otol Rhinol Laryngol 2009;118(4):276-80.

33. Mendenhall WM, Riggs CE Jr, Cassisi NJ: Treatment of head and neck cancers. In: DeVita VT Jr, Hellman S, Rosenberg SA (Eds). Cancer: Principles and practice of oncology. 7th edn. Philadelphia, Pa: Lippincott Williams and Wilkins, 2005.pp.662-732.

34. Meyer- Lueckel H, Kielbassa AM. Use of saliva substitutes in patients with xerostomia. Schweiz Monatsschr Zahnmed 2002;112:1037-58.

35. Motamed M, Laugharne D, Bradley PJ. Management of chronic parotitis: A review. J Laryngol Otol 2003;117(7):521-6.

36. Nederfors T. Xerostomia: Prevalence and pharmacotherapy. With special reference to beta-adrenoceptor antagonists. Swed Dent J Suppl 1996;116:1-70.

37. O'Connell AC. Natural history and prevention of radiation injury. Adv Dent Res 2000;14:57-61.

38. Porta M, Gamba M, Bertacchi G, Vaj P. Treatment of sialorrhoea with ultrasound guided botulinum toxin type A injection in patients with neurological disorders. J Neurol Neurosurg Psychiatry 2001;70:538-40.

39. Rajendran R, Sivapathasundharam B. Diseases of salivary gland. In: Shafer's textbook of oral pathology, 5th edn. Elsevier, 2005.

40. Rauch S, Herzog D. Parotidectomy for bulimia: A dissenting view. Am J Otolaryngol 1987;8:376-80.

41. Roh JL, Park CI. Gland-preserving surgery for pleomorphic adenoma in the submandibular gland. Br J Surg 2008;95(10):1252-6.

42. Scarpini M, Bonapasta SA, Ruperto M, Vestri A, Bononi M, Caporale A. Retrograde parotidectomy for pleomorphic adenoma of the parotid gland: A conservative and effective approach. J Craniofac Surg 2009;20(3):967-9.

43. Shott SR, Myer CM, Cotton RT. Surgical management of sialorrhea. Otolaryngol Head Neck Surg 1989;101:47-50.

44. Spiro RH. Factors affecting survival in salivary gland cancers. In: McGurk M, Renehan AG (Eds). Controversies in the management of salivary gland disease. Oxford, UK: Oxford University Press, 2001. pp.143-50.

45. Valdez IH, Fox PC. Diagnosis and management of salivary dysfunction. Crit Rev Oral Biol Med 1993;4:271–7.

46. Von Lindern JJ, Niederhagen B, Bergé S, et al. Frey syndrome: Treatment with type A botulinum toxin. Cancer 2000;89(8):1659-63.

47. Wasserman T. Radioprotective effects of amifostine. Semin Oncol 1999;26:89-94.

Index

Page numbers followed by *f* refer to figure and *t* refer to table